Additional Titles for New Parents From the American Academy of Pediatrics

Baby and Toddler Basics: Expert Answers to Parents' Top 150 Questions

Baby Care Anywhere: A Quick Guide to Parenting On the Go

Caring for Your Baby and Young Child: Birth to Age 5*

Dad to Dad: Parenting Like a Pro

Food Fights: Winning the Nutritional Challenges of Parenthood
Armed With Insight, Humor, and a Bottle of Ketchup

Guide to Toilet Training

Mama Doc Medicine: Finding Calm and Confidence in Parenting,
Child Health, and Work-Life Balance

My Child Is Sick! Expert Advice for Managing Common Illnesses
and Injuries

The New Baby Blueprint: Caring for You and Your Little One

New Mother's Guide to Breastfeeding

The Picky Eater Project: 6 Weeks to Happier, Healthier Family Mealtimes

Raising an Organized Child: 5 Steps to Boost Independence, Ease
Frustration, and Promote Confidence

Raising Twins: Parenting Multiples From Pregnancy Through
the School Years

Retro Baby: Cut Back on All the Gear and Boost Your Baby's Development
With More Than 100 Time-tested Activities

Retro Toddler: More Than 100 Old-School Activities to Boost Development

Sleep: What Every Parent Needs to Know

Understanding the NICU: What Parents of Preemies and Other
Hospitalized Newborns Need to Know

Your Baby's First Year*

For additional parenting resources, visit the HealthyChildren bookstore at
https://shop.aap.org/for-parents.

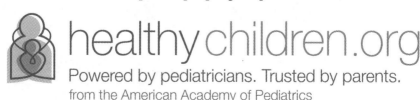

healthy children.org
Powered by pediatricians. Trusted by parents.
from the American Academy of Pediatrics

*This book is also available in Spanish.

7/5

Heading Home With
Your Newborn
From Birth to Reality
FOURTH EDITION

Laura A. Jana, MD, FAAP & Jennifer Shu, MD, FAAP

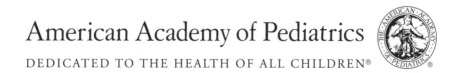

American Academy of Pediatrics
DEDICATED TO THE HEALTH OF ALL CHILDREN®

American Academy of Pediatrics Publishing Staff

Mary Lou White, *Chief Product and Services Officer/SVP, Membership, Marketing, and Publishing*

Mark Grimes, *Vice President, Publishing*

Kathryn Sparks, *Senior Editor, Consumer Publishing*

Shannan Martin, *Production Manager, Consumer Publications*

Amanda Helmholz, *Medical Copy Editor*

Sara Hoerdeman, *Marketing Manager, Consumer Products*

Published by the American Academy of Pediatrics

345 Park Blvd
Itasca, IL 60143
Telephone: 630/626-6000
Facsimile: 847/434-8000
www.aap.org

The American Academy of Pediatrics is an organization of 67,000 primary care pediatricians, pediatric medical subspecialists, and pediatric surgical specialists dedicated to the health, safety, and well-being of infants, children, adolescents, and young adults.

The information contained in this publication should not be used as a substitute for the medical care and advice of your pediatrician. There may be variations in treatment that your pediatrician may recommend based on individual facts and circumstances.

Statements and opinions expressed are those of the authors and not necessarily those of the American Academy of Pediatrics.

Any websites, brand names, products, or manufacturers are mentioned for informational and identification purposes only and do not imply an endorsement by the American Academy of Pediatrics (AAP). The AAP is not responsible for the content of external resources. Information was current at the time of publication.

The persons whose photographs are depicted in this publication are professional models. They have no relation to the issues discussed. Any characters they are portraying are fictional.

The publishers have made every effort to trace the copyright holders for borrowed materials. If they have inadvertently overlooked any, they will be pleased to make the necessary arrangements at the first opportunity.

This publication has been developed by the American Academy of Pediatrics. The contributors are expert authorities in the field of pediatrics. No commercial involvement of any kind has been solicited or accepted in the development of the content of this publication. Disclosures: Dr Jana reports a publisher/author relationship with National Center for Youth Issues; an advisory board member relationship with Owlet, Ingenuity Foods, Yoee Baby, and BabyNoggin; a consultant relationship with Primrose Schools; and an author relationship with Hachette.

Every effort is made to keep *Heading Home With Your Newborn* consistent with the most recent advice and information available from the American Academy of Pediatrics.

Special discounts are available for bulk purchases of this publication. Email Special Sales at nationalaccounts@aap.org for more information.

Printed in the United States of America

9-452/0820   1 2 3 4 5 6 7 8 9 10
CB0120
ISBN: 978-1-61002-424-2
eBook: 978-1-61002-425-9
EPUB: 978-1-61002-426-6
Kindle: 978-1-61002-427-3

Cover design by LSD DESIGN, LLC
Publication design by Linda J. Diamond
Pencil drawings by Anthony Alex LeTourneau

Library of Congress Control Number: 2020930658

Praise for Previous Editions of *Heading Home With Your Newborn*

One of the "best guides to the first year of your baby's life."

—*Parents* magazine

This book packs the advice of a parenting class, a doctor's visit,
and a best friend into one indispensable package.

—*Library Journal*

Funny yet sage…having this book in the house is like having
a doctor on call (without the co-pay).

—*ePregnancy* magazine

I LOVE, LOVE, LOVE the humor in *Heading Home*! Very entertaining
and informative. I am now recommending that all my new parents
get a copy, whether they are on their first or fourth baby.

—Dan Brennan, MD, CLC, FAAP
Sansum Clinic, Santa Barbara, California, and contributing writer for
Santa Barbara Parent magazine, the *Daily Sound,* and the *Goleta Voice*

Heading Home With Your Newborn is one of the very best books
for parents that I've run across in the 24 years that I have been reviewing
parenting books. Written with great heart and soul, it provides up-to-date
medical information. These two pediatrician authors are both smart
and compassionate, and it's obvious that they remember just
what it feels like to bring home a brand-new baby.

—Bobbi Conner
Creator and host of *The Parent's Journal*
nationwide public radio program

★

A special book that new parents will want to read cover to cover before their little one arrives. No matter what challenges new parenthood throws your way, Drs Jana and Shu are sure to leave you feeling both confident and competent. *Heading Home* is the perfect shower gift!

—Barton Schmitt, MD, FAAP
Professor of Pediatrics at the Children's Hospital of Denver

In short, easy-to-read chapters, these pediatrician-authors explore all the topics…which are part of every new baby's life. Their sections on car seat safety and traveling with an infant are especially informative and up-to-date. The authors' supportive reassurances and sensitive advice will be particularly helpful to parents whose baby does not fit the norm. Without a false note anywhere, the authors have made a gift to parents of their own confidence and experience. This book is a fresh contribution to adults just beginning the parenting journey.

—Molly Frederick
Senior Associate Editor, formerly of *Contemporary Pediatrics*

This book will lower your stress about raising your child. It is a wonderful narrative that reads as if it was a conversation among friends…. You can have a shared learning experience with the authors who are moms, docs, and daughters and really do know.

—George A. Strait
Former Medical Correspondent, *ABC News*

In an era of one-size-fits-all parenting advice, this book truly stands out. Doctors Jana and Shu offer the kind of advice that will help new parents keep their expectations reasonable, while giving them the confidence and encouragement they need to be great parents, and to have fun at the same time.

—Armin Brott
Author of *The Expectant Father* series

A family-friendly, easily read…guide to the unique experience of caring for a newborn that is both practical and medically sound.

—Lillian Blackmon, MD
Former Chair, American Academy of Pediatrics
Committee on Fetus and Newborn

The advice you'd get from your sister or best friend,
if she had her baby only last year.

—Gil Fuld, MD
AAP News Editorial Advisory Board

Its spirited, light, and conversational tone makes readers feel like they are talking to a trusted good friend who just happens to be a pediatrician.

—John C. Nelson, MD, MPH
Obstetrician-gynecologist
Past President, American Medical Association

As an ER doctor, I've cared for countless infants in a clinical setting. But nothing can truly prepare you for bringing home your own baby! Informative, realistic, and reassuring, this book answers all of your questions, from changing diapers to burping to traveling with baby, and it became my own go-to resource. *Heading Home With Your Newborn* not only empowers moms with the knowledge to raise a happy and healthy baby, but also—and most importantly—gives us the confidence to believe that we can.

—Darria Long Gillespie, MD, MBA
ER Physician, Emory University Healthcare; EVP, Sharecare.com

To everyone who humored us when we told them we were writing a book,

to those who actually took us seriously, and most important,

to all of you who welcome us into your homes and share this

unforgettable part of parenthood with us.

—LJ and JS

Contents

Section 3
ACTIVITIES OF DAILY LIVING

Section 4
ACTIVITIES OF DAILY LEARNING

Acknowledgments

As we marvel that *Heading Home With Your Newborn* has touched the lives of more than a million families since the very first edition was published more than 15 years ago, we realize just how fortunate we've been to be able to share in what we truly consider to be one of the most momentous occasions of parenthood. We are also reminded of how grateful we are for our own family, friends, and colleagues. As cliché as it may sound, this book wouldn't exist without their love, support, understanding, and ongoing reassurances that what we have to say continues to be worth putting into print. For that, they are deserving of both recognition and our sincerest thanks.

First and foremost, we are thrilled to be in this long-standing partnership with the American Academy of Pediatrics. After years of hard work and climbing our way up the steep learning curve together in the world of publishing, we couldn't have found a more perfect fit. Special thanks to past Executive Directors Errol Alden, MD, and Joe Sanders, MD, who offered us an incredible opportunity to work with the American Academy of Pediatrics, which we continue to believe represents the gold standard in caring for children.

We also owe our gratitude to all the many expert colleagues who reviewed our text for technical (and practical) accuracy over the years.

Laura A. Jana, MD, FAAP

I have been fortunate to have crossed paths with several people whose faith in my abilities has helped me to get to where I am today. Perhaps one of the most influential people early in my career was Benjamin Spock, MD, who not only took me seriously years before I had an MD behind my name but was an incredibly insightful man whose love of life and understanding of both children and parents continue to inspire me. I also want to thank pediatricians Robert D. Needlman, MD, FAAP, who first demonstrated to me how to practice the art of pediatrics, and Barton D. Schmitt, MD, FAAP, whose kind words of support meant far more to me than he probably realized. And finally, I owe a special thanks to Georges Peter, MD, whose commitment to involving young pediatricians and women in the American Academy of Pediatrics is what serendipitously brought me back in touch with my coauthor, Jennifer, years after we trained in pediatrics together at the University of California, San Francisco.

My 3 children—Bethany, Alex, and Ryan—help remind me every day what is truly important in life, and I am forever grateful for their willingness to let me test out (and fine-tune) my parenting techniques before sharing them with others. While many others played impactful roles in making this book come to life, I especially want to acknowledge my best friend and husband of 25 years, Ajoy Jana, MD. Ajoy has given me not only his unwavering support but his unconditional love. It is the life and family we have created together that define who I am and represent my greatest accomplishments.

Jennifer Shu, MD, FAAP

Space prevents me from personally listing all the important people with whom I have crossed paths in life. Many of you have given me the encouragement and confidence to become the person I am, and for these, I am most grateful. I would like to give my utmost appreciation to my husband and children, who patiently supported a book that took several years to come to life. Thanks to my parents, who taught me to believe that I could be anything I wanted to be. A big shout-out goes to my sisters, who have been my peppiest cheerleaders. To my extended family of in-laws, thanks for welcoming me into your lives as a daughter, sister, and friend. My tenth grade English teacher, Paul Lankford, told me I would be a star no matter where I went, and I was naive enough to believe him. I know he has similarly influenced many other students in a tremendously positive way, and I would like to recognize the effect he has had. My heartfelt thanks go to my pediatric colleagues, coworkers, and mentors, who have guided me in this ongoing quest to be a better pediatrician. My friends from all stages of my life have been incredibly supportive and tolerant of my quirks and tendency to share my excitement about our books. I would also like to extend my gratitude to all my patients, who have taught me just about everything I know about newborns. And last, a big woo-hoo to my coauthor, Laura. We not only finally finished the first edition but have been able to watch it grow to the fourth edition (and I hope more!). I'm glad we get to go through this amazing experience together!

Introduction

The Current State of Parenting Affairs

We'd like to start out by acknowledging that we are by no means the first authors to write about the wondrous but admittedly daunting journey called *parenthood*. We live in a time when parenting experts all but grow on trees, and parenting books, blogs, and social media posts are overflowing with advice. Given the sheer magnitude of information already available, you may wonder why we ever decided to toss our hats into this overcrowded ring and set out to write on the subject of raising children in the first place. To be perfectly honest, we almost didn't.

A Journey of Our Own

Originally, we set out in search of what we knew parents (our patients, our friends, and ourselves) wanted—easily accessible parenting advice that was informative and practical, that offered explanations right alongside recommendations, and, most of all, that was firmly grounded in the realities of modern-day parenting. At the end of the day (or several years later, to be more exact) and hundreds of parenting books, patient visits, baby showers, and playgroups later—not to mention several children of our own—we still hadn't found a book that reflected our unique perspective on parenting. In fact, what we discovered was that new parents were reading "all the baby books" and were still left with questions about the realities of caring for their newborns. It was then that we decided there was room for at least one more parenting book on the shelf, and we set to work on creating a book that would specifically focus on the first few weeks of parenthood. More than 15 years and 4 editions later, a lot has changed. Books are now as likely to be found on virtual shelves as real ones. Children are inherently growing up digitally in a world very different from the one we were born into. What remains *un*changed, however, is that we still see the need for practical, reassuring evidence-based information to help you make a confident, enjoyable entrée into parenthood.

Following the Rules: Parenting by the Book

Nowadays, it's easy to find well-defined rules about everything from feeding and sleeping schedules to dressing, diapering, and discipline. As convenient as it may seem to have someone write out for you an exact recipe for parenting success, we believe there is not just one right way to do things. As with diapers and baby clothes, we are convinced that parenting techniques are not simply one size fits all. Our goal is to help familiarize you with the basics of baby care and, even more important, to build your confidence as a parent right from the beginning during what many consider to be an overwhelming time—the newborn period. With a little knowledge and a positive attitude, you will find that you are very capable of anticipating and reasoning your way through even the most challenging aspects of what lies ahead. It's a great feeling to find yourself comfortable enough in your parenting abilities that you don't have to live life with a quick reference guide or an e-book—ours or anyone else's—tucked into your back pocket.

Parenting With Style

We have found that it is a rare parent—new or seasoned—who isn't also on the constant lookout for good, practical parenting advice to make life a bit easier, a bit less expensive, a bit safer, or simply more fun. We like to think of these little pearls of wisdom as parenting revelations—the "wow, what a good idea…I never thought of that" or "you know what, that really makes sense; I wish I had thought of that sooner" kind of revelation that comes when fellow parents share their insights or, in this case, when we share ours. After all, we firmly believe that parenting not only is a lifestyle but can be done in style.

From Birth to Reality

As parents ourselves, with 5 children between us, we have firsthand knowledge of what parenting questions tend to arise and what dilemmas have a way of presenting themselves in the course of a typical day—or night—with a newborn. Opportunely enough, we both also happen to be pediatricians. The years we have spent in pediatric training and practice in interacting with children and parents have provided us with an added understanding of babies, children, and parents—not to mention what obstacles they (and you) are likely to run into along the way. Add to that background Laura's 10 years of owning a 200-student educational child care center and between us, we have had the opportunity to talk with and listen to thousands of parents just like you—and believe us, we have listened! We have not only listened to concerns about first fevers, flat heads, and breastfeeding, as well as helped parents sort out their babies' common (and not so common) medical ailments, but answered questions about everything from the family bed, infant attire, and choosing child care to first airplane trips and car seat installation.

Parent Tested, Pediatrician Approved

And now we're honored to have the opportunity to help guide you through the transition from birth to the reality of being a parent. In this fully updated fourth edition of *Heading Home With Your Newborn,* we share with you what we've learned not just in our professional lives but also from our 50 years of combined experience in interacting with everyday parents just like you. While we have complete faith in your ability to figure things out for yourself, we thought you might find it helpful to hear our thoughts *before* you have to do it all on your own! *Heading Home With Your Newborn* represents a blending of our experiences and brings you the best of both worlds—a book that presents the reality of parenting from a parent's perspective but with a pediatrician's stamp of approval. Instead of being "kid tested, mother approved," this book is "parent tested, pediatrician approved," with all its pearls wrapped into one convenient package.

Anticipating Change

You may have heard people say that life is never the same after having a baby. Until you have lived through the experience yourself, it may be difficult to imagine exactly what heading home with your newborn will mean for you and your family. One thing you can count on, though, is that your life *will* certainly change—physically, emotionally, and financially. By this change, we're referring not just to the shedding of pregnancy pounds, the psychological stress of sleep deprivation, or the cost of baby gear (not to mention the cost of college, which is forever looming in the distance) but also to your general perspective on life. The phrase "Toto, we're not in Kansas anymore" springs to mind.

Adopting a Growth Mindset

How you deal with the inevitable changes and challenges of parenthood is likely to be colored by your initial expectations of what life with your newborn is going to be like. While we will provide the information to help prepare you for the day-to-day tasks of life with a newborn, in the end, it will be up to you to create a positive mental attitude. After all, we firmly believe that an important part of preparing for life with a newborn involves getting into the right mindset, a mindset that will allow you to grow into and adapt to your new role as a parent.

Rude Awakenings

Fairly often, we find that new parents expect too much of their newborns (and themselves). While we've dedicated entire chapters of this book to the topics of breastfeeding and sleep, they make for perfect examples of unrealistic expectations. In the case of breastfeeding, suffice it to say that although the "textbook" pattern may be 15 minutes on each breast every 3 hours, a newborn who nurses sporadically and frequently throughout the day and night (up to 8 to 12 times in any given 24-hour period) is much more the norm during the newborn period. And if you're expecting a full night's sleep right from the start as opposed to being grateful for a 4-hour stretch, we're sorry to say, you're likely to be in for many rude awakenings. We could use any number of similar examples to support our belief that expecting too much inevitably sets parents up to *feel* as if they've derailed when, in reality, they are usually still right on track. Instead, we simply plan to help you understand and set realistic goals and expectations.

Keeping It Real

Whether you are heading into the homestretch of your pregnancy or are already homeward bound, take a minute to ask yourself how you feel about your parenting abilities. Some people find themselves to be petrified. Others maintain a cool confidence. As you get ready to go from birth to the sudden reality of parenthood, we suggest you adopt the mantra "I think I can, I think I can, I think I can…" long before you ever formally become acquainted with *The Little Engine That Could* (much less find yourself reading this timeless children's book aloud for the hundredth time). Whether your expectations of yourself and your newborn simply need some fine-tuning or a major readjustment, we hope you'll head home confidently and soon be saying, "I *knew* I could, I *knew* I could, I *knew* I could…."

SPECIAL DELIVERIES: PREMATURE BABIES, MULTIPLES, AND MORE

We've been asked over the years what new-parent advice *Heading Home With Your Newborn* offers for parents of preterm babies, multiples, or babies requiring a stay in the neonatal intensive care unit. The reality is that these sorts of special deliveries require special attention to details that are beyond the scope of this book. Fortunately, plenty of good resources are out there, devoted completely to these specific topics. That said, it is our hope that much of the information we provide about newborns and new parenthood will be relevant, at least in part, to all parents of new babies.

High Hopes and Great Expectations

We have the highest hopes and sincerely believe that you and your baby will settle into a manageable lifestyle. After all, millions of parents before you have had newborns and still chose to have a second, a third, a fourth…. In the short term, we encourage you to set your sights not so much on the day-to-day challenges but on the more intangible aspects of parenthood—the joy, pride, and sense of awe and accomplishment that are the essence of parenthood. These should be your great expectations. We can all but guarantee that the joy will outweigh the fatigue, and your overall sense of accomplishment will erase many of the doubts you may have.

THE PRICE OF THINGS TO COME

Labor and delivery . . . . .Daunting

Furnishing, decorating, and stocking the nursery . . . . .Expensive

Keeping up with your newborn's eating
and (not) sleeping schedule . . . .—Tiring

Forgetting to brush your teeth or shower .Unhygienic

Being a parent . . . . .Priceless

Brave New World

While you have many years ahead to familiarize yourself with the nuances, joys, and responsibilities of raising a happy, healthy child, we want to help make the first baby steps you take up the new-parent learning curve a little less wobbly. We decided that the most logical way to begin this wondrous journey from birth to the reality of becoming a parent is with a look at one of the most unforgettable events of parenthood—when new parents like you pack up their things at the hospital, take a deep breath, place their precious new babies into carefully installed car seats, and boldly go where they have never been before. We call it "heading home with your newborn."

getting ready to head home

Making the Transition From Hospital to Home

In earlier editions of this book, we jumped right in to how to take care of your baby after packing up your things, taking a deep breath, and leaving the hospital. We figured the doctors, nurses, and other hospital staff responsible for helping you welcome your new baby would also send you out into the brave new world of parenthood as armed with a congratulatory pat on the back and helpful information about this hospital-to-home transition. We soon realized, however, that we had overlooked one important fact: many of you are likely reading this book *before* delivery. We thus decided it would be most helpful to include some additionally useful nuts-and-bolts information about what needs to happen *at* the hospital, in anticipation of heading home. After all, for many new parents, the life-altering transition from 24/7 supervised hospital-based baby care to what seems like home-alone parenthood can be a bit daunting. So we decided to take a small step back into the hospital and share a quick overview of what you should do, know, and expect before you set foot out of the hospital.

HOSPITAL DELIVERIES: TIMING YOUR STAY

The practice of delivering babies in the hospital began nearly 200 years ago and has become a standard of care today. Just how long new mothers and their babies stay in the hospital, however, has changed considerably. With the average length of stay steadily declining and a trend toward early newborn discharge, the US Congress in 1996 passed The Newborns' and Mothers' Health Protection Act. This federal law helped ensure that hospital stays up to 48 hours following vaginal delivery or 96 hours after birth by cesarean delivery (C-section) would be covered by insurers.

Today, the American College of Obstetricians and Gynecologists and the American Academy of Pediatrics also support average hospital stays for uncomplicated deliveries of full-term newborns (at 37 to 40 weeks' gestation) of 48 to 96 hours. Early discharge, especially within 24 hours of delivery, is approved only with careful consideration.

Hospital Happenings: Checks and Balances

When it comes to who will help prepare you and your baby for hospital discharge, rest assured that there is likely to be an entire team of health care professionals responsible for making sure you're both in tip-top condition. This cast of characters will most likely include

- **Obstetrician or midwife.** Success at home depends on checking to make sure that both baby and mother are ready to leave the hospital. That need for readiness is why leaving typically requires sign-off from the obstetrician or midwife.

- **Nurses.** Newborns are generally weighed and have other vital signs, such as temperature, heart rate, and respiratory rate, taken during their stay in the hospital. Before babies are deemed ready to leave, it is recommended that all babies have documentation of normal vital signs that have been stable for at least 12 hours before discharge.

- **Pediatrician, nurse practitioner, or another pediatric professional.** In addition to a double check of routinely measured weight, routinely measured vital signs, and any test results, your newborn's in-hospital routine will most likely include a daily head-to-toe check.

- **Lactation specialist.** In many hospitals, lactation specialists are available to evaluate how a newborn is feeding and able to assist with the all-important breastfeeding skills of latching on, positioning, and more (see Breastfeeding on page 5).

Taking the Necessary Steps: Tests and Procedures

In addition to getting checked out by a team of doctors, nurses, and other health care professionals, newborns generally have to complete a handful of important tests and procedures before discharge (many of which we discuss in more detail in Just for the Health of It on page 277). These include the following procedures and actions and assessments.

Standard Procedures

Erythromycin eye ointment application. Most hospitals are required by state law to put drops or ointment into a newborn's eyes to protect against potentially serious forms of newborn pinkeye (*conjunctivitis*). Erythromycin has, for the most part, replaced the silver nitrate that was more commonly used in days past.

Vitamin K injection. It is recommended that all newborns receive a single injection of vitamin K before discharge to protect against an uncommon but serious and preventable bleeding problem. All babies are born with low levels of vitamin K, which is necessary for blood clotting. The shot is considered safe and effective for newborns.

Oxygen saturation testing. This quick and painless, needle-free test is typically done before discharge to check for low levels of oxygen in a baby's blood that might identify any significant but fortunately rare heart defects. Measuring oxygen in the blood simply involves placing a Band-Aid–like sensor onto the baby's right hand and one foot.

Newborn screening. All babies in the United States are checked for a set of medical conditions soon after birth, usually before leaving the hospital. While the specific conditions tested for vary by state, they all involve taking a few drops of blood from a newborn's heel. Be aware that it can take a few weeks for these results to come back, so plan on asking your baby's doctor about them at one of your upcoming visits.

Hearing screening. Because it's important that all babies be screened for hearing loss within 1 month post-birth, most hospitals routinely do a hearing screening before newborns are discharged. This test is painless and does not even require newborns to be awake during the procedure.

Hepatitis B vaccination. Children typically need three doses of the hepatitis B vaccine to be protected against the hepatitis B virus, with the first shot recommended within the first 24 hours after birth. The shot is very safe and generally has no adverse effects. (See Your First Shot at Prevention: Hepatitis B on page 348.)

Additional Actions and Assessments

Baby's blood type test. While all pregnant women are routinely tested to determine their blood type and whether they are Rh positive or negative, only the newborns born to moms who are Rh negative or O blood type must be tested. In both instances, blood from the umbilical cord is used for testing. Other babies may also get tested, depending on individual circumstances. (For more information, see It's in the Blood on page 336.)

Measurement of bilirubin level. Some, but not all, newborns require a check of the level of bilirubin (the substance in the bloodstream responsible for causing jaundice). For more information, see Measuring Bilirubin Levels on page 340.

Other blood tests. Depending on circumstances, these can include measurements such as blood glucose ("blood sugar"), blood counts, and blood cultures.

Circumcision. Although circumcision is not required before discharge, or at all, for that matter, most baby boys who get this procedure have it done before going home. (For more information, see Penis Care on page 317.)

Removal of umbilical cord clamp. The umbilical cord clamp plays an important role in stopping the umbilical cord from bleeding immediately after delivery. By the time newborns leave the hospital, however, the umbilical cord stump should already be drying out so that the clamp no longer serves any useful purpose. Because cord clamp removal is occasionally overlooked, we recommend you double-check to make sure your baby's clamp is removed so that it doesn't prove to be a nuisance at home.

All Systems Go

In addition to passing specific laboratory tests, newborns must prove that all their "systems" are in good working order. Along with physical examination and in-hospital observation, one of the most reassuring ways for them to do this is simply by demonstrating their ability to eat, pee, and poop well. Once they do, this should help instill confidence in you and the hospital staff that your newborn is ready to set out on her own (with your assistance, of course).

AT-HOME RECORD KEEPING

Rest assured that transitioning from the clinical setting of the hospital to caring for your baby at home generally means getting a feel for how your baby is doing overall without needing to record lots of numbers to back you up.

After spending time in the hospital with what can seem like nearly constant poking, prodding, and monitoring of your baby, it's understandable why you might feel the need to continue documenting everything in comparable detail. But unless there are special circumstances or you or your baby's doctor has concerns about how your newborn is faring, it's generally unnecessary to do so—especially after your baby has settled into reassuring patterns of feeding, peeing, and pooping (see Into the Mouths of Babes on page 1 and What Goes In Must Come Out on page 71).

Simply making check marks on a piece of paper can help you keep track of the basics, such as number of wet and poopy diapers and number of feedings per 24 hours. Of course, for those of you who prefer, you can use any one of a zillion baby-tracking apps that are currently available.

On that note, we are well aware that some pretty cool and convenient new baby apps are out there. And it's perfectly fine to use them to record your baby's detailed data, if you're so inclined or if your baby's doctor is interested in having you track something in particular. Just be aware that while technology can be appealing and serve a useful purpose, especially for sleep-deprived new moms and dads and other caregivers who are otherwise too bleary-eyed to remember the most recent time their baby fed or had a diaper change, make sure you don't spend more time digitally documenting than you do attuned to your baby.

Hands-on Training

Classes. New parents are often given the opportunity (and may even be required) to take a hands-on class or watch a going-home video covering the basics of feeding, diapering, bathing, and safety, before discharge. Required or not, as well as regardless of how tired you are from recent events of the day, we strongly suggest you take advantage of any such offerings. Be sure to participate actively (assuming you feel up to it), and ask any questions you may have.

Rooming-in. Many hospitals now encourage having newborns stay right in your hospital room rather than separately in the newborn nursery. This room sharing not only is great for bonding and getting better acquainted with your newborn but also allows those of you who are nervous about soon being solely responsible for a newborn a valuable opportunity: to watch and learn how trained new baby professionals with vast experience diaper, dress, undress, bathe, weigh, and otherwise handle your newborn.

Fine dining. Expect to put on a dinnertime "show" during your hospital stay. According to recommendations from the American Academy of Pediatrics, all newborns should be required to prove themselves as capable of successfully feeding at least twice before being discharged. For breastfed newborns, this process should include observation by someone knowledgeable in breastfeeding to verify that they have the fundamental "skills" necessary for at-home success (ie, latch, suck, and swallow). (See Catching On to Latching On on page 17.)

Ready for the ride. As you head into the homestretch and pack up your things, be aware that placing your precious new baby into a carefully installed car seat is not optional when you are leaving any US hospital. In other words, don't let lack of an appropriate infant car seat stand between you and taking your baby home. (See Before Leaving the Hospital on page 220.)

Planning for Follow-up

With the hospital discharge checks and balances complete, the last step before you confidently step into your new parent-of-a-newborn life is to make sure (and, in some instances, show proof to those in charge of your discharge) that you have arranged follow-up appointments for mom and baby. This arrangement should give you additional peace of mind that you're not going to be on your own for long. Newborns generally are seen by their pediatricians within one to three days of discharge. As for new moms, a follow-up visit is typically scheduled for two weeks after a vaginal delivery or six weeks after a cesarean delivery, or C-section.

Homecoming

Once you've cleared all hospital hurdles and are ready to head home, you may feel like celebrating. While we certainly don't want to dampen your enthusiasm, you may want to consider waiting a bit to adjust to life at home before you commit to any major homecoming celebrations. Some new parents jump right in and adapt quickly. But far more often than not, it takes at least a few days (or, more likely, weeks) to adjust to caring for a newborn without the benefit of 24/7 nursing support. We suggest you give yourself plenty of time to rest, recover, and enjoy your new baby—and, of course, to read the rest of what we've put together for you.

into the mouths of babes

introduction

· · · · · · · ·

As the parent of a newborn, you'll undoubtedly be spending a good deal of time paying attention to what goes into your baby's mouth. Whether by breast or by bottle, the frequent task of feeding a newborn has the potential to raise a whole host of questions ranging from how to know whether your breast milk has "come in" or how to prepare your baby's formula to the facts about sucking and whether it's okay to use pacifiers.

Before we dive in, let us first point out that birth to about 18 months of age isn't referred to as the *oral stage* for nothing. What goes into your baby's mouth during this stage of the game is going to be a big part of her life experience (not to mention yours). Not only will eating and growing be her biggest and most important responsibilities for many months to come, but her mouth will play a valuable role in allowing her to comfort herself and interact with the world around her long before she learns to use her hands and other senses to explore.

With that mouthful in mind, you may find that you look at your baby's cute little lips with new respect and awe. In this first section of the book, we offer a hands-on look at the reality of feeding your newborn—not only as a nutritional necessity but as a wonderful opportunity for you to bond with your baby. Our ultimate goals are to help you settle into a comfortable routine and give you a clear idea of what you can expect, as well as what to look out for.

Now to turn our attention to the substance of the matter at hand—breast milk and formula. For the sake of convenience, we have tried to separate breastfeeding from formula feeding—a well-defined separation in print that is not always so clear-cut in real life. That's because quite a few parents ultimately find themselves relying on some combination of the two. Once you've finished the relevant chapter(s)—whether that's breast, formula, or both—we encourage you to keep reading because later in this section we address subjects that are likely to be of interest to all of you. They include pacifiers, feeding schedules (or lack thereof), and nipple confusion. You'll also brush up on the basics of bottle-feeding—from supplies to technique and cleanup—in a chapter meant to be useful to any one of you who plans to use a bottle, regardless of what you choose to put in it.

DOLLARS AND SENSE

If the decision about whether to breastfeed or formula feed were based solely (or even partly) on finances, breastfeeding would win hands down. As one of the more obvious and largest potential expenses, it's worth noting that not all breastfeeding moms actually need or use a breast pump. For those who do, they're almost always provided by insurance, the Women, Infants, and Children (WIC) program, or many state Medicaid programs. In other words, breast pumps don't need to be an additional cost to mom. As for the other potential expenses of breastfeeding, they are generally limited to the cost of a few extra calories breastfeeding moms typically need (estimated to be just under $20 a month), as well as the cost of nursing bras, breast pads, or any of the other optional supplies you may pick up along the way. With formula feeding, on the other hand, most of the inherent costs are not optional. As some of you may have already discovered, formula tends to be quite costly. Twenty years ago, the average cost of formula was estimated to be more than $1,500 a year. It's safe to assume that the cost of formula, like the cost of everything else, has gone up since then. When we pieced together a ballpark calculation of our own, we came up with a very approximate but realistic amount of more than $1,600 a year (ranging from as low as $1,000 per year for generic formula using coupons or close to $3,000 for high-end formula). As a point of interest, if you consider a global birth rate of 131.4 million babies born each year, it would cost more than $210 billion to NOT breastfeed.

CHAPTER

1

breastfeeding

• • • • • •

As with most aspects of parenting, the most significant contribution we stand to make to your breastfeeding success is to start you off with realistic expectations. To do that, we address many of the common breastfeeding myths and misconceptions that tend to weigh on the minds of new parents. We have found it's particularly helpful for you to start by reminding yourself of two reassuring facts.

- Millions of mothers have been able to breastfeed their babies successfully.
- The first couple weeks of breastfeeding are by no means representative of what the entire breastfeeding experience will be like.

A handful of fortunate new moms are able to ease into breastfeeding as if they were born to do so and are quickly rewarded with an overwhelming sense of accomplishment. In reality, however, there is usually a period of self-education and on-the-breast training. Consider this time to be one of trial and error—a "get acquainted with and accustomed to the process" phase during which breastfeeding your baby may take a bit more time, thought, and effort than it will in your not-so-distant breastfeeding future. With a few safety precautions in place and your eyes on the prize, you will most likely be able to dodge many common obstacles—both perceived and real. If you're coming to us already frustrated and all but resigned to giving up any hope of breastfeeding altogether, we hope to offer you a new lease on your breastfeeding life.

A Comment on Breast Is Best

As you enter the world of parenthood, you will undoubtedly encounter the phrase "breast is best." This encounter is likely because that phrase has become an almost universal slogan prominent in parenting advertisements, websites, textbooks, and formula packaging alike. Given that breast milk has thus far proven impossible to duplicate, and the health benefits it offers are invaluable, we wholeheartedly support the recommendation of the American Academy of Pediatrics (AAP) to feed your baby breast milk for as long as possible—

exclusively for about the first six months and ideally continuing for one year and as long thereafter as both you and baby would like to do so. With that as a backdrop, what we have to say about your decision to breastfeed may therefore come as a bit of a surprise—especially from two pediatrician-moms who are fully aware and in support of the idea that there are great benefits to breastfeeding. We feel the need to mention that we have come across instances in which breastfeeding has not always worked out for the best. Now lest the preceding statement be regarded as a letdown to breastfeeding advocates everywhere, let us explain.

The standard consideration in favor of breast milk is very straightforward. Breast milk has long been and continues to be unrivaled as the ideal food for infants. Not only is it considered to be a perfect mix of nutrients, including the fatty acids DHA (*docosahexaenoic acid*) and ARA (*arachidonic acid*) that are thought to play an important role in brain and eye development, but it contains infection-fighting antibodies that can't be bottled in even the most expensive of commercial formulas. Breast milk has also been shown to reduce a newborn's chance of developing everything from ear and respiratory tract infections, asthma, allergies, diarrhea, and eczema to diabetes, obesity, lymphoma, leukemia, sepsis, and even sudden infant death syndrome (SIDS). There are some pretty compelling big picture health benefits for breastfeeding mothers as well. They include a decreased risk for heart disease, diabetes, and several types of cancer (breast, ovarian, endometrial, and thyroid). Just about the only caveat we feel compelled to mention is that for some caring and devoted new mothers, when it comes to putting recommendations into practice, breastfeeding sometimes just doesn't work out right. Whether it's a matter of modesty, attitude, medically related issues, or disappointment of unsuccessful attempts, breastfeeding can be a potential source of frustration for some new moms. Worse yet, difficulties with breastfeeding can cause some serious feelings of parental inadequacy, leaving some mothers questioning their overall ability as parents. Too many of these new parents are led to believe—by convincing themselves or by being told by others—that to be a good mother, breastfeeding is an absolute requirement.

We now say to you what we suggest to every new or expectant mother who comes to us with questions or concerns about the early days of breastfeeding. First, decide for yourself whether you are looking for breastfeeding help or secretly hoping someone will tell you it's okay not to breastfeed. On the one hand, if you've already made the *informed* decision (ie, understanding all the facts and options, including those we lay out for you in the next several pages, and ideally discussing them with a qualified health care provider) that breastfeeding is not for you, you have our full support in flipping directly to the formula-feeding discussion of this book (see Formula for Success on page 45) without experiencing unrelenting pangs of guilt. If, on the other hand, you've never given much thought to breastfeeding, you find yourself questioning your ability to do it successfully, or you have run into a few bumps in the road to what will almost surely be breastfeeding success, we hope you read on. Breastfeeding admittedly can be challenging in the beginning. Thankfully, there are a lot of breastfeeding resources available to you. For our part, we hope that this book serves as one of them and that we can help boost your confidence and make sure your breastfeeding experiences are not only successful but also enjoyable.

BREASTFEEDING'S BUDDING POPULARITY

Both the popularity of breastfeeding in the United States and the numbers of women who choose to do so have grown tremendously over the past several years as compared to some 40 years ago when essentially no new moms in the United States attempted to breastfeed. According to the Centers for Disease Control and Prevention (CDC) 2019 breastfeeding data, a vast majority of new moms (more than 8 in 10) at least try their hand (or breast) at it, more than half are still breastfeeding at 6 months, and more than one-third continue to do so through the first year. This represents a significant change for the better if you consider what is clearly known about the health benefits of breastfeeding.

How Far We've Come and How We Got Here

Anyone looking at breastfeeding popularity in the United States over past decades is sure to notice some major shifts. After a marked decline extending from the 1930s through the 1960s, public awareness campaigns aimed at promoting breastfeeding beginning in the 1970s resulted in a steady increase over the remainder of the 20th century. And, of course, what was considered to be "best," not to mention socially acceptable, has varied considerably not only over time but also because of many other factors such as what area of the country parents live in, their ages, and their backgrounds. Fortunately, over the past couple of decades, we have seen a steady increase in the numbers of women choosing to breastfeed. Despite having come a long way from the days when breastfeeding moms were the exception to the rule and ostracized for their choice, we have not come so far that there isn't an occasional outdated, hard to believe, or even downright comical law that prohibits public displays of breastfeeding still on the books.

BREASTFEEDING WITHIN YOUR LEGAL RIGHTS

Laws in most states protect a woman's right to breastfeed. With a final 5 states coming on board since we wrote the previous edition of *Heading Home With Your Newborn,* we are happy to be able to say that all 50 states, as well as the District of Columbia, Puerto Rico, and the US Virgin Islands, make it clear that it's legal for mothers to breastfeed in public. In addition, there are now laws on the books that

- Include provisions for workplace pumping, requiring employers to provide breastfeeding mothers reasonable break time, albeit not necessarily compensated, to express breast milk. Even those with fewer than 50 employees must comply unless able to show undue hardship (federal law). Given that the law makes explicitly clear the specific provisions to which all nursing mothers are entitled, we want to share with you the exact wording as found in the Affordable Care Act, which amended Section 7 of the Fair Labor Standards Act (FLSA): *An employer shall provide a reasonable break time for an employee to express breast milk for her nursing child for 1 year after the child's birth each time such employee has need to express the milk and a place, other than a bathroom, that is shielded from view and free from intrusion from coworkers and the public, which may be used by an employee to express breast milk.*

- Specifically exclude breastfeeding from public indecency laws (30 states).

- Address workplace breastfeeding (29 states).

- Exempt breastfeeding mothers from jury duty or allow it to be postponed (17 states plus Puerto Rico).

- Exempt breastfeeding products from being charged sales tax (thanks to Maryland and Louisiana leading the way).

- Establish a Breastfeeding Mothers' Bill of Rights (New York).

Slowly but surely, the numbers, as well as the breastfeeding-friendly laws they represent, are improving. If we've piqued your interest and you somehow manage to find yourself with some spare time, you can check out the National Conference of State Legislatures website (www.ncsl.org) to brush up on additional breastfeeding rights and regulations and watch for more progress to come.

Getting Started

What's Natural Doesn't Always Come Naturally

Yes, the act of breastfeeding is "natural," but the truth of the matter is that it doesn't always come naturally. All too often, new parents expect to be handed a newborn who gracefully latches on, nurses no more than 15 minutes on each breast every 3 hours, and delights in a plentiful supply of breast milk within a few short days. We can only wish this scenario for all of you. But clinging to this idealistic picture of breastfeeding bliss, especially during the newborn period, is all but guaranteed to set you up for perceived failure. If in the introductory weeks of breastfeeding, however, you prepare yourself for the distinct possibility that your newborn may lack interest or sucking stamina, that each feeding may be different, and that your nipples may be a little worse for wear early on, well then, you only stand to be pleasantly surprised. The most likely scenario: breastfeeding may be natural, but expect it to be a learning process for you and your baby over the first few weeks or possibly longer. While some new moms do experience nipple irritations, others experience nothing more than some slight and short-lived tenderness. Some babies are quick learners. Others take their own sweet time.

Advice Abounds

As you educate yourself and start your on-the-job training, you're almost certain to find that anyone who has ever breastfed (or been remotely involved in breastfeeding) considers themselves a full-fledged expert. Some of the advice you get will undoubtedly prove to be helpful. But be aware that you'll probably get your fair share of unsolicited suggestions and contradictory, confusing, or just plain wrong advice—even when it comes from moms who have breastfed many children, are highly intelligent, and have the best of intentions. Just keep in mind that, at the end of the day, there are only a few universally accepted facts about breastfeeding (which we've made a point of including throughout this chapter). The rest of what you do and how you do it will be a matter of establishing your own breastfeeding style.

Sending Out an SOS (In Search of Support)

Breastfeeding has amazing rewards, but it can also be a demanding and tiring 24-hour-a-day job. If you find yourself experiencing feelings of frustration, isolation, or even entrapment, one of the worst things you can do is try to cope alone. Of course, it's not any better to find yourself in the company of a well-meaning colleague, friend, or family member who is just waiting for the opportunity to tell you how easy formula feeding would be in contrast. Please take a moment and reassure yourself you are absolutely not alone and don't need to figure out the tricks of the trade the hard way! We strongly suggest that if what you really need is a supportive shoulder to lean on, put down this book and find one (or several). It may seem like yet one more thing you don't have time for, but reaching out for support, when needed, can make all the difference in the world.

- **Get help from your hospital.** Labor and delivery staff (including your obstetrician, midwife, or doula), nurses in the mother-baby unit, and hospital lactation specialists are a great place to start exploring what types of support are available in your community before, during, and after you deliver.

- **Turn to your pediatrician for advice or assistance.** As pediatricians, we routinely observe newborns breastfeeding and are very accustomed to providing practical advice and troubleshooting tips. Increasingly, pediatricians are also providing more in-depth lactation support services in their offices, and some pediatricians themselves are even IBCLCs. Be sure to ask your pediatrician for advice, what additional services they offer, and, when necessary, a referral to a lactation consultant or other breastfeeding resources in your area.

- **Find a certified lactation support provider.** The term *lactation support provider* encompasses a wide range of providers (and abbreviations), some of whom may also be nurses, doctors, or other health care providers. Perhaps the most familiar, international board-certified lactation consultants (IBCLCs) are credentialed breastfeeding specialists with the knowledge and training in breastfeeding support necessary to support even those breastfeeding mothers facing significant challenges. However, IBCLCs are not always available or necessary, since other types of providers (eg, certified lactation counselors, or CLCs; certified lactation educators, or CLEs) can help with more routine aspects, challenges, and questions about breastfeeding. Ask your hospital, baby's doctor, or insurance company for the name(s) of a local lactation support provider, or visit www.ilca.org to find an IBCLC near you. You may even find one who makes house calls.

- **Check out peer counselors** such as La Leche League International (LLLI), which has local chapters throughout the world and offers valuable mom-to-mom support, as well as other breastfeeding resources. Check their website (www.llli.org) to find area leaders and meeting places and times. LLLI offers a Breastfeeding Hotline as well (800-525-3243). In addition, the Women, Infants, and Children (WIC) program offers support for low-income breastfeeding women, who are at nutritional risk, up to their infant's first birthday.

- **Call the National Women's Health and Breastfeeding Helpline.** Through this resource, the national Office on Women's Health reportedly makes available trained breastfeeding peer counselors for phone support. Although it's not a substitute for direct medical attention or advice, feel free to access this support or find additional breastfeeding answers and resources at www.womenshealth.gov/breastfeeding or by calling 800-994-9662.

- **Don't be afraid to enlist your spouse, partner, friends, family members, or neighbors**—anyone you think might be able to lend a hand or offer emotional support. Even though no one else can breastfeed for you, we've never met a new mother who doesn't appreciate the offer of help with other items on the family's daily to-do list, whether it's in the form of cleaning, cooking, running errands, doing laundry, or simply holding the baby for a bit.

- **Join a support group.** In today's connected world, in-person and virtual breastfeeding support groups abound and are easily found through a quick search on the internet. Of course, as with any internet activity, be careful about any private information you divulge online, and look for credible sources of information, such as from hospitals, trained consultants, or LLLI chapters. It's always a very good idea to discuss any concerns, advice, and/or information you read about related to your baby's safety, health, and development with your baby's pediatrician.

A BREAST A DAY KEEPS THE DOCTOR AWAY

Based on many studies done in the United States and elsewhere around the world, we know that breastfeeding not only is nutritionally sound and decreases the risk of sudden infant death syndrome (SIDS) (see The Reality of SIDS: Creating a Safe Sleep Environment on page 103) but can translate into fewer respiratory tract infections, allergies, ear infections, hospitalizations, and visits to the doctor's office. That's because protective proteins called *antibodies,* along with other infection-fighting cells found in breast milk, are continually transferred from you to your baby for as long as you breastfeed. This added level of defense against bacteria and viruses is particularly beneficial during the first several months when babies' immune systems aren't yet functioning at full speed.

My Baby, My Breasts, and I

Becoming a new breastfeeding mother really does involve a fundamental shift in one's view of the world—a shift that is not only lifelong in the sense of awe you get from nurturing a child of your own but more immediate in a practical, concrete way. That is, you are suddenly thrust from a world primarily focused on "me, myself, and I" (or perhaps "me, my spouse/partner, and I") to one inevitably structured around "my baby, my breasts, and I." As you set out to master the fine art of breastfeeding, you are likely to look at your breasts in a whole new way, giving them far more consideration than ever before (regardless of how significant they were to you in your pre-breastfeeding past). In fact, we are of the strong belief that if your baby's health care provider doesn't ask you how you, your baby, *and* your breasts are doing in your early days of breastfeeding, he or she has, for lack of a more tactful description, missed the boat.

First Attempts

Assuming all goes well with the birth of your baby and both of you are doing well in the minutes and hours immediately following delivery, the best time to attempt your first breastfeeding is as soon as possible, ideally within the first hour after birth. While this may seem obvious, it's easy to find yourself feeling as if you have little to no say or control in what takes place during your hospital stay, much less in your delivery room. If you simply wait for someone to tell you what to do and when, whether you are encouraged to breastfeed right away will depend on your hospital's attitudes toward breastfeeding. In contrast, showing up at the hospital with a good general understanding of what to expect and a birth plan that can be modified as need be can be both empowering and make it more likely that your breastfeeding and bonding efforts will get off to a great start.

Helping Hands at the Hospital

Your goal for breastfeeding in the delivery room (and throughout your stay at the hospital) should be to make sure you and your baby work out the concept of latching on correctly. Ideally, the labor and delivery nurses bring mothers their newborns within minutes of delivery (if not immediately) and offer plenty of breastfeeding instruction and encouragement. While fortunately less common than in days past, sometimes a baby may be cleaned up, weighed, and have any number of procedures before mom gets to hold much less breastfeed for the first time. If you want to get breastfeeding off to a good start, don't be afraid to take things into your own hands and give it a try while you're still in the delivery room. Don't let routine hospital procedures keep you from taking advantage of your baby's temporary state of alertness (which we liken to a honeymoon period). Put more strongly, it's actually considered critical to breastfeeding success for the first attempt to occur in the delivery room or as soon as mom is alert, in the case of a caesarean section, unless other medical issues take precedence. Having just been through a pretty eye-opening experience, many babies tend to be temporarily wide-awake right after delivery, but within a matter of hours, you may well find you have a very sleepy baby on your chest.

Getting Comfortable

Given that just about all new moms are prone to focusing their attention on their breasts (and their babies) when they first sit or lie down to nurse, we also want to remind you to take a moment and make yourself comfortable. Support yourself with extra pillows, making sure you have on convenient and comfortable clothing. Have anything you might want or need within arm's reach (a glass of water, a book, the phone, or the TV remote control) *before* getting down to business. These small details can definitely make the experience more enjoyable. When it comes to the actual position you try, the choice is up to you. In case you aren't aware of them, we briefly describe several of the most popular options.

- **Cradle hold (Figure 1-1).** This is the position most novice breastfeeders start with and the one that many moms prefer. The most common exception is new moms who have just had cesarean deliveries and want to avoid having their newborns press on their bellies or those whose babies need a bit more guidance while still learning how to latch on correctly. While sitting up (preferably with lots of comfy pillows and good back support in place), you simply lay your baby across your lap sideways so she is facing you with her head in line with your breast. In the typical cradle hold, you use your right arm to support your baby's head and body while she nurses on your right breast (her head resting in the crook of your right arm as your hand supports her bottom). Use your left arm for support while she is nursing on your left breast. To help ease strain on your back, shoulders, and neck, try putting a regular or specially designed breastfeeding pillow or two across your lap to help raise your baby up to the level of your breast. While you may be content with cradling your baby in your arm(s) as she breastfeeds, trust us when we tell you a few well-positioned pillows placed under your arms can work wonders and spare you some unnecessary aches and pains. As you get into the finer points of positioning, or if you find the traditional cradle to be difficult, you can also try what is referred to by breastfeeding experts as the *cross-cradle hold*. With your baby lying across your lap ready to nurse on your left breast, you can use your right arm (ie, opposite side) instead of your left, as in the typical cradle hold, to support your baby's head and body. This will allow you to support your left breast with your left hand—something new moms often find more helpful in the early days of breastfeeding when babies have not yet mastered latching on and need a bit more guidance. For either type of cradle hold, whichever arm you are not using to support your baby's head and body is free to help position your baby's mouth onto your nipple.

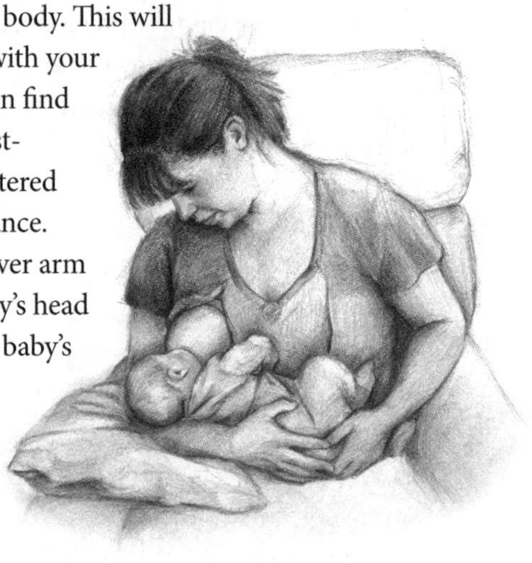

Figure 1-1. The cradle hold

- **Football (or clutch) hold (Figure 1-2).** To position yourself for breastfeeding by using the so-called football hold, some parenting books suggest you picture a football player holding a football under his arm as he runs downfield. We're willing to bet that conjuring up this mental image won't be enough to help many of you prevent some initial fumbling. As you sit down and try to replicate the position with your baby, here's an explanation we hope you find more practical: unlike the cradle hold, during which your baby lies across your lap, the football hold involves laying your baby to one side of you or the other. If you're going to start nursing on your right breast, position your baby so that her face is level with your breast while her body rests against your right side (with her legs to the back). You can then use your right arm to support her body. Well-placed pillows under your baby—this time, along your side instead of across your lap—can take a lot of strain off your supporting arm, shoulder, and neck. We ourselves never had much success with this hold, but for your purposes, all that really matters is that it works well for some moms and not so well for others, so feel free to try it out for yourself.

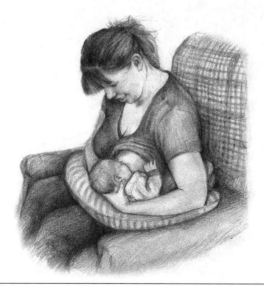

Figure 1-2. The football (or clutch) hold

- **Side-by-side (or lying down) position (Figure 1-3).** In this position, you and your baby lie down facing each other. Have your baby's mouth in line with your breast. You'll probably find yourself using your lower arm to support your head, leaving the upper part of your arm to help adjust your baby (or breast) as needed. While most women seem to prefer nursing from their lower breast (ie, when they are lying on the right side, they offer their right breast), there are no hard-and-fast rules. If you find yourself recovering from a cesarean delivery, or if you're just plain exhausted and don't feel like sitting up, you may decide this is a great way to breastfeed with less effort—especially once you get the hang of it.

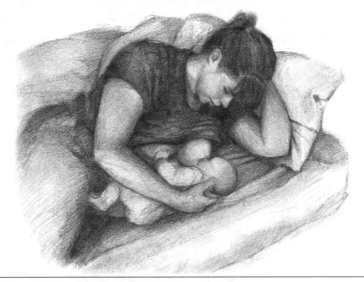

Figure 1-3. Side-by-side (or lying down) position

Breathing Room

Regardless of what breastfeeding position works best for you, a couple of fundamental "rules" apply to all positions. Once you've brought your baby to your breast, make a point of allowing him to move his head as needed by supporting his neck with your thumb and index finger behind his ears rather than holding the back of his head firmly against your breast. Yes, his head needs support, but you can relax your hold (and yourself) a bit once your baby has latched on and is breastfeeding. This allows him to adjust himself as necessary. You'll just want to make sure to continue to provide enough head and neck support that he doesn't start "slipping off" and latching on improperly, which can lead to sore nipples for you and less success for him. You can also help make sure he has adequate room to breathe at all times by making sure at least one nostril is always visible (ie, not completely covered by your breast).

COLOSTRUM: IT'S WHAT'S FOR DINNER

Your breasts are likely to start producing thick, yellowish milk called *colostrum* even before your baby is born—as early as the second trimester. Colostrum provides most newborns with everything they need for the first several days, including both nutrition and infection-fighting antibodies. Frequent small feedings in the early days are normal and adequate for most babies, and your pediatrician will monitor your newborn's weight at least daily. By the end of your baby's first week, if not sooner, your body should begin to make a larger volume of milk that is less yellow and more watery, known as *transitional milk*. This milk is more likely to satisfy your baby's hunger and help him settle into somewhat of a more predictable pattern of feeding. We suggest you put a positive slant on this transitional period and view your colostrum-producing breasts as half full rather than half empty, and of course, discuss any concerns about your baby not getting enough in these early days (or at any time, really) with your baby's pediatrician.

Catching On to Latching On

Anyone who's ever breastfed can tell you there's a big difference between getting babies to latch on and getting them to latch on *correctly*. For nursing mothers everywhere, this can mean the difference between smooth sailing and choppy waters, as defined by sore, cracked, blistered, or otherwise irritated nipples. For babies, it can mean the difference between actually getting some milk in return for their efforts and the equivalent of sucking on the closed end of a straw. To nurse effectively, babies need to use their tongues to essentially lap or massage milk out of the breast. This requires that the tongue be positioned under the breast in such a way that the baby can draw the nipple *and* the darker colored area around it (*areola*) into her mouth as she sucks. Remember that hugging your baby onto your breast instead of leaning into your baby's face can help facilitate a better latch. If your baby starts out nursing by simply pursing her lips around your nipple incorrectly and sucking away, you'll very quickly realize two important facts: the harder she sucks, the less likely she is to get anything and the more likely your nipples are to suffer the consequences.

Lending a Helping Hand

With any luck, you will find that there is at least one nurse or other health care provider present in the delivery room or available on the mother-baby floor of your hospital who is skilled at assisting new mothers with getting newborns to latch on correctly. Even if there's not, you can play an active role and facilitate.

- **Express interest.** Gently expressing a few drops of breast milk onto and around your nipple can help your baby hone in on his intended target.

- **Root for success.** If your baby still doesn't seem interested in opening his mouth, try lightly stroking his cheek just to the side of his mouth or to his lips to stimulate what's known as the *rooting reflex*—a reflex that should cause him to open his mouth in search of your nipple.

- **Open wide.** If he doesn't open his mouth wide enough, you can help him open it further by gently pushing down on his chin.

- **If at first you don't succeed…** If your baby doesn't get it right the first time, don't be fooled into thinking that any latching on is better than none. If it seems your baby's mouth didn't open wide enough to assume the necessary position on your breast, don't hesitate to take him off and encourage him to try again. The same advice applies if he seems to have only gotten your nipple into his mouth, or it continues to hurt when he sucks.

- **Don't get tongue-tied.** Be aware that a few (an estimated 0.02% to 4.4%) babies are born with their tongues a bit tethered. This so-called tethering is caused when the piece of tissue under the tongue limits the tongue's ability to stick out and move around freely (a condition known as *ankyloglossia*). The vast majority of babies with tongue-tie will be able to breastfeed without any problems. Given that the tongue plays a very important role in latching on and breastfeeding, just be sure to have your baby's doctor assess the degree of tethering, especially if you and your baby are experiencing breastfeeding difficulty. If lactation support alone does not help, a minor procedure to correct partial or complete ankyloglossia may make a difference in breastfeeding success (see Tongue-Tied on page 308).

GOING FOR THE GUSTO

Newborns have been shown to have an amazing inborn drive to nurse. In one study, newborns demonstrated their impressive ability to inch their way up from their mothers' bellies all the way to their breasts in search of food within mere minutes of being born. Quite impressive to witness, but given that this is a book about practicality, we don't suggest you sit around waiting for your newborn to propel herself up to your breasts before offering her the opportunity to breastfeed.

Getting It Right

We are well aware that telling you to take your baby off your breast and getting him to try again until he latches on correctly is sometimes easier said than done. For lack of a better analogy, many babies can admittedly seem a bit like leeches when it comes to latching on. Once they're on, they're on tight and holding on for dear life. Getting them to let go by attempting to pull them off is therefore a misguided and potentially painful prospect. There is, however, a relatively easy solution (that does not involve the use of salt or matches commonly recommended for leech removal). Before removing your baby from your breast, gently slide one finger into his mouth to break the seal of his lips around your nipple. Once the seal is broken, you'll find it much quicker, easier, and less painful to take him off and have him start over again. You can also use this technique whenever you need to interrupt or end a feeding. While it's true that most babies don't like being taken off the breast in the middle of a feeding, this interruption can actually work in your favor. If your baby subsequently cries in disapproval, he's all but guaranteed to open his mouth wider, increasing the likelihood that he'll latch on correctly during his next attempt. Bottom line: if the latch is painful, it is not correct, and time to try again and seek help, both for you and for the baby.

NOT ALL NIPPLES OR BREASTS ARE CREATED EQUAL

To get straight to the point, nipples come in all shapes and sizes, as do breasts themselves. That said, new and expectant moms often wonder whether flat or inverted nipples or a past history of breast surgery will affect their ability to breastfeed. The good news: as long as a baby can latch on enough to get a good portion of the breast into his mouth (which may take a little extra assistance or consultation), most types of nipples don't inherently interfere with breastfeeding success. As for women who have had any prior breast surgery, the important underlying factor is going to be whether the milk ducts or major nerves were affected. The best way to find out? You can simply clarify with the surgeon who performed the surgery. In addition, your baby's health care provider can help make sure all is in working order by assessing your baby's weight gain and nursing abilities.

Breastfeeding Irritations

During the first days and weeks of breastfeeding, it's entirely normal for mothers to experience a certain degree of mild tenderness as their nipples grow accustomed to repeated sucking and stimulation and to feel a "tug" with suckling. How then, you might wonder, are you supposed to know the difference between discomfort associated with starting out anew and pain and irritation resulting when a baby doesn't latch on correctly? Beyond paying close attention to how your baby latches on, try also to figure out whether the irritation tends to subside as your baby gets into a rhythm of sucking. Mild irritation or discomfort that occurs only at the start of each feeding is generally associated with the newness of nursing. As you and your nipples toughen up over the days and weeks to follow, you're likely to find that this type of irritation quickly fades away (thank goodness!). Nipple pain that persists or worsens as your baby nurses, on the other hand, is more likely to be a sign that she is not latched on correctly and may be accompanied by cracked or blistered nipples—the thought of which is enough to make anyone (especially breastfeeding moms) cringe.

Nurturing Your Nipples

In the spirit of being honest and preparing you for what may lie ahead, the bad news is that cracked or blistered nipples can appear after even just one breastfeeding session gone wrong. The good news is that nipples heal. With proper care, patience, and a little extra attention, they can get better within a matter of days. Given that this never seems fast enough to those of us who've experienced such nipple pain and misery firsthand, here are some temporizing measures you can try if you happen to find yourself with sore, dry, cracked, or blistered nipples.

- **Hang in there.** Pain and misery are not what breastfeeding is ultimately about. As the saying goes, "This too shall pass."

- **Focus on the latch.** First and foremost, readdress how your baby is latching on. Rather than having your baby latch straight onto your nipple like a target, you may find more success by using what's called an "asymmetrical latch," during which your baby's mouth centers more on the lower part of your areola.

- **Go for the lesser of two evils.** If one breast feels any less sore than the other, by all means, go with the lesser of two evils and offer that one to your baby first because babies tend to suck harder when they first start nursing.

- **Smooth things out.** Consider the use of specially designed nontoxic creams such as lanolin (available in most stores that sell baby products) after breastfeeding, or even use a little dab of your own breast milk on your breasts. Then expose them to open air.

- **Bare yourself if need be.** If the pain doesn't start to resolve despite your best efforts or if you have any questions, seek professional help sooner rather than later—as in within a day or so at most—to get things back on track. This should be from someone accustomed and qualified to be offering breastfeeding advice. Ideally, you can find someone you are comfortable baring your nipples to if need be (refer back to Sending Out an SOS: In Search of Support on page 10).

- **Options are out there.** It's well worth remembering that many more options, techniques, and tricks of the trade available to breastfeeding mothers who find themselves sore, frustrated, and with seemingly uncooperative breasts. They include but are not limited to pumping, breast shells, nipple shields, and supplemental nursing systems. While these additional options can be very helpful to ensuring your breastfeeding success when used appropriately, be sure to ask your baby's doctor or see your local lactation consultant to make sure they're actually indicated. In the case of nipple shields, for example, they can actually limit the amount of milk a baby gets and require pumping after feedings and should therefore only be used under the careful guidance of a lactation professional.

WHAT'S BEHIND BURNING NIPPLES

If you happen to experience nipple irritation that is best described as a tingling, burning sensation lasting more than a few days, it's always worth discussing with your (or your baby's) health care provider. While there are several potential causes, a yeast infection may occasionally be to blame. Yeast like moist areas and don't discriminate between your baby's mouth (see Thrush Attack on page 307), your baby's rear end (see A Word on Diaper Rash on page 147), and your nipples. Letting your nipples air-dry before stuffing them back in your bra or under breast pads can help lessen your chances. If yeast do take up residence on your nipple(s), you'll want to discuss appropriate yeast-fighting measures with your baby's doctor. Sometimes all it takes is a little appropriately applied medication—on your nipples and in your baby's mouth—to clear things up and get your nipples on the fast track to full recovery.

Cramping

While you may have heard plenty of tales of sore breasts and nipples from others who have breastfed before you, they may have forgotten to forewarn you about the associated cramping of the uterus that some new mothers experience during the early days of breastfeeding. By this point in the chapter you may be asking yourself if the fun ever stops, but trust us when we say that breastfeeding isn't all about enduring pain. When you sit down to breastfeed, your uterus may cramp (described by some as resembling a contraction) in response. That's because the signal that is known to cause contractions is the same one responsible for triggering the milk letdown reflex (see The Letdown Tingle on page 25). So while the cramping itself isn't exactly pleasant, you can consider it a good sign that your baby is latching on correctly and sending your body all the right signals. In fact, this dual response also plays a signifi-cant role in helping your body recover more quickly from pregnancy and childbirth, decreasing the likelihood of uterine bleeding and shortening the amount of time it takes your uterus to shrink back down to its normal size. Of course, any ongoing, increasing, or otherwise concerning cramping or bleeding needs to be discussed with your obstetrician or another qualified health care provider.

Going With the Flow

A Simple Matter of Supply and Demand

Once the latching-on part of breastfeeding is squared away, many parents find themselves worrying about whether their newborns are getting enough to eat. If you want to know the truth, in many ways the answer would seem to be no, but that answer doesn't tell the whole story. Allow us to explain. Yes, your baby will be getting enough to live on until your full volume of milk comes in. But what he is getting is a relatively small volume of a milky, yellowish white substance called *colostrum* (see Colostrum: It's What's for Dinner on page 17). While colostrum is rich in protein, it is lacking in fats, sugar, and overall calories, as well as sheer volume. The fact that a new mother's body comes equipped with colostrum makes perfect sense in the grand scheme of things. Nature has made it so newborns get just enough nutrients to get them through the first few days. The fact that newborns naturally want to breastfeed frequently in the early days helps ensure that their mothers' milk production will increase in response. During your first few days of breastfeeding—and for as long as you continue to breastfeed your baby—the more he breastfeeds, the more your body will sense his increased demand and respond by stepping up the milk production, increasing your supply of breast milk accordingly. Conversely, whenever supplemental formula is offered in lieu of nursing (and without any pumping or emptying of the breasts to compensate), this sends your body the signal that less is needed. As you might imagine, the perceived decrease in demand that results from this sort of supplementation eventually leads to a decrease in supply.

SIZE MATTERS

You may be relieved to know that breast size doesn't really matter when it comes to milk production, as it is not proportional to breast size. While everyone's bustline tends to expand during pregnancy, rest assured that when it comes to breastfeeding success, mothers who barely fill their A cups can rival their D-cup colleagues.

The Turning Point: How Will I Know When My Milk Comes In?

You may think that knowing when your milk has "come in" is another one of those "you can't relate until you experience it yourself" scenarios. But chances are good that when your breasts have gotten the message and respond by making larger volumes of milk, it will be an occurrence unlikely to go unnoticed. We can't think of any clearer way to describe it than how my (Laura's) husband put it the day my milk came in. He matter-of-factly said, "Wow! You definitely did not have those when I married you." In other words, one's milk coming in is more often than not accompanied by a not so subtle change in breast size.

Some new mothers find that the initial change from producing colostrum to producing transitional milk takes place over a couple of hours. For others, the course of change becomes noticeable over a few days as the breast milk supply goes from transitional milk to mature milk. In either case, most moms experience a noticeable increase in breast size accompanied by a feeling of fullness during the first week. That said, new moms can sometimes be deceived into thinking they've started producing a full supply of mature milk before their breasts actually get the hang of it. If you don't experience a reassuringly noticeable change, or if there's any question in your mind as to whether your milk has started to flow and your newborn is getting enough—especially during these early days and weeks—take your questions or concerns to your baby's doctor without delay. In fact, this is one of the most important topics (along with weight gain) that serves to justify the recommendation for all newborns to be seen by their pediatrician within three to five days following discharge.

Progressive Production

The change from colostrum to transitional and then to mature milk that takes place over the first week or so is an important one. It gives you and your baby's doctor reassurance that all is going well. Because the transition to an increased milk supply is not always so clear-cut for some women, it is useful to be aware of several other clues that can help you figure out that everything is moving ahead as it should. They include

- Your breast milk turns white instead of remaining yellow in color. It also appears thinner or clearer.
- Your baby makes more obvious gulping and swallowing noises when nursing.
- Your baby begins to pee and poop much more frequently (see What Goes In Must Come Out on page 71).
- Your baby begins to gain weight relatively noticeably on *and* off the scale instead of losing weight or just holding steady (see Weighing in on page 33).

The Letdown Tingle

The sensation that typically accompanies letdown isn't exactly the same for everyone. For that matter, it isn't present at all for some breastfeeding moms. That said, most women experience what is often described as a "tingling," a "prickling," or even an electric-like feeling in their breasts. Such sensations at the start of a feeding are helpful but not necessary in signifying that your milk has started to flow. As an aside, you may find (if you haven't already) that there are plenty of other potential triggers of milk letdown besides a latched-on baby at your breast. These can include but are not limited to the sound of a crying baby (yours or someone else's), a breast pump, nipple stimulation, sexual arousal, a warm shower, or, on occasion, nothing at all.

GETTING THE GOOD TIMES TO ROLL

New mothers who breastfeed typically experience a noticeable increase in milk production, commonly referred to as having their milk "come in," anywhere from two to five days after the birth of their babies (usually on the later side for moms who've had a caesarean delivery, commonly referred to as a "C-section"). How well you keep up with your fluid intake and your baby's ability to latch on correctly, how often you are able to nurse in the first few days, and many other factors can all play a role in the timing of this much anticipated turning point. This is a major reason why pediatricians want to see all newborns within a few days of discharge from the hospital. If your milk supply hasn't come in yet or you're unsure as to whether it has, your baby's doctor will evaluate your baby and offer reassurance or additional assistance to get your milk supply going.

Alleviating the Discomfort of Engorgement

For some of you, breast "fullness" will be a purely euphemistic way of describing *engorgement,* a word familiar to many new breastfeeding moms defined as "being filled to the often-painful point of capacity or congestion." Yes, your body may well have some work to do in the first days and weeks of breastfeeding before your breasts learn to control how much milk they make and spare you the discomfort of overdistension. Until your milk production matches your baby's needs—your breasts making as much as needed, when it's needed, without going overboard—you may find yourself in some uncomfortable positions. Frequently feeding your baby goes a long way toward avoiding engorgement. For those who still find themselves in the uncomfortable position, fortunately, there are things you can do about engorgement.

The two mainstays of managing engorgement are

1. Wear a supportive bra (to help carry the extra weight).
2. Express a little milk whenever necessary to allow your baby to more easily latch on and/or to relieve the discomfort of very full breasts.

When it comes to the latter, be sure to think about the concept of supply and demand (mentioned in A Simple Matter of Supply and Demand on page 23) before expressing a lot of milk. You'll find there's a fine line between expressing enough breast milk to relieve the pain and expressing so much that you give your body the unintended message to produce even more. Using a warm compress or taking a warm shower and then expressing a little milk, as well as feeding your baby a bit more frequently, may also help relieve your symptoms.

MASTITIS

If you are a breastfeeding mom, it's going to be well worth your time to be on the lookout for mastitis (pronounced mast-EYE-tiss). Be forewarned that this type of breast infection has a way of sneaking up on breastfeeding mothers. It's sneaky because the more obvious signs of breast-specific infection may not be apparent until a day or two after you start to feel run-down, achy, sick, or feverish. In mastitis, bacteria infect the breast ducts that store milk, resulting in painful, red, swollen breasts. By familiarizing yourself with mastitis, you stand a fighting chance of noticing it early on, getting necessary medical advice, and getting appropriately treated with antibiotics sooner rather than later. Although mastitis may be uncomfortable, it's good to know that you can (and should) take the following measures:

- The most important step in managing mastitis is frequent and effective milk removal. Continue to breastfeed on the affected side as much as possible (as often as every two hours) to keep the breast from becoming overly sore. If it is too sore to feed on that side, try emptying the breast by pumping or hand expression, or start feeding on the unaffected side. Then progress to the affected side once milk is flowing.

- Make sure your baby has latched on well and try to aim your baby's nose or chin toward any specific areas of tenderness (ie, blockage) to help drain the affected area.

- Apply a warm compress to get milk flowing if needed.

- Wear a supportive but not constricting bra.

- Carefully massage the affected part of the breast. This can potentially help speed up the healing process.

- Take comfort in the fact that most antibiotics can be safely taken while breastfeeding.

- Consider taking an over-the-counter medicine such as ibuprofen (the active ingredient in Advil and Motrin) to help reduce inflammation and control pain.

    While it's easy to become very focused on one's breasts when mastitis sets in, remember that treatment of mastitis also involves rest, hydration, and nutrition. In other words, take care of yourself as best as you can (and be sure to enlist others' help as well!).

Leaky Breasts: It's Not Worth Crying Over Spilled Milk

Having also experienced leaky breasts firsthand, we readily admit that they all too often come with the territory as your body adapts to breastfeeding. While they may represent a mild nuisance for some, they can be a source of considerable frustration or great embarrassment to others. It's not clear why some women's bodies seem to control milk flow more "conveniently" than others. Some experience only minimal leakage limited to the few days after milk comes in. Others face a more pervasive problem that can last for weeks (or even months) into the course of breastfeeding. If nothing else, we offer you some words of advice and encouragement that we hope help you take this potentially leaky fact of breastfeeding life in stride.

- **Gain the power of perspective.** You may hear an occasional account of someone whose breasts never quite contained themselves and proceeded to leak the entire time she breastfed. Statistically speaking, your own chances of "recovery" are actually good. Any leakage you may experience at the outset will most likely subside or resolve completely over time. And just because you leak a lot with your first baby doesn't mean you are destined to leak a lot with every subsequent child. Okay, so it may not be that much of a consolation this time around, but at least there's light at the end of the next tunnel!

- **Invest in breast pads.** Breast pads are a very useful invention. Feel free to try out the thin cotton disposable ones if you have only minimal leakage. Just be ready to head straight for the washable, reusable, and generally more absorbent type if the disposable ones don't do the trick. For those of you whose breasts really haven't gotten the hang of holding the milk in until feeding time, you wouldn't be the first to decide to stuff a burp cloth or hand towel or even a clean cloth diaper into your bra to keep things under control while sleeping or lounging around in the privacy of your own home.

- **Provide pressure.** If you start to leak (or are blessed with some warning of impending leakage in the form of a letdown tingle), put pressure on your breasts to slow or stop the flow. When in public, you can subtly fold your arms across your chest and squeeze firmly. Often effective, at least temporarily, this gives new meaning to assuming an arms-crossed power pose.

- **Contain yourself.** Take extra measures to contain yourself, so to speak. Wearing a supportive bra during the time when you are breastfeeding is said not only to decrease your odds of being left with saggy breasts after your breastfeeding days are over but to help decrease the likelihood of engorgement and leakage. While it may not be a common topic of public discussion, believe us when we tell you that plenty of new moms (particularly those who are prone to leakage or engorgement) take up the habit of wearing a well-fitting but not too tight bra 24/7 for as long as it takes for the flow to be better controlled.

If the Bra Fits…

As a general rule—even before pregnancy and breastfeeding are factored in—we firmly believe that splurging on comfortable bras and underwear is well worth whatever it costs. You've probably already discovered that pregnancy is often responsible for increasing one's bust size. So is breastfeeding. By how much varies, but it's relatively safe to say that bras that once fit you in your pre-pregnancy days are not going to be of much use for a while. With that in mind and the task of bra shopping at hand, we suggest you

- **Consider comfort and convenience.** Above all else, look for bras that offer comfort and convenience. After all, you'll be breastfeeding your newborn as many as 12 times a day, and this is a garment that you may well find yourself wearing 24 hours a day! You'll have enough going on with your breasts that the last thing you'll need is to add another potential source of discomfort or irritation from a poorly fitting bra.

- **Expect expansion.** Expect that you'll keep expanding until your milk supply comes in. While you may have already invested in some new, bigger bras during your pregnancy, you may find that your cup size "runneth over" as you start breastfeeding, thus requiring yet larger bras to accommodate. Of course, this means that you should also be ready for a reduction in breast size as your body adjusts to your baby's needs over the first weeks. A decrease in size does not inherently mean that you've stopped producing enough milk (assuming that everything else is going smoothly) but rather that you might just need to go back to a previously smaller size bra.

- **Evaluate for ease of use.** Nursing bras nowadays come with all sorts of modern-day conveniences—not the least of which are flaps that can be opened on each cup to allow easy and more discreet access. Be sure to try on a couple to see not only if they are comfortable and fit well but also if the flaps are easy to fasten and unfasten.

- **Go with what works.** Regular bras are also an option. Some women find wearing a regular bra and simply pulling the shoulder strap (and therefore the cup) down to work well. Partially opening a front-fastening bra is another option, as some find it as easy as wearing a true breastfeeding bra, not to mention less expensive and in some cases more comfortable.

BIG GIRLS DO CRY

On a more serious note, many a new mother has, in fact, cried over spilled milk, as well as the absence of milk, an inadequate milk supply, or just about anything else to do with breastfeeding or new parenthood. The fact of the matter is that the "baby blues" and postpartum depression are very real (and can, in fact, affect new mothers *and* new fathers). While it's perfectly okay for "big girls" to cry too, if you find yourself frequently frustrated, more teary than usual, or feeling persistently sad, anxious, overwhelmed, or moody, don't be afraid to ask for support from your spouse, family members, or friends, and be sure to talk with your doctor or another qualified health care provider about your feelings right away.

How Much Is Enough? How Much Is Too Much?

Unlike their formula-feeding counterparts, who rely on the ounce-by-ounce markings displayed on the sides of their babies' bottles, breastfeeding parents typically have questions and concerns about exactly how much breast milk their newborns are getting and whether it is enough.

To address this understandable but often unnecessary concern, it's helpful to first distinguish between the several days *before* your milk comes in and the period *after* this turning point. As we've already discussed (see Getting the Good Times to Roll on page 26), the 2- to 5-day period preceding your milk coming in is inherently going to be a different breastfeeding experience—for you and your baby—than what you should expect as soon as the tide has come in, so to speak. By breastfeeding as often as you can during the first few days, without letting yourself become *too* irritated or sore by making sure you get a good latch every time, you can help ensure that your baby doesn't become dehydrated before your body reaches full milk production. Practically speaking, we recommend that you breastfeed more frequently during the day (at least every 2 to 3 hours but more often if your baby is ready, willing, and able). While it's okay to let up a little at night, set your alarm for every 4 hours at the most if your baby will sleep that long. Overall, it's still good to aim for an initial 8 to 12 feedings within each 24-hour period. Over the course of the first month, the number of times babies feed each day typically decreases. While the actual number can vary considerably from one baby to the next, ending up in the ballpark of 7 to 9 feedings per day sometime between the first and fourth weeks is fairly common. If your baby has jaundice (see Seeing Yellow: Jaundice on page 335) or you suspect he may be getting dehydrated (peeing less, dry mouth, etc), you'll definitely want to have him checked out, as well as discuss specific feeding recommendations and expectations with his doctor.

Settling Into a Routine

Once your milk supply comes in, be prepared to enter into a new phase of breastfeeding that more closely resembles the mental image many new parents have about breastfeeding—one that includes frequent feedings accompanied by lots of wet diapers and soft, if not outright watery, poop (for more on this subject, see What Goes In Must Come Out on page 71). What you should not expect, however, is that you and your baby will gracefully fall into a predictable routine defined by a set feeding schedule. Even after the first week or so, you may still find there are days when your baby wants to breastfeed every hour or so—a pattern that often signals a growth spurt (see Growth Spurts on page 65). At other times, she may sleep her way through four or more hours and still show no signs of waking up to eat. These considerations are what make the strictly defined patterns of feeding touted in some parenting books so unrealistic. That said, a somewhat predictable feeding schedule would not be misguided unless you try to get your baby to adhere to it without exception from day 1. Overall, it is reasonable to expect to feed your baby at least every two to three hours as a baseline, with the possibility of one longer stretch of four or more hours (preferably at night) within a few weeks. Remember that this schedule is a work in progress over the next several weeks or possibly months.

Breastfeeding On the Go

While a handful of new moms seem to be as comfortable baring all on a bench at the park, in the center seat on an airplane, or at the home of a friend as they are in the privacy of their own homes, there's nothing wrong or prudish about you if you aren't so sure about breastfeeding in public—now or ever. It's all about your comfort level. There's certainly a sense of liberation that comes with learning some of the tricks of the trade that will ultimately allow you to breastfeed discreetly in public places (see, for example, Breastfeeding in Restricted Airspace on page 258). But unless you're ready, don't worry about mastering them now. For many mothers, this is but one of the many differences between first and subsequent children.

BREASTFEEDING IN THE AGE OF SOCIAL MEDIA

In an era of Facebook, Instagram, Snapchat, Twitter, and more that offers new moms greater access to social support, it should come as no surprise that breastfeeding-related discussions abound. At the heart of the matter? Whether there's such a thing as overexposure when it comes to the sharing of breast-baring images of nursing mothers. Facebook, for example, faced a year of protest over gender-based discrimination for deeming photographs depicting topless breastfeeding mothers and images of exposed nipples—all in the context of breastfeeding—to nevertheless be in violation of policies restricting nudity and obscenity. A year and tens of thousands of tweets and emails later, Facebook's so-called nipple ban was lifted in mid-2014.

Breastfeeding by Numbers

You can use the following handy definitions and rules of thumb to establish your own approach to a breastfeeding routine:

- **Feeding intervals.** If you haven't started breastfeeding yet, it's probably hard to imagine how this can be a source of confusion. The issue at hand has to do with the starting point—whether to use the *start* of a feeding or the time at which your baby actually *finishes* the meal to determine when it's time to feed again. The pokier your newborn is at breastfeeding—with some babies seeming to take upward of an hour to complete a feeding— the more this subject will apply to you. The standard convention is to use the time from the start of the first feeding to the start of the next. Yes, this may well mean starting a second feeding within an hour or so of finishing the previous one. What this means in real life: if you are attempting to make sure your baby eats at least every 2 to 3 hours and he starts nursing at 10:00 am, has to be woken up several times along the way, "requests" a diaper change at 10:30 am, and requires your active encouragement to latch back on to the second breast before finishing at around 11:00 am, you may still be looking at sitting down for another feeding no later than noon or

1:00 pm. It is worth noting that babies who seem to take an hour to complete a feeding are often not actually latched on and feeding the whole time but rather taking intermittent breaks, not latching correctly, or even sleeping on the job—all of which are appropriate topics to discuss with your baby's pediatrician. While there are plenty of new moms who understandably find this schedule a bit daunting, take comfort in knowing it is likely to last no more than the first few weeks of your breastfeeding experience.

- **Breastfeeding frequency.** The most commonly recommended schedule for newborn breastfeeding is every 2 to 3 hours, which translates into a minimum of 8 to 12 feedings during any given 24-hour period. The reason it's so important for you to focus on fitting in this many feedings a day is to make sure your baby gets enough to eat to gain weight and avoid getting dehydrated. Newborns who are still waiting for their mothers' milk supply to come in or those who are slow to catch on, latch on, or nurse even after milk is made abundantly available to them may end up having less energy and become increasingly more interested in sleeping. Newborns who start to go longer periods between feedings—especially when they have yet to establish themselves as good eaters and regain their birth weight—run the risk of getting even less to eat and becoming even more fatigued. A vicious cycle can ensue with a decrease in your milk production due to decreased stimulation. It is this cycle that you should be aware of and your seemingly round-the-clock feedings will help prevent.

BREASTFEEDING STRIKES

Conventional wisdom tells us that it's not a nutritionally great idea to skip meals. This belief certainly holds true when it comes to newborns. Anytime a newborn decides to go on strike and, as a result, misses two or more "meals" in a row for any reason—whether out of disinterest, lethargy, or difficulty feeding—you need to take heed and consult your baby's doctor without hesitation to find out why.

- **Weighing in.** You will find that just about everyone tends to focus on how much babies weigh in the days and weeks after they are born. That's because how much newborns weigh is a measurable, objective way of determining if they are getting enough to eat. Although all newborns are expected to lose some amount of weight after birth (mostly in the form of water weight), breastfed newborns may lose 7% to 10% of their birth weight before gaining it back by about two weeks of age. Your pediatrician may use a resource such as the Newborn Weight Tool (also called NEWT) at www.newborn-weight.org to identify babies who are losing too much weight.

One Breast or Two

The often-debated question of whether it is better to breastfeed a baby on one or both breasts at each feeding does not, in fact, have a single right answer. Some experts in the field recommend one, allowing babies to drain the breast fully and therefore get to the dessert equivalent of breast milk, known as *hind milk,* that has been shown to be richer in the fat that babies need to grow and develop. Others recommend the double-breasted approach, noting that 15 minutes of breastfeeding on each side typically drains most of a breast's total milk volume and offers the more practical benefit of preventing women from becoming temporarily lopsided after each feeding. Some women choose to drain the first breast fully to be sure their baby gets the hind milk and then nurse as long as possible on the second. From a practical standpoint, we've found that either approach is reasonable, with the added point that instead of just focusing on the clock to figure out when to switch sides, it's best to pay closer attention to your baby—watching for him to slow down to a few suckles before a pause, for example, to determine when to switch sides. Should you notice your baby has green, frothy poops, this could be a sign he's getting an abundance of foremilk compared to the amount of hind milk. In this instance, the recommendation is to try offering one breast per feeding (assuming your baby doesn't object) in order to more fully empty it.

- If your baby is a poky eater who can hardly be woken up to tackle the second breast after nursing from the first, well then, the "one breast per feeding" approach may better suit your needs. This is especially true if she happens to have a hard time latching on, is finicky, or rebels when- ever you attempt to take her off the first and switch her to the second. Just remember to keep track of which side your baby last nursed on and alternate breasts at each feeding. This routine may require you to use a newborn tracking app or write down which breast your baby fed from last because many a new mother has found that her memory isn't quite what it used to be before being in a chronic state of sleep deprivation. Or simply put a bracelet on your wrist or an extra breast pad on the side you need to breastfeed on first, an easy reminder of which side to start on the next time. Also, just remember that it's always a good idea for pokey eaters to be assessed by their pediatrician and weighed frequently to make sure they're actually getting enough.

- If your baby is content switching from one side to the other during the course of a feeding, or if you find that your "neglected" breast becomes uncomfortably engorged when you alternate, the two-breast routine may be better for you. Depending on how your baby acts at any given time of day, you may just want to follow her lead and try to keep each side as even as possible. As we mentioned earlier, this is more of a consideration when it comes to engorgement, leaking, and milk production in the first couple weeks of breastfeeding than it is down the road.

When all is said and done, your body and breasts will learn to accommodate whatever pattern you and your baby settle into, and you will have more flexibility in deviating from your standard routine.

Falling Into Bad Habits?

Even though you may be a relative newcomer to the world of parenthood, you've nonetheless probably been warned to not let your baby use your breasts as a pacifier or a snack bar; to not let him fall asleep while breastfeeding lest he become dependent on doing so for months, if not years, to come; and to try to get him onto a set feeding schedule as soon as you can. Well, here's news that will make your life easier: these warnings and recommendations don't apply to you during the first several weeks after birth. Spoiling is not and should not be a concern at this stage. In fact, resisting the urge to follow the scheduled approach to feeding, especially early on, and instead offering your newborn the opportunity to nurse frequently can actually help establish breastfeeding in such a way as to ensure future success. Once you and your baby have gotten comfortable and settled into the breastfeeding routine, you can more appropriately consider your options when it comes to feeding schedules and nursing as a pacifier substitute, if you so choose. Let us just add that trying to keep a newborn from falling asleep while breastfeeding is, in our experience, nothing short of an exercise in futility. All these things will come in time, but you don't need to worry about them for several weeks.

Nipple Confusion Defined

With respect to breastfeeding success, the overarching concern to keep in mind is that hungry babies who are inadvertently given pacifiers in lieu of being fed end up with poor weight gain and decreased milk supply. A good deal of attention has thus been paid to the notion that babies who are in the process of learning to breastfeed can sometimes be led astray by the introduction of artificial sucking devices—whether in the form of a nipple on a bottle or a pacifier (see also Practical Pacifier Principles on page 67). Even the experts seem to be divided when it comes to supplementing with a bottle or offering pacifiers to breastfed babies. We have found that it is entirely feasible to do either or both without sabotaging your chances for breastfeeding success, so long as you understand a few simple concepts and follow a few basic rules.

Remember, your baby's mouth is and will continue to be the center of her universe. Quite simply, babies naturally want to suck—and some more than others. In the first days and weeks, this urge to suck can certainly work to everyone's advantage in speeding up a breastfeeding mother's milk production. But once the milk is in and breastfeeding is well established, some new mothers find themselves in the challenging and sometimes uncomfortable position of having a baby who *constantly* wants to suck (or so it seems). That's because for some babies, sucking is not just about getting fed. This additional interest is referred to as *nonnutritive sucking* and is the reason why pacifiers (or fingers) can and often do come in handy in consoling a fussy baby. While there's nothing inherently wrong with letting your young infant nurse even after your breasts are drained and in between feedings (unless it is causing you undue pain), it is perfectly acceptable to use a pacifier instead. That said, it may help to limit pacifier use to times when your baby really wants it, has been adequately fed, and is falling asleep (see Sleeping Like a Baby on page 101) instead of offering it to her all the time. Be sure to talk with your baby's doctor if you have more questions about the use of pacifiers.

The Confusion About Nipple Confusion

The problem that some experts have with artificial nipples is that they have the potential to confuse a baby who is being breastfed. During the time when a baby is learning to breastfeed, sucking on the nipple of a bottle to get milk is thought to be considerably easier than the effort required to effectively lap milk out of a breast. The concern, therefore, is that babies not yet fully accomplished at breastfeeding may either opt for the "easy way out" or become confused about the necessary way to suck when returning from bottle to breast. Although pacifiers aren't responsible for supplying an alternative source of milk, they, too, require a baby to suck differently than he would on his mother's breast. That said, we have found that most breastfed babies do just fine with the introduction of a bottle or pacifier if their parents wait long enough to introduce it. How long is long enough? The practical answer is long enough to let your baby get the gist of breastfeeding first but not so long that he will accept no substitute. There's definitely a fine line between long enough and too long. While the exact timing is debated, somewhere in the vicinity of three to four weeks is generally accepted as a reasonable time to introduce an artificial nipple onto the sucking scene. If your baby is latching on, nursing, peeing, pooping, and gaining weight well, then we have found that many babies can successfully take a pacifier even within the first week without it interfering.

VITAMIN D FOR BREASTFED NEWBORNS

With only a few exceptions, most healthy full-term newborns get all the vitamins they need from breast milk or formula. One of the most notable exceptions is vitamin D—an important nutrient that helps prevent rickets and promotes general bone health. The American Academy of Pediatrics (AAP) recommends vitamin D supplementation for all exclusively and partially breastfed newborns beginning in the first few days (400 IU [international units] per day). Breast milk alone does not provide infants with an adequate amount unless moms take 6,400 IU of vitamin D daily, even if mothers are taking vitamin D–containing vitamins.

From a practical standpoint, you can give vitamin D drops by squirting them directly into your baby's mouth with the dropper or syringe that comes with the product (this may be less messy if you do it during bath time) or mixing them into a small amount of breast milk or formula.

Supplementing Scenarios

The decision to give a breastfed baby additional breast milk or formula from a bottle—better known as *supplementing*—may be strictly a matter of choice and convenience for some mothers. For others, it's born out of nutritional necessity. In reality, something as simple as needing to get a single stretch of sleep longer than three hours in the course of several tiring weeks motivates some exhausted new and experienced moms to supplement. Other motivating circumstances typically include babies who have latching or feeding problems, dehydration, or jaundice, as well as mothers who are struggling to increase their milk supply or have physical and/or medical limitations or work responsibilities that affect their ability to breastfeed. In any such scenario, supplementing is an acceptable option. Tempting though it may be, we want to make sure, however, that those of you who are struggling to breastfeed and beginning to question your abilities don't find yourself reaching for a bottle for lack of perceived alternatives. Instead, we urge you to enlist the help of your pediatrician or a local lactation consultant to explore your breastfeeding options first.

Pump It Up

With only occasional exception, it's technically never too soon to start pumping your milk and storing it for present or future use. Pumping can help stimulate a new mom's milk supply to come in, increase her milk production, or relieve engorgement once the supply has been established. That said, adding pumping into the already rigorous newborn feeding schedule can be quite challenging and a lot of extra work. Unless you are eager to get started, used to pumping, or need to pump out of necessity, we suggest waiting until you are comfortable with breastfeeding and your milk supply is well established. If you plan to pump infrequently, you may get by with a manual pump (or even manual expression). For anything more frequent, we highly recommend an electric version. Let us also mention that some women (Jennifer included) have little luck with pumping (much less manual expression) and are perfectly content to supplement their nursing with a bottle of formula when deemed necessary or convenient. In this case, just remember that for each feeding replaced with formula, your body misses the signal to make more milk. If done frequently and/or over time, this can result in decreased production and weaning. For all of you who are met with pumping success, you'll want to note the following breast milk storage recommendations from the Centers for Disease Control and Prevention (CDC):

- Freshly pumped breast milk can remain in room temperature for up to 4 hours or be refrigerated for up to 4 days before being used.
- Breast milk fares okay in the freezer (0°F or colder) for up to 12 months, but up to about 6 months (if in 24°F or less) is best.
- Previously frozen breast milk thawed in the refrigerator is considered safe to use for up to 24 hours, whereas thawed breast milk kept at room temperature should ideally be used within 1 to 2 hours.
- Once thawed, previously frozen breast milk should not be refrozen.

We recognize that it can be hard to keep all these expiration dates straight. For those interested, you can find a copy of these recommendations by going to the CDC's breastfeeding website at www.cdc.gov/breastfeeding. Bottom line is that if the breast milk looks or smells bad, it's best to toss it, regardless of how long it has been stored. Also, reality tells us that most babies tend to finish up their supply of frozen breast milk long before it has the chance to expire in the freezer.

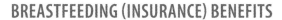

BREASTFEEDING (INSURANCE) BENEFITS

According to HealthCare.gov, health insurance plans must provide what we consider to be really valuable breastfeeding-related coverage. This includes

- Breastfeeding support, counseling, and equipment for the duration of breastfeeding. These services may be provided before and after birth and apply to all health insurance plans except those that are grandfathered, so be sure to check with yours!

- The cost of a breast pump. It may be a rental unit or a new one, and your specific plan may have guidelines on whether the covered pump is manual or electric, the length of the rental, and when you'll receive it (before or after birth). For mothers who qualify, it's worth mentioning that WIC can also be helpful in providing breast pumps for exclusively breastfeeding mothers.

Overall, however, remember that it's ultimately up to you and your doctor to decide what's right for you. Fortunately, insurance plans often follow doctors' recommendations on what's medically indicated and appropriate, so definitely remember to talk with and enlist your doctor's help (and potentially insurance pre-authorization) regarding potential breastfeeding support and supplies!

Into the Mouths of Moms

Newborns are not the only ones whose food intake is of particular interest during the newborn period. In addition to potentially finding yourself thirstier and with an increased appetite once you enter the milk production business, you may also find yourself the recipient of a whole lot of advice about exactly what *you* should and shouldn't be eating and drinking—all given in the best interest of your milk. We've found that most moms who are new to breastfeeding benefit a great deal from our practical perspective on this subject.

- **The scoop on eating for two.** Some breastfeeding moms figure they can eat just about anything they want. Others become overly focused on quickly regaining their figures and set out to diet. As a breastfeeding mother, you may have had others suggest that you take advantage of eating for two. However, just as in pregnancy, breastfeeding should not serve as an open invitation to let your cravings run wild. Rather than doubling how much you eat and overindulging in desserts and empty calories with little nutritional value, you'll be better served by focusing on your body's hunger cues and trying to eat a relatively balanced eating plan. As a general reference, the Institute of Medicine (now the National Academy of Medicine) suggests that breastfeeding women need approximately 330 additional calories per day (above their pre-pregnancy needs). For women who've been given the medical go-ahead to lose some weight, this may be a bit less, with the cautionary note that total caloric intake should not go below 1,800 calories a day and that trying for weight loss during these first few months is not recommended.

- **The good, the bad, and the spicy.** Given that much of what a nursing mother eats or drinks has the potential to ultimately end up affecting her breast milk, you might be convinced that you are in for many months of a bland diet. You may be relieved to know, then, that most breastfed babies happily tolerate a lot more variety than you'd think—even if your favorite foods include garlic, onions, cabbage, broccoli, or spicy foods. Unless you have a strong family history of certain food allergies or can pinpoint a particular food that seems to upset your baby, there's no inherent need to take the spice out of your life—or your food. After all, your baby is already used to the different flavors you ate while you were pregnant. Perhaps more important, exposing infants to a variety of flavors while they're young may actually lead to better acceptance of a broader variety of foods later on. Of course, should your baby give you reason to suspect that a certain food (or food group) is causing problems, just be sure to talk with your pediatrician and, should you choose to cut it out, make sure you and your baby are still getting all the nutrients you need.

- **Staying well hydrated.** While there is no truth to the old wives' tale that you need to drink milk to make milk, drinking enough liquid to quench your thirst and stay well hydrated can definitely help keep things flowing. Some moms actually experience strong pangs of thirst associated with milk letdown each time they breastfeed, conveniently ensuring that they remember to take time to drink. Even if you don't, use your breastfeeding times as regular reminders throughout the day to make sure you take time to drink and stay well hydrated. In other words, drink while your baby is drinking.

LET THEM EAT FISH

Seafood, which includes fish and shellfish, is one of the most beneficial foods for your baby's developing brain and eyesight. Seafood is a source of high-quality protein, vitamins, minerals, and healthy omega-3 fatty acids that cells in the brain and the retina require.

Despite what we know about its benefits, unfortunately, there's a lot of misunderstanding about eating seafood during the childbearing years, especially among those who stand to benefit most. As a result, many pregnant and breastfeeding women simply don't eat enough seafood.

The source of this confusion comes, in large part, from the fact that certain types of seafood contain excessive levels of methyl mercury, which may prove harmful to a child's development. To help clarify and encourage safe seafood consumption, the US Food and Drug Administration and the US Environmental Protection Agency in July 2019 issued updated guidelines for seafood consumption by pregnant women, breastfeeding mothers, and young children.

According to these latest evidence-based recommendations,

- *All* breastfeeding mothers should eat 8 to 12 ounces (two average servings) of fish and shellfish each week. Fortunately, there are a lot of options (ie, lower mercury-containing), including cod, crab, lobster, tilapia, freshwater trout, shrimp, canned light tuna, salmon, pollock, and catfish.

- Only a handful of relatively uncommon types of fish should be avoided altogether during pregnancy and breastfeeding. They include king mackerel, marlin, orange roughy, shark, swordfish, Gulf of Mexico tilefish, and bigeye tuna.

- Fish still deemed safe for consumption when limited to just 4 ounces per week include grouper, halibut, mahi-mahi, snapper, and albacore (white) tuna, which contains more mercury than canned light tuna.

- Although pregnant women and young children are advised to avoid raw fish or shellfish, breastfeeding moms who miss their sushi may be glad to know that it's fine (at least from a mercury standpoint) to resume eating these delicacies so long as you heed the limits above.

Medications

Regardless of whether you are going to be taking herbal remedies, supplements, prescriptions, over-the-counter medications, or homeopathic preparations, it's a good idea to assume that *any* type of medication has the potential to affect your breast milk and harm your baby or decrease your milk supply. In reality, many prescription medications are safe for use in breastfeeding. Even though package inserts often warn that they're not for use in lactation, some medications don't actually find their way into the breast milk at all. Others do but have been determined to be perfectly safe, with little or no effect on breastfeeding babies. Don't leave it up to chance to find out which is which. Check with your doctor to know what medications are safe to take while breastfeeding. An excellent resource for physicians, pharmacists, and parents alike is the National Library of Medicine Drugs and Lactation Database (LactMed), which can be found online.

Indulgences and Vices

As we shift our focus to discussing caffeine, nicotine, marijuana, and alcoholic beverages, we're clearly not talking about nutritional or health benefits. Yet the fact of the matter is that a mom's use of such substances can have a significant impact on a baby's health and well-being. That's why we've pulled together the latest recommendations and concerns pertaining to each.

- **Caffeine.** If you didn't already quit caffeine cold turkey when you were pregnant—or you did but now can't wait to welcome caffeine back into your life—you may be relieved to know that breastfeeding and enjoying a little caffeine every now and then aren't mutually exclusive. In fact, by some estimates, the level of caffeine measured in breastfed babies may be about only 1% of that in their mothers. While the AAP proposes that up to 2 or 3 cups of coffee per day poses no inherent harm to nursing mothers or babies, the amount of caffeine can range considerably and is based on how big a cup you use. Instead, consider simply looking up the caffeine content of your favorite caffeinated beverages and aiming for a total of no more than 200 to 300 milligrams of caffeine a day. If you notice your baby is irritable or fussy, you might want to try decreasing or gradually eliminating your caffeine intake.

- **Tobacco and electronic cigarettes.** If you were able to quit smoking during your pregnancy, congratulations! Now is most definitely not a good time to restart. And if you didn't attempt or manage to quit before, now is as good a time as any (if not better) to succeed, for your baby's health and your own. While you undoubtedly know that smoking cigarettes isn't good for you, it still comes as an occasional surprise to some that doing so while they are breastfeeding allows chemicals to pass into breast milk and cause dangerous side effects. Secondhand smoke increases a baby's risk of infections, asthma, and SIDS. For breastfeeding moms who smoke, the AAP recommends several ways to minimize its negative impact. These include never smoking inside the house or car and changing clothes after smoking. Trying to reduce the amount of smoking and limiting it to the period of time immediately after breastfeeding are also thought to help minimize the transmission of nicotine and other by-products to your infant. As for electronic cigarettes, such as vaping devices or JUULpods, they are not only harmful to users' lungs but contain liquid solutions that can be poisonous to young children who touch or ingest them.

- **Alcohol.** An old wives' tale—fortunately, becoming less familiar over time—suggests that drinking alcohol increases a breastfeeding mother's milk supply. According to the AAP *New Mother's Guide to Breastfeeding,* "Contrary to popular myth, drinking beer does not increase your milk supply…." Apparently, it's not the alcohol in the beer that's thought to stimulate milk production but rather a component of barley, which might explain why nonalcoholic beer has been shown to have the same effect on lactation as alcoholic beer. What we know for sure, though, is that alcohol consumed in large amounts by pregnant or breastfeeding mothers can harm babies, not to mention significantly impair their mothers' ability to care for them. If you choose to occasionally drink alcohol, it is best to do so right after you finish breastfeeding, knowing it will show up in your breast milk soon thereafter (within 30 to 90 minutes) and will most likely be cleared within 2 to 4 hours. It's not uncommon, however, for lactation consultants and other health care providers to suggest that if you're sober enough to hold your baby, you're okay to nurse. If you're concerned about having consumed too much alcohol when it's time to feed your baby, you can simply use the "pump and dump" approach to getting rid of alcohol-affected breast milk.

- **Marijuana.** While findings from studies looking at the isolated effects of marijuana use during pregnancy are fairly limited, what is known is that marijuana has the ability to reach the fetus, by crossing the placenta, and to potentially affect breastfed infants. This effect is possible because its active chemical (*tetrahydrocannabinol,* or THC) can make its way into breast milk. Marijuana may also impair a mother's ability to care for her child, and exposure to secondhand smoke from marijuana can be harmful to babies. Because of the potential health effects of cannabis products on babies, the wisest advice is for all breastfeeding moms to avoid all cannabis products, including medical marijuana, edibles, and cannabidiol (CBD) products.

2

formula for success

· · · · · ·

We admit it. In many ways, feeding your baby formula can seem much easier than breastfeeding, especially in the beginning weeks. On the one hand, one doesn't have to wonder about having enough of a supply, it's rather painless (if you don't count the sleep deprivation that comes with round-the-clock feeding), and it's easy to monitor your baby's intake. On the other hand, formula can be costly, you have to wash a lot of supplies, and, on occasion, babies can be finicky about which nipples or formula they are willing to accept. Either way, most parents today end up using formula at some point during their child's first year. With that in mind, we intend to give you a practical approach to selecting formula, buying and cleaning bottles and nipples, and troubleshooting for newborns who don't seem to play by the rules.

Sifting Through the Formula Facts

In this day and age, all it takes is a casual glance down the formula aisle to become overwhelmed by the number of customized formula options available to you and your baby—a little "ultra lipid powder" here, some "lactose-free concentrate" there—all marketed in the name of formula feeding without fussiness, gas, colic, spitting up, or other unwanted problems.

We therefore thought it might be useful to simplify the world of formula a bit by giving you a quick overview. It's easiest to start by categorizing formula into the three most commonly used types.

1. Cow's milk–based
2. Soy-based
3. Specialized (such as lactose-free) or partially or extensively hydrolyzed (sometimes called *gentle, sensitive,* or *hypoallergenic*)

The hydrolyzed formula's components are broken down to be more easily digestible. Some parents choose soy formulas because of personal preference, such as to maintain a vegetarian-based diet for their baby. Others turn to soy formula when their infants are thought to have lactose intolerance. Regardless of the type, you're sure to find modern-day add-ins in all of them, including essential fatty acids such as DHA (*docosahexaenoic acid*) and ARA (*arachidonic acid*), prebiotics, probiotics (the so-called friendly gut bacteria), lutein, and choline—all of which are meant to increase formula's nutritional value and similarity to breast milk.

A BRIEF HISTORY OF FORMULA AS WE KNOW IT

In addition to being a prominent mainstay of modern-day parenthood, formula is big business. Despite many options that make their way to the grocery-store shelves, only a handful of major manufacturers are in the United States, all of whom must meet the same well-defined standards established by the US Food and Drug Administration. As you might imagine, a quick look back tells us this availability was not always the case.

Mid-1800s	Most attempts to create a substitute for breast milk before this time were met with disastrous results. Almost everyone stuck to breastfeeding.
1867	In the mid-19th century, researchers began to analyze breast milk in an attempt to create a reasonable substitute, and the first in today's formula lineage was introduced. A liquid containing wheat and malt flour was mixed with cow's milk, cooked with bicarbonate of potash, and billed as the "perfect infant food." We're not exactly sure what potash is or if this primitive formula was met with open mouths, but by the late 1800s, the foundation of modern-day formula had been laid, and the marketing of artificial infant formula had begun.
1951	The first non-powder infant formula hit the shelves and rapidly became the most popular product available on the infant formula market.
1950s	The developed world fully embraced artificial infant formula, and it soon became the feeding method of choice.

There is no evidence, however, that using a soy-based formula instead of a cow's milk–based one will prevent allergies or colic. While you may have heard a lot of talk about babies needing to be switched from one formula to the next, most babies are started on cow's milk–based formulas and do just fine. In fact, most babies spend their entire formula-consuming careers drinking the same formula they were given on day 1. That most babies do well with cow's milk– and soy-based formulas is financially fortunate because while these two types of formula tend to be comparable in price (with soy typically costing only pennies more per ounce, if that), extensively hydrolyzed formulas can be significantly more expensive (as in nearly 50% more). Thankfully, this category of formulas is generally reserved for babies who have significant reactions to cow's milk– or soy-based products (see Tales of the Truly Intolerant on page 48) and better tolerate the broken down, easier-to-digest proteins found in hydrolyzed formulas.

SWEET ON ORGANIC FORMULA?

With the word *organic* often perceived as synonymous with *healthier,* it came as no real surprise that organic infant formula was well received after its introduction in 2006. What came as a surprise to many health-conscious parents and pediatricians alike was a *New York Times* article a couple of years later suggesting that the reason babies seemed to be so sweet on their organic fare was because the leading brand of organic formula contained cane sugar (sucrose), which is significantly sweeter than sugars used in other formulas. Despite the apparent increase in the number of organic formulas on the market since that time—some of which do not contain sucrose—it's still not easy to determine whether there are clear health benefits to buying organic formula. That said, if you prefer your baby's formula to be certified as "organic" by the US Department of Agriculture, there are plenty of options.

Formula Intolerance

While cow's milk–based formulas account for an estimated 80% of all formula sold today, some babies have a clear preference for one type or brand of formula over another. Some prefer the smoothness of ready-to-feed formula to the consistency of prepared powder formula. Others demonstrate a penchant for cow's milk–based formula over soy-based (or vice versa). In many instances, preferences are subtle. For a handful of babies, however, the word *preference* can prove to be a bit of an understatement. In search of a formula cure for a lot of extra fussiness, gas, spitting up, or any number of other ways that babies "reject" certain types and voice their opinion, parents are prone to a fair bit of formula trial and error. The good news is that most newborns do quite well with whatever form, brand, or type of formula they are given. While many even tolerate being switched back and forth without any problems, we want to caution you that it is probably best to pick one and stick with it. If, however, you find yourself with a finicky eater on your hands, we suggest you talk with your baby's doctor to discuss a reasonable approach to formula switching and determine whether your baby happens to be one of the few who might truly benefit from any of the assorted "specialty" formulas.

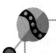

TALES OF THE TRULY INTOLERANT

An estimated 2% to 3% of infants are truly intolerant of formula with cow's milk and/or soy—a condition sometimes referred to as *cow's milk or soy protein intolerance* during which the intestinal tract is irritated by proteins found in both types of infant formulas. Babies with this type of food intolerance may have blood or mucus in their poop from time to time. If you suspect that your baby may have a formula intolerance, be sure to discuss your suspicion with your pediatrician. By running a quick test on your baby's poop and looking for traces of blood and other incriminating substances, your pediatrician can help determine whether your newborn's intestinal tract is reacting to formula. If your baby is truly intolerant, your baby's doctor will recommend an alternative formula and discuss with you the game plan for future feeding. Fortunately, babies often outgrow their intolerances after several months.

The Importance of Being Iron Fortified

It is very important that your baby gets enough iron, especially during the many months before he starts eating iron-rich foods. Iron is a mineral that plays a key role in growth, development, and delivery of oxygen to muscles and other tissues. The reason we consider this role to be important to mention is because it's still possible to find "low-iron" infant formulas online, if not in your local store. Because of the common misconception that iron in regular formula was to blame for everything from constipation and stomach pain to colic and reflux, low-iron formulas used to seem like a reasonable solution. While this assumption is understandable, especially coming from any woman who has ever experienced the uncomfortably constipating side effects while she is taking prenatal iron supplements, the fact of the matter is that the amount of iron in regular iron-fortified infant formula (approximately 12 milligrams of iron per liter) is the amount necessary for healthy growth and development. Fortunately, it is well tolerated. Nearly 20 years after the recommendation was made to either discontinue the manufacture of low-iron formulas (which contain as little as 2 milligrams of iron per liter) altogether or label them as "potentially nutritionally inadequate," it's still possible to find them. If you do, it's best to avoid them, as the American Academy of Pediatrics (AAP) currently recommends that all newborns and infants who are not breastfed (or are partially breastfed) be given iron-fortified formula. Your pediatrician may also recommend iron with appropriate laboratory tests to check your baby for iron-deficiency anemia, if needed.

CHEWING THE FATTY ACIDS (DHA AND ARA)

Two fatty acids, known as DHA (*docosahexaenoic acid*) and ARA (*arachidonic acid*), have become a mainstay in infant formulas. In their naturally occurring form, these fatty acids are thought to be crucial for a baby's development—especially of the eyes and brain. According to the government agency that oversees production of infant formula (the US Food and Drug Administration), the addition of fatty acids is known to be safe. In fact, given the potential benefits and lack of any known draw- backs to this addition, the American Dietetic Association (now the Academy of Nutrition and Dietetics) recommended in 2007 that "all infants who are not breast- fed be fed a formula containing both ARA and DHA through at least the first year." Given that most, if not all, brands of formula sold in the United States are fortified with them, you're sure to find these fatty acids on your next stroll down the for- mula aisle—by reading the ingredients list; checking for references on labels such as "immune support," "immunity protection," and "brain and eye health"; or simply looking for prominently displayed words such as *lipids* or *DHA and ARA*.

Formula Form and Function: Powders, Concentrates, and Ready-to-Feed

Infant formulas generally come in three forms.

1. Ready-to-feed liquid
2. Concentrated liquid
3. Powder

Which type is going to work best for you is likely to depend on how much formula you plan to use, where you plan to use it (ready-to-feed is definitely convenient when you're out and about), and how much you want to spend. Just as pregnancy taught most of you to think in weeks instead of months, bottle-feeding your baby will require you to think in ounces. For you to com- fortably adopt it as your standard unit of measurement, we want to first clarify the basic measurements you'll need for formula success.

MEASUREMENTS YOU'LL NEED FOR FORMULA SUCCESS

1 ounce = 30 cc (cubic centimeters) = 30 mL (milliliters)

8 ounces = 1 cup

32 ounces = 1 quart

Now that you have the necessary frame of reference, we'll move on to the actual substance of formula preparation.

- **Powder.** The simple concept is that you add powder to pre-measured water and shake a lot. In what we can only assume was an enlightened attempt to eliminate room for mixing errors, most powdered formula is mixed according to the same recipe: 1 scoop of powder to every 2 ounces of water (**Figure 2-1**). Powdered formula comes in cans containing enough powder to make anywhere from 90 to more than 200 ounces of prepared formula. It is certainly your most economical choice and, quite frankly, works well for most babies. You can decide whether to mix it up as you go or prepare a full day's worth at a time, since formula prepared from powder can be kept in the refrigerator for up to 24 hours.

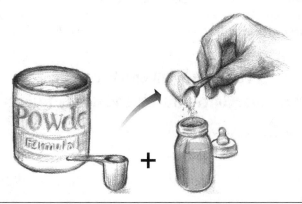

Figure 2-1. *Preparing powdered formula.* 2 scoops + 4 ounces of water = just over 4 ounces of mixed formula

- **Liquid concentrate.** This is the "just add water as directed and shake" formula option. Mixing and measuring are again straightforward because all brands of concentrate call for equal amounts of water and concentrate. If you intend to end up with a total of 4 ounces of prepared formula, you'll need to mix 2 ounces of concentrate with 2 ounces of water (**Figure 2-2**). Of course, many people choose to mix an entire can of concentrate (13 ounces) with an equal amount of water. The resulting 26 ounces of now-ready-to-feed formula can be covered and put into the refrigerator to be used over the next 48 hours. While some parents find concentrate to be easier, neater, and more convenient than powder, it is a convenience for which you will pay more.

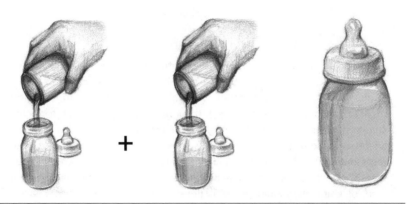

Figure 2-2. *Preparing concentrated formula.* 2 ounces of concentrated formula
+ 2 ounces of water = 4 ounces of mixed formula

- **Ready-to-feed.** This is your no-mixing, no-measuring, no-mess option.
  Typically sold in 2-, 6-, or 8-ounce containers (with anywhere from 4 to
  24 to a pack) or 1-quart (32-ounce) containers, the use of ready-to-feed
  formula is hopefully self-explanatory: what you see is what you give
  (**Figure 2-3**). While the fairly small "Ready-to-Feed" caption isn't always
  prominently displayed on the label, you'd be hard-pressed to miss the
  distinguishing price tag (see Comparing Ounces to Ounces: For What
  It's Worth on page 54). While buying ready-to-feed formula inevitably
  costs the most, it leaves almost no room for error (if we assume you
  don't mistake it for concentrate and dilute it with water). Unopened
  ready-to-feed formula can be conveniently stored at room temperature.
  Once it is opened, unused portions can be covered and refrigerated for
  up to 48 hours.

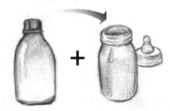

Figure 2-3. *Preparing ready-to-feed formula.* Pour 4 ounces of ready-to-feed formula
into a 4-ounce bottle

VITAMIN D FOR FORMULA-FED NEWBORNS

According to the Centers for Disease Control and Prevention (CDC), most healthy full-term newborns get all the vitamins they need from breast milk or formula, with the notable exception of vitamin D. Vitamin D is an important nutrient that helps prevent rickets and is thought to help strengthen the immune system, decrease the risk of diabetes and other chronic diseases, and even lessen the risk of some types of cancer. The American Academy of Pediatrics (AAP) recommends that all exclusively and partially formula-fed babies who drink less than 32 ounces of formula a day (which essentially means all newborns and many older infants) should get 400 IU (International Units) of vitamin D daily.

From a practical standpoint, you can give vitamin D drops by squirting them directly into your baby's mouth with the dropper or syringe that comes with the product (this process may be less messy if you do it during bath time), or mix them into a small amount of breast milk or formula.

Formula-Buying Tips

Buying formula is a significant expense of parenthood, so we've put together a little list of ways you might save along the way.

- **Do the math.** We realize it's not always easy, fun, or feasible, but it can be quite worthwhile to take the time to figure out how much you're paying per ounce (see Comparing Ounces to Ounces: For What It's Worth on page 54). You may be surprised by what you find after comparing prices of brands, types, and sizes. Per ounce will hopefully be listed for you right next to the total price posted on the display shelf. If not, you can calculate it yourself. Just look at the label to figure out how many total prepared ounces you'll be getting in any given can or container. Then simply divide the price by the total number of prepared ounces.

- **Stock up.** Before stocking up, you'll want to make sure your baby is content with the formula he's getting. Then take advantage of any sales and coupons you may spot along the way. Be sure to check the expiration dates. While some expiration dates on formulas extend well in excess of a year, others can be much shorter, and you definitely don't want to get stuck with a bunch of formulas whose time will be up before you are able to use them.

- **Save receipts.** Early on, it's more difficult to know for sure that the formula you buy now is going to be the formula you buy forever after (ie, through the end of the first year). While you're still settling in over the next several weeks, we suggest tucking your receipts—for formula and all your other new baby purchases—away somewhere for safekeeping and easy retrieval.

Mixing It Up

Be sure to read the instructions carefully when you are preparing formula. Any incorrectly prepared formula, whether it's too concentrated or too diluted, has the potential to cause serious problems. Ready-to-feed formula makes preparation easy. You just pour the room-temperature contents directly into a bottle, screw on the nipple, and have your baby feed away. All other formulas require accurate mixing. As for the water you use, you'll want to pay attention to fluoride concentration because regularly mixing powdered or liquid formula concentrate with fluoridated water may increase the chance of fluorosis (ie, faint white markings on the teeth in the future). Because the amount of fluoride in tap water can vary considerably, the best way to find out how much your tap water contains is to contact your local water utility. Because too much fluoride can have a negative effect on developing teeth, you can use low-fluoride bottled water at least some of the time when you are preparing liquid concentrate or powdered infant formula. If you find that you want (or need) to limit your baby's fluoride exposure, most grocery stores sell low- or no-fluoride bottled water typically labeled as "purified," "demineralized," "deionized," or "distilled." It's also possible to remove fluoride from tap water with a reverse osmosis filter.

COMPARING OUNCES TO OUNCES (FOR WHAT IT'S WORTH)

By using a recent check of prices at the local retailer, we thought it would be helpful to give you a general idea of how the different types of formula stack up ounce for ounce at the checkout counter. To do so, we compared one particular type and brand of formula and did not factor in sale prices (which can unquestionably save you a lot of money). Also, keep in mind that the ounces we are comparing—and that you can easily compare for yourself—are of *prepared* formula once it is ready to feed your baby.

Type	Size	Prices per Prepared Ounce
Ready-to-feed	Six 8-ounce cans = 48 ounces prepared	$0.29
Ready-to-feed	1 quart = 32 ounces prepared	$0.23
Concentrate	13-ounce can = 26 ounces prepared	$0.19
Powder	Small (12.5-ounce) can = 90 ounces prepared	$0.18
Powder	Large can	$0.16 (or as low as $0.07 for a popular generic/store brand)

To compare ounces to ounces for yourself, first look at the formula container and figure out how many ounces you'll be able to make from the formula once it is properly prepared. You can usually find this number on the back of the label. Then divide the total price by the number of prepared ounces and you're guaranteed to be a better-informed formula-buying consumer in no time!

For most healthy babies, regular tap water with fluoride levels below
2 milligrams per liter (sometimes listed as "2 ppm") is perfectly acceptable.
Check with your pediatrician or water department before using well water
(which can contain dangerous nitrates) or if you have any concerns about
the purity of your tap water supply. In general, according to the Centers for
Disease Control and Prevention (CDC), you may want to consider boiling
water for babies younger than three months, who were born prematurely,
or who have a weakened immune system. If you have any questions about
mixing your formula, don't hesitate to contact your baby's doctor for recommendations. Although they are rare, mixing mistakes can, in fact, cause very
serious problems for babies in a period of only days.

FOCUSING ON FOOD SAFETY

Keeping your baby's formula clean and germ-free is relatively easy so long as
you follow a few simple recommendations.

- Before preparing formula for your baby, wash your hands thoroughly with
  soap and water and dry them well.

- Because babies can get very sick otherwise, it is important to carefully follow the instructions on the product label for preparation, use, and storage.

- Do not use prepared formula if it has been left unrefrigerated for more than
  two hours.

- Once you have fed your baby from a bottle, resist the urge to refrigerate it
  in hopes of offering it again later, as bacteria from your baby's mouth can
  multiply even in the refrigerator.

- Instead, discard remaining formula at the end of each feeding if it has been
  more than an hour from the start of the feeding.

3

bottles and nipples

· · · · · ·

Whether you plan on bottle-feeding your newborn with formula or pumped breast milk, you will obviously need to properly equip yourself with a supply of bottles and nipples. Nowadays, you can choose from lightweight plastic bottles, glass bottles, collapsible (disposable) plastic-bottle bags, angled bottles, colored bottles, contoured bottles, and countless shapes, sizes, and consistencies of nipples. Although we're certain that many of you would like to have all your bottles in a row in anticipation of your baby's arrival, there's really no good way to know ahead of time whether your baby will agree with your initial choices. Just be aware that when it comes to nipples and even the bottles you choose, one size does not always suit all. If your baby happens to be less than tolerant of the type/brand you've so carefully selected, you may be faced with a trial period as you test out different shapes, sizes, and brands of bottles or nipples in an attempt to find a good match. We therefore recommend starting off with the basics and waiting to buy in bulk until you find a keeper. If you are set on stocking up on a particular type of bottle in advance, simply hang on to your receipts. Once a sample bottle and nipple have been met with your baby's approval, you'll be all set.

The Model Bottle

We've found that in reality, most babies go along with their parents' taste in bottles and there isn't such a thing as a single "model bottle"—one that outshines all the rest. Nevertheless, we have found the following considerations to serve bottle-buying parents well:

- In general, a clear 4-ounce bottle is the most practical choice for newborns. These may also have ounce (oz) or milliliter (mL) markings so you can tell you much your baby has fed.

- Slow flow are generally considered a better choice for breastfed babies. Although labeled "slow flow," most bottles still provide faster flow than the baby will get at the breast.
- Larger (6- or 8-ounce) bottles are okay if you don't mind using them half full until your baby is bigger.
- Angled bottles and those with disposable bags, built-in vents, or flow and control systems may help decrease the amount of air your baby swallows (although regular bottles held at the proper angle will also).
- Disposable bags have the added benefit of, well, being disposable. That leaves you with only a nipple to wash after each feeding. These may be especially useful when you are away from home.

A BIT ABOUT BPA

As you make your baby-bottle selections, you're likely to find many advertised as "BPA-free." BPA (bisphenol A) is a chemical that has been used since the 1960s in all sorts of plastic products. Up until recently, this included baby bottles made of polycarbonate, as well as the plastic linings used in cans of ready-to-feed formula. Notice, however, our use of past tense. Baby bottles no longer use BPA because in July 2012, the US Food and Drug Administration (FDA) banned its use in both baby bottles and sippy cups. The reason? Studies suggested that this potentially toxic chemical could leach out into food and pose a potential health risk—especially to infants and young children. As a result, BPA-containing bottles (generally marked with the number "7") were already being shunned by parents and prohibited by individual cities and states even prior to the US FDA formal ban.

4

going with the flow: all things bottle-feeding

• • • • • •

Nearly all babies will receive an "artificial nipple" at some point in their lives, even if they are exclusively given breast milk as their beverage of choice. Surprisingly, some infants can learn how to cup feed by lapping it up with their tongue even as a young infant, and others can learn to use a sippy cup, a straw, or another device without a nipple as early as six months of age. However, since many infants are more successful using bottles in the first year, we've listed some highlights of the bottle-feeding process for newborns in addition to thoughts on another artificial nipple—the pacifier.

Nipple Considerations

One of the most useful things for you to consider when you are choosing a nipple is finding one that allows the right amount of milk flow for your baby. Because babies can handle different flows at different ages and stages of development, you'll find that there are literally dozens of nipples from which to choose. Typically marketed according to a baby's age, the "preemie" and 0- to 3-month nipples allow for slower flows than nipples designed for use by six- to nine-month-olds. As mentioned in the previous chapter, slower-flow nipples are also thought to be better suited for breastfed babies. Voracious newborns, however, may do perfectly well with a faster-flow nipple. Others may take months before they are able to drink from the age-recommended nipple without having large volumes of milk streaming down the sides of their mouths. As for the openings, you will find yourself with a choice of not only 1-, 2-, and 3-hole nipples but also nipples that are crosscut and who knows what else. For practical purposes, all you really need to pay attention to is how fast the milk flows—too fast, too slow, or "just right."

It is worth mentioning that nipples also come in a variety of shapes and sizes, from basic round nipples to "angled"(slanted nipple), "vented" (tiny hole or holes in the nipple prevent your baby from swallowing too much air when he is sucking), and "orthodontic" (flattened nipple). It's not convincingly clear whether the orthodontic shape adds much, if any, benefit. While neither of us had to spend much time in search of a suitable nipple for our babies, if your baby is finicky, you'll want to pay more attention to the vast array of nipples and choose whichever shape your baby most readily accepts.

Heating Things Up

While there is no inherent medical, nutritional, or even comfort-related need to warm your newborn's bottles, if you're like many new parents, you'll be spending the next several months heating expressed breast milk or formula for your baby. The good old-fashioned way to do this was and still is to put a bottle of breast milk or formula into a bottle warmer or saucepan of warm water until the milk is warm. When thawing a bag of frozen breast milk, consider placing it into a second, outer bag before heating it in warm water. That way, if the bag leaks, the breast milk will not be lost into the water. You can also hold a bottle under running warm water for a few minutes. Alternatively, you can also warm up the water you're going to use to mix the formula first, before you mix it with the formula. While these are all straightforward methods, you would not be the first parent tempted to microwave your baby's bottle. Before you succumb to temptation, you need to be aware that microwaves are known to heat unevenly, creating potentially dangerous "hot spots" in the middle of the liquid. In addition, microwaving breast milk destroys the protective infection-fighting antibodies it contains. For these reasons, we recommend that you avoid using the microwave altogether for the purpose of warming bottles.

If you decide to use a baby-bottle warmer, dozens are on the market. You'll find digital bottle warmers, car-charger bottle warmers, and even dual-purpose heating and cooling ones and ones that double as baby food warmers (for later on, down the road). Known for their convenience factor, baby-bottle warmers make use of a few basic warming methods—warm water, steam, and electric. All are designed to conveniently provide you and your baby with an evenly heated, just right bottle of warm milk. In general, they are able to accomplish this goal in roughly three to five minutes, with some doing a better job of evenly heating (and not overheating) than others. If you plan on using a baby-bottle warmer, be sure to put it to the test by seeing how long it takes to heat a refrigerated bottle of milk (because this will obviously take longer than one that is room temperature). Remember to also consider ease of use; for example, does the water bath need to be refilled, and does it automatically turn off if it is left on?

While many parents love their baby-bottle warmers, in all honesty, if it's ease of use you're looking for, we also suggest a simple trial run of unwarmed formula or breast milk before you convince yourself that you and your baby can't live without the latest in milk-warming technology. You might be pleasantly surprised to find that your baby learns to drink bottles straight out of the refrigerator. After all, those are what most toddlers drink without a second thought when they switch to drinking refrigerated milk from a cup.

Finally! The Feeding Part

Once you've found a good bottle-nipple combination and have formula or breast milk on hand that's not too warm, or not too cold, but just right, you are ready to bottle-feed your baby. One of the most helpful things to remember when bottle-feeding is to angle the bottle almost fully inverted (ie, unless you're using an angled bottle, in which case it's already done for you). By holding the bottle fairly upright in your baby's mouth instead of more horizontally, you'll minimize the amount of air she swallows along with her milk. To do so,

1. Hold your baby in an upright position or lean her back at a slight recline while you are supporting the back of her head and neck.
2. If she isn't already openmouthed in eager anticipation, you may find it helpful to stroke the side of her mouth or cheek with the nipple to get her to open her mouth (see Root for success on page 18). Untuck her lips so they are flared, as this makes the baby more efficient.
3. Insert the nipple into her mouth, and hold the bottle with the end tilted up enough that the milk completely fills the nipple as your baby drinks.
4. You may find you need to hold some types of bottles almost upright as the bottle empties.
5. Avoid "bottle propping." Leaving babies to feed on their own before they are able to hold their own bottles (which doesn't happen until many months down the road) is frowned on. It should be avoided because feeding time is an important time to interact and bond with your baby. Equally concerning, the hands-off approach of simply propping up a bottle can lead to choking, an increased risk of ear infections, or both.

Bottle-feeding by Numbers

You've probably read enough by now to know that we have no way of telling you exactly how many ounces your newborn will take. However, it's always useful to have some sense of what is typical. For those of you coming from the breastfeeding chapter (page 5) who may have skipped over the formula chapter (page 45) to get here, it's worth our briefly sharing (again) the commonly used terms of measurement so as to make sure we're all on the same page.

1 ounce = 30 cc (cubic centimeters) = 30 mL (milliliters)

8 ounces = 1 cup

32 ounces = 1 quart

As you get a feel for feeding your baby (and the associated peeing and pooping that should accompany it), here are a few numbers for you to use as general guidelines.

- **First feedings.** Newborns typically take anywhere from 0.5 to 1.5 ounces at each of the first few feedings.

- **Later feedings.** By the end of the first month, most babies take about 4 ounces per feeding—an amount that for some babies increases to 6 to 8 ounces by 6 months of age. That said, it's worth noting that breastfed babies may not increase past 4 to 4.5 ounces per feeding even at a year of age.

- **Daily totals.** After the first several days, most newborns drink 12 to 24 ounces during the course of each 24-hour day. By 6 months, infants reach a maximum of 32 to 40 ounces per day.

- **Feeding frequency.** On average, formula-fed babies drink every 3 to 4 hours, while those given bottles of breast milk still tend to eat every 2 to 3 hours. Regardless of feeding frequency, any newborn who refuses feedings 2 or more times in a row should be brought to the immediate attention of his doctor.

- **Weighing in.** The true test of whether a baby is drinking enough is if he is gaining weight as expected. This holds true for both breastfed babies and formula-fed babies (see Weighing in on page 33).

DOUBLE SIPPING

We recommend filling each bottle with only as much as you think your baby will take, with a little extra for good measure in case she happens to be particularly hungry; that way, you can minimize the amount you end up having to discard at the end of each feeding. The party line is that it's okay to hang on to leftover formula or breast milk for a little while in hopes that your baby decides to finish it off, especially if you've got a grazer on your hands or your baby decides to drink less than you expected. However, plan on keeping leftovers around no longer than about an hour before throwing them away because bacteria from a baby's mouth are known to multiply fairly rapidly in milk (or just about any other food or drink that's been subjected to double-dipping or "double sipping").

Keeping It Clean

Sample nipples obtained from the hospital or doctor's office conveniently come in sterilized packages for the earliest feedings and are meant to be disposed of after a single use. Aside from that, the standard recommendation is that all feeding supplies and pacifiers should be washed and, whenever possible, sterilized before first use.

- You can easily sterilize your supplies by placing them into boiling water for about five minutes. A whole host of convenient sterilizer options are also available for this purpose, from microwave steam sterilizer bags or containers to stand-alone electric steam sterilizers.
- In general, many parents are content to hand wash bottles and nipples in hot, sudsy water and rinse. This is best done right after feedings to keep the remaining contents of the bottle from sticking and drying to the sides, nooks, and crannies. Fortunately, this approach should kill or remove most germs.
- Bottle and nipple brushes are inexpensive and invaluable for cleaning even the hard-to-reach places.
- You can either re-sterilize your bottles and nipples between uses or wash them in a dishwasher that uses heated water and has a hot drying cycle.
- Plenty of dishwasher-safe plastic baskets are on the market and specially designed to serve the sole purpose of holding all the small items involved in bottle-feeding—the nipples, lids, and other baby accessories that will most likely take up a sizable chunk of your dishwasher's upper rack. A small mesh laundry bag can also serve this function.

STERILIZING STRATEGIES

While baby-bottle sterilizers aren't always a necessity, a variety are on the market that offer a fair degree of convenience when it comes to keeping your baby bottles, nipples, and related accessories extra clean. And by *a variety,* we mean a variety: big ones and small ones, steam-based electric and microwave sterilizers, and ones that use hot water. Whichever you choose, the basic principles are going to be the same: sterilizers offer the added (but not inherently necessary) protection by sanitizing whatever is put into them. While the heat of a dishwasher run with hot water and a heated drying cycle is, in reality, all that you'll most likely need, sterilizing at least once a day is thought to provide extra germ removal. According to the Centers for Disease Control and Prevention (CDC), this is likely to be most useful during the first few months, as well as for premature (preterm) newborns and infants or those with weakened immune systems.

Schedules and Routines

Setting a Schedule or Going With the Flow

Getting babies to follow some semblance of a feeding schedule is a subject of great interest to many parents of newborns, ranking right up there with longing for predictable sleep schedules (see Sleeping Like a Baby on page 101). You should know it is also a topic that inspires great debate. You'll find many differing opinions depending on whom you ask, what you read, and where you look. While we certainly don't presume to have the one and only answer to the eternal question of whether one should feed on demand or follow a set schedule, we can give you the background you'll need to choose a practical and safe approach to the whole issue of when and how much to feed your baby.

Schedules Gone Awry

As you might have already gathered, we are not advocates of strict feeding schedules—at least not in the true sense of the phrase. That's because more often than not, babies aren't either. While there are some general feeding rules of thumb, babies aren't exactly aware of them and often choose not to play by the rules. The following several more common and normal variations in newborn feeding habits are all too often perceived as schedules gone awry.

Day-to-Day Variability

We feel compelled to point out that nobody (with rare or eccentric exception) eats the same thing, in the same amount, at the same time, every day—day in and day out. Babies are no exception, so prepare yourself for a reasonable amount of variation in the amount your baby drinks on any given day. Focus your attention instead on making sure your newborn is waking up every few hours to feed, getting enough to drink, and growing as expected.

Growth Spurts

Until we had our own children, growth spurts were merely a concept we learned about as pediatricians. They sounded logical enough—involving intermittent brief periods of rapid growth accompanied by increased hunger—but they didn't seem to us to have that much bearing on reality.

And then reality set in (as it does for most new parents). Your first introduction to a growth spurt will probably come when your baby is two or three weeks old. Everything will seem to be going just fine, you'll have just started to feel as if you have control of things (and of your milk supply if you are breastfeeding), and out of nowhere your baby will let you know otherwise. Almost overnight, he's likely to be less easily satisfied, more frequently fussy, and seemingly hungry all the time. While formula-feeding parents can certainly be thrown for a loop by growth spurts, adding an extra ounce or two to their babies' bottles or feeding them more frequently can quickly settle everyone back into a comfortable new routine. For breastfeeding moms, accommodating growth spurts can take a little more time and flexibility. During the several days it may take for your breasts to adjust to your baby's increased needs and demands, try not to question your breastfeeding abilities. Instead of letting growth spurts shake your confidence, remind yourself that it is only natural for newborns to be fussy and seem as if they're temporarily not getting enough milk. When you consider the concept of supply and demand as it applies to breastfeeding (see A Simple Matter of Supply and Demand on page 23), this fussiness is the only way your baby will be able to tell you to increase the amount of milk you are producing to meet his growing needs.

Cluster Feeding

Cluster feeding is just as it sounds—when a baby decides to eat several times in a relatively short period of time, even more frequently than the every two hours typical for breastfed babies in the first month, and in seeming defiance of those who dare to suggest bottle-feeding no more than every three hours. This pattern is sometimes referred to as *grazing*—especially when a baby is a frequent feeder with seemingly little stamina and takes the snackbar approach to feeding in general. In your newborn's first days and weeks, we strongly recommend you follow your baby's lead, whether that means feedings that are evenly spaced or clustered together, long sessions or short. That said, it's worth keeping in mind that breastfed infants should be "kept on task" while feeding (as best you can), rather than allowed to get into the habit of sleepy partial feeding. Even after your baby's feeding patterns become relatively predictable, it's worth mentioning that many babies still choose to cluster feed, most commonly in the evening before bedtime. Without scientific data to support it, let us just say that some parents swear by cluster feeding in the evening as a way to "top off the tank" in the hopes of buying everyone involved a longer stretch of nighttime sleep before hunger strikes again.

Routine Considerations

The Merits of an All-Liquid Diet

For the next several months, your baby will get all the nutrition he needs from breast milk or formula. While we are well aware that babies of generations past were given rice cereal as young as a few weeks of age, giving any form of solid food to babies before four or even six months of age is no longer recommended except under certain circumstances, such as significant reflux. Starting solids before four months of age is thought to increase a baby's risk of developing allergies, constipation, overweight, and even choking. Even if you find yourself pressured by well-meaning grandparents or friends who swear by it, we suggest you suppress the urge to give your baby any type of solid food and follow the American Academy of Pediatrics recommendation to exclusively breastfeed until your baby is at least four, if not a full six, months of age, unless you discuss extenuating circumstances with your pediatrician and get the go-ahead to start sooner.

Where Does Water Fit In?

In response to a question many parents ask: yes, water is a liquid, but no, your newborn does not need any. They get plenty of water from formula or breast milk, and giving them extra water not only stands to fill them up without offering nutrients but actually has the potential to make babies ill.

No Milk (for Now)

Until your baby reaches one year of age, you should continue to reach for the breast milk or formula instead of introducing regular, grocery-store cow's milk. This recommendation is based on the fact that cow's milk is less easily digested, contains higher concentrations of certain proteins and minerals, offers inadequate amounts of vitamins and iron, and has the potential to place unrealistic demands onto your baby's kidneys and intestinal tract.

Sucking Sense and Sensibility

It's a rare parent who doesn't find the classic "baby sucking thumb in utero" ultrasound picture worthy of framing or at least showing off to friends or around the office. But the ability to suck is more than just cute. It's important for other reasons as well. While babies are sometimes caught sucking their thumbs as early as 18 weeks or sooner, the sucking and swallowing efforts necessary to drink from breast or bottle don't become coordinated until closer to 34 weeks. Not only do babies perfect their sucking skills once they are born in the name of good growth and nutrition, but most of them rely on sucking to soothe themselves as well, with some relying on it more heavily than others. The fact that babies don't have enough control over their fingers and hands to reliably get them to their mouths to suck on for many weeks after they are born naturally leads many parents (and us) into a discussion of pacifiers.

Practical Pacifier Principles

Pacifiers have proven themselves to be yet one more source of parenting controversy. Breastfeeding purists say stick to your convictions and keep them out of your newborn's mouth—even when your baby is not yet able to use his own fingers as an alternative. (We would note that if and when your baby is able to find his own fingers, it's okay to let him continue using them as natural pacifiers.) This advice is not without reasons, as pacifiers have been associated with missed feedings in breastfed infants, so it is better to avoid them in the first three to four weeks until milk supply is established (and even then, only offered after a feeding). See Nipple Confusion Defined and The Confusion About Nipple Confusion on page 36. Others forewarn that pacifiers are simply a bad habit waiting to happen. Well, fear not as long as you understand a few practical pacifier principles and pitfalls. Most important, be aware that pacifiers have been recognized as a valuable ally in the fight against sudden infant death syndrome (see The Reality of SIDS: Creating a Safe Sleep Environment on page 103). Whether you choose to breastfeed, bottle-feed, or a combination of both, here are some tips for if and when you decide to give your baby a pacifier.

- **Soothing through sucking.** Pacifiers can be invaluable in soothing babies, as well as in satisfying those who want to suck all the time. You need not worry about your baby developing a lifelong dependency on them. Just be very careful not to offer your newborn a pacifier at times when he really should be fed instead, because pacifiers can inappropriately pacify hungry babies in addition to those who are looking for comfort. If you want to follow the advice to wait until breastfeeding is well established before introducing one, make sure your pacifier-free preference is known during your initial days at the hospital.

- **Picking out the perfect pacifier.** These days, picking the perfect pacifier may seem like a considerable task, given all the various brands and styles on the market. Size matters to the extent that you don't want to offer one that's too big. Latex pacifiers are known to wear out and need to be replaced faster than the silicone kind. Other than that, to the best of our knowledge, there's no correlation between price or marketing strategy and pacifier effectiveness. We simply recommend trying one out and seeing whether your baby likes it.

- **If at first you don't succeed...** When you first offer your baby a pacifier, don't be surprised if he seems disinterested, gets downright angry, or spits it out even when you know he's not hungry and just wants comfort. For breastfed babies, sucking on a pacifier inherently requires a different technique, one that may take a few tries. For breastfed and bottle-fed babies alike, a nipple that does not provide milk may not be quickly welcomed. As you offer your baby a pacifier, try lightly stroking just to the side of his mouth and then gently holding the pacifier in his mouth for a moment as he starts sucking to keep it from popping right back out.

- **A practical pacifier substitute.** The cheap, easy, and ever-present pacifier substitute: your pinky finger. If you find yourself in the position of wanting to soothe your baby by giving him something to suck on other than your breast, you can always use your (clean) little finger. Simply turn your hand palm side up and let your baby suck on your pinky finger, allowing it to rest gently in the roof of his mouth. As a word of caution for anyone with longer fingernails than ours: you may want to rethink how much you value your long nails or at least the one on your little finger. You'll likely find that it's a small sacrifice to make to clip it shorter for the sake of having a contented baby. Some babies find their own fingers to suck on earlier than others, so do your best to be prepared by making sure those fingers are clean and have clipped nails too!

- **Passing on pacifiers.** If your baby isn't that much of a "sucker," he may not need to be soothed by sucking on a pacifier at all. Just be thankful that there's one less thing to keep track of and keep clean during the day, and simply consider offering one as he is falling asleep (see The Reality of SIDS: Creating a Safe Sleep Environment on page 103).

what goes in must come out

· · · · · · ·

introduction

· · · · · · ·

This section is devoted to a subject that, if nothing else, helps you realize just how far you're about to come—from your days as an expectant parent to your days as a master of bodily fluids and functions. A very basic understanding of how your baby's body works, combined with some reflection on your own life experiences, should be more than enough to tell you that a good deal of what goes into your baby's mouth will eventually come out in one form or another. A significant portion will undoubtedly go toward your baby's growth and development. But a fair bit of indigestible, unnecessary, or undesirable stuff—be it solid, liquid, or gas—is all but certain to make its way out regularly. First and foremost, pee and poop will soon be in abundant supply, at least after you've made it past the first few days during which your baby's system is still gearing up for bigger and better things. Don't be surprised if these and other previously less than tasteful subjects indiscriminately make their way into your casual (and not-so-casual) conversations. In fact, we consider the contemplation and shared discussion of pee, poop, and related topics to be a defining feature of parenthood.

Looking Into What Comes Out

In this section of the book, we take a close look at the inner workings of newborns and what's behind all the peeing and pooping, not to mention the gas, hiccups, burps, spit-up, and vomit that come along with having a baby. Your task of tending to these commonplace "events" may leave some of you scratching your heads in wonder, confusion, or amazement. Don't worry if this closer look doesn't sink in right away. Trust us when we say it soon will (refer to Stain removal on page 171).

Peeing and Pooping

If we were attempting to write a medical textbook, we would now be turning our focus to the topics of urine, stool, and bowel movements. The facts of the matter are that

1. This book is not in any way meant to resemble a medical textbook.
2. Once you've been buried in a sea of diapers over the first weeks, months, and years of parenthood, just nothing is academic about that situation.

Given that most parents we've talked with over the years simply refer to these topics as good old "pee" and "poop," we will too. With our choice of words thus briefly explained, let's get to the real substance at hand. To give you some context, the reason why pediatricians seem to care so much about whether a baby is peeing and pooping normally is because it is one of the easiest and most reassuring ways we have to determine whether a baby is getting enough to eat. It also serves as a reassuring sign that all systems are in good working order, and he is generally healthy.

As you settle into your own daily feeding *routine* (a term we use loosely, as we explain in Schedules Gone Awry on page 64) and attempt to gauge if your own baby is getting enough to eat, drink, and be merry, you'll find that pee and poop play a leading role. First, to figure out whether your baby's plumbing is working normally, you'll need a good understanding of what is meant by the word *normal*.

to pee or not to pee

● ● ● ● ● ●

How Wet Is Wet Enough?

The answer to the question "How wet is wet enough?" depends on how you're feeding your baby (by breast or by bottle) and how old your baby is. The number of wet diapers in the first few days can be far fewer than the by-the-book 8- to 10-plus wet diapers a day that comes later. For formula-fed newborns who are taking well to the bottle, it's perfectly reasonable to expect a good 5 or more wet diapers a day within the first day or two. Breastfed newborns, however, can be a bit more variable during the first several days until their mothers' milk supply has "come in" (see Breastfeeding on page 5). While breastfed babies get their necessary calories from the early milk (*colostrum*), this first form of breast milk comes in a much smaller volume. It therefore stands to reason that breastfed newborns pee less frequently— sometimes only 2 or 3 times a day—and in much smaller amounts until their mothers' full-volume milk supply comes in (typically 2 to 5 days after delivery). Once you reach this breastfeeding milestone of milk production, you can expect your baby to catch up to her formula-fed colleagues and have at least 5 (if not 8 or 10) wet diapers in any 24-hour period. When everyone's drinking and peeing are up to full capacity, the standard 8 to 10 wet diapers a day applies. If at any time you are concerned that your baby is not peeing as much as she should, this is as good a reason as any to enlist the help and expertise of your pediatrician.

IN SEARCH OF A LITTLE PEE IN A BIG DIAPER

Detecting small amounts of pee in a newborn's superabsorbent disposable diaper can at times be likened to finding a needle in a haystack. If you're having difficulty determining whether your newborn's diaper is wet, some diapers make your job a little easier by including moisture-sensing strips that change color when wet. Although we haven't tried it, for a higher-tech option, a smart diaper is now available that connects to an app to let you know when baby has a wet diaper and can even track sleep. For the tried-and-true low-tech option, however, simply put a cotton ball or folded tissue inside a regular diaper—toward the front of the diaper near the penis for baby boys and lower in the vaginal area for baby girls. Then be patient. Any subsequent pee will now be much easier to detect; the challenge of detecting it, most likely short-lived. It shouldn't be more than a few short days before you find yourself faced instead with the problem of overly soaked diapers and laughing at the thought of cotton balls and tissue. For additional information on difficult-to-identify diaper contents, see UDOs: Unidentified Diaper Objects on page 146.

CHAPTER

6

poop happens

· · · · · ·

When it comes to newborn poop, it helps to be aware that a normal and expected poop progression takes place over the first week or so. Most doctors expect newborns to demonstrate their pooping ability before sending them home from the hospital. And most newborns happily oblige—doing so without much difficulty or delay. The first newborn poops you'll see, usually in the initial 24 hours or so, are typically thick, tarry, and black. This lovely, gooey mess, referred to as *meconium,* is simply the poop that accumulated before your baby was born.

The Scoop on Poop

As breast milk or formula begins to make its way through your baby's system over the next few days, expect your baby's poop to become more of a pasty brown color (the so-called transitional stool). Ultimately, it will become either the standard mustardy yellow, seedy poop typical of breastfed babies or the pastier, more formed, and variably colored poop of formula-fed babies. For all babies, but especially for those who are breastfed, the establishment of frequent poop that has gone through this predictable change in color and consistency is a good indication they are getting enough to eat. For breastfed babies, it also suggests that the eagerly anticipated full-volume milk supply has arrived. (See The Turning Point: How Will I Know When My Milk Comes In? on page 24.)

The Many Colors of Poop

Long after adjusting to parenthood and your role as principal poop watcher and wiper, you may still find yourself fretting over changes in the color of your baby's poop. In reality, once your baby has pooped enough to get rid of the tarry meconium, all the varying shades of yellow, brown, and even green that may follow are considered perfectly acceptable. Mustardy yellow is the color of choice for most breastfed babies. For those who are formula fed, it's yellow-tan with hints of green. Being presented with a changing palette of colors is not uncommon, however, particularly later on when your baby is introduced to solid foods and snotty nose colds, both of which can add new shades and substance to the mix.

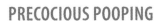

PRECOCIOUS POOPING

In some instances, babies actually poop before they are born. This allows meconium to mix into the amniotic fluid that all babies bathe in before exiting their uterine home. While the passing of meconium is a reassuring sign that all's well in the poop department, anytime it occurs in utero, it requires babies to be a bit more closely observed in the period immediately after being born just to make sure the meconium didn't make its way into their lungs.

Black, White, and Shades of Red

A few colors of baby poop, should you see them, always warrant discussion with your baby's doctor.

- **Red.** Seeing red can mean blood, especially in the newborn period when your baby isn't eating or drinking anything red colored that could be mistaken for blood when it comes out the other end. Blood should not signal you to panic immediately, but you should bring it to the attention of your pediatrician, who will be able to help you sort out the cause. It is not uncommon for babies to swallow some blood during delivery that presents itself shortly thereafter—in either the baby's spit-up or poop. Additionally, in the case of blood-streaked spit-up, remember to consider whether your own sore, cracked nipples might be the source. In any case, any amount of bloody poop should be evaluated because it can be a sign of a problem.

- **Black.** Black-colored poop is worth paying attention to because blood typically turns from red to black over time in the intestinal tract. Remember that this black color alert does not apply to your baby's first few meconium bowel movements, which you can fully expect to be black and tarry looking without having to be concerned about blood.

- **White.** White poop is quite rare but needs to be brought to the attention of a doctor as soon as possible. Pale poop that's lacking in color can be caused by an underlying liver problem. The earlier it is assessed, the better, for peace of mind or for important medical management.

The Eating-Pooping Connection

You'll find that for many young babies, a little thing called *the gastrocolic reflex* (*gastro-* referring to the stomach and *colic* referring to the colon—the end of the road in the intestinal tract) is responsible for causing eating and pooping to occur nearly simultaneously. In fact, many newborns have such a strong gastrocolic reflex that they poop just about every time they eat, sometimes even in anticipation of being fed before any milk has graced their lips. If you stop and think about it, you may find that you're already quite familiar with this particular reflex because it is not, in fact, unique to infancy. While this gastrocolic reflex is generally less exaggerated and hopefully less immediate in adults, many adults never fully outgrow it. Unlike newborns, however, most adults are able to control the urge long enough to finish their meals before needing to excuse themselves to the bathroom to take care of business.

FULL SPEED BEHIND

Once your baby has gotten the hang of eating—especially if you have chosen to breastfeed and your milk is fully in—don't be surprised to find yourself faced with poop that can be described as nothing less than explosive. In fact, it brings to mind the problems Southern Californians once had with paintball shooting sprees: wayward teenagers drove around with paintball guns, terrorized neighborhoods by firing off blobs of paint at high speeds, and targeted whomever and whatever happened to cross their paths. That's the best analogy we've come up with to date to convey the potential forcefulness (and subsequent mess) that can result when a breastfed baby's intestinal tract is fully up to speed. Having now forewarned you, we suggest you review The Art and Science of Diapering on page 133 to make sure you're comfortable with your diapering technique. And remember to keep your baby's back end securely contained whenever possible, or be prepared to run for cover or suffer the consequences!

Consistency: A Word About Diarrhea and Constipation

Many parents are concerned (usually unnecessarily) that their new babies have diarrhea. With the definition of *diarrhea* typically involving the words *frequent* and *watery,* it's certainly not hard to understand. In fact, most young babies simply have well-functioning gastrocolic reflexes, and everything that goes in one end comes flying out the other. That said, if you are concerned

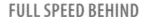

or simply want a reality check that what you're seeing in your baby's diaper is normal, go right ahead and grab a poopy diaper (if you have one available to submit as evidence), stick it into a plastic bag, and head over to check things out with your pediatrician.

TRULY INTOLERANT POOP

On occasion—studies currently show that somewhere on the order of 2 to 3 out of every 100 babies, to be exact—a baby's intestinal tract reacts to a component in formula or breast milk. This type of intolerance is worth being aware of, as it is caused by inflammation of the rectum or colon (food protein–induced *proctitis* or *proctocolitis*). It is commonly referred to as *milk protein intolerance, cow's milk sensitivity, soy intolerance,* or *milk-soy protein intolerance* (MSPI for short). Babies with symptoms of intolerance typically appear healthy, but every now and then, blood or mucus will turn up in their poop. For parents, it is admittedly not always easy to recognize food protein intolerance from your more run-of-the-mill baby poop. And you shouldn't feel as though you have to. If you have questions about whether the formula or breast milk you are feeding your baby is not being well received by his intestinal tract, pack up your baby and a recent poop sample, if you can, and head into your pediatrician's office. The diagnosis may be confirmed by simply removing the offending protein(s) from your baby's diet (or your own, if you are breastfeeding); any blood in the poop should disappear within a few days, and the sensitivity itself usually resolves by one year of age.

Pooping by Numbers

Once babies have proven themselves capable of clearing out their intestinal tracts of any meconium and moved on to dishing out the real thing, you can be relatively assured that their plumbing is in good working order and can turn your attention to the so-called normal pooping patterns of infancy. What's considered normal at this stage of the game (and for months to come) ranges anywhere from one poop every several days to several poops every day. Some babies are like the sprinters of the pooping world—fast and furious—while others are more like distance runners—slow and steady. In general, breastfed babies poop more than formula-fed ones, and younger babies poop more than older ones. Newborn babies and young infants also tend to have several tiny poops in succession. As a point of practicality, we therefore recommend waiting a few minutes until your newborn is convincingly finished rather than jump into diaper-changing action after the first signs of activity. From your pediatrician's perspective, the actual number of poops is likely to be less important than the fact that everything is generally moving along.

ENOUGH IS ENOUGH?

In the spirit of helping you distinguish between the healthy but fast and furious pooper and those newborns pooping beyond the limits of acceptability, experts in the field of newborn care suggest the following rule of thumb: anytime a newborn's poop becomes progressively watery or outpaces feeding frequency, it's time to seek medical advice.

When the Pooping Gets Tough

On the flip side of loose or watery poop, many parents end up with questions about constipation as soon as their babies begin to grunt, strain, or get red in the face while pooping or the first time they go several days without a poopy diaper. Fortunately, true constipation—as defined by hard, difficult to pass, or infrequent poop—isn't a big issue for most young infants. Believe it or not, going as many as five to seven days between poops is not inherently a problem for babies who have already proven themselves fully capable of pooping during their first couple of weeks and are eating and growing well. As long as your baby's poop is fairly soft and comes out easily, you can breathe with relative ease despite the exaggerated degree of discomfort your baby seems to display. Even if your baby occasionally seems to have difficulty getting the poop out, remind yourself that pooping while lying flat on one's back isn't exactly natural. Given that your baby won't have many options for a while, you can try to facilitate by pushing your baby's knees up toward her chest while she's lying on her back to give her some resistance against which to strain. If, however, your baby consistently seems to have problems pooping—she does so infrequently or with apparent pain, or you notice blood or poop that just doesn't seem right to you—be sure to check in with your baby's doctor about what (if anything) you can do to remedy the situation.

IRONING OUT ANY MISUNDERSTANDINGS

The iron found in formula is often given undue blame despite its unquestionable benefit. Given that iron supplements are well-known to make adults constipated (a side effect with which some of you may have had recent firsthand experience), it's no wonder that concerned parents are prone to blaming the iron in their infant's formula for perceived problems with constipation. In reality, the iron in infant formula is rarely, if ever, responsible for causing constipation, while the risk of becoming iron deficient is a reality for more than 1 in 10 infants. In addition, the iron you see listed on the label isn't actually the amount your baby gets. Yes, they technically "get" it, but iron in infant formula is not absorbed all that well. The seemingly large amount of iron contained in most infant formulas is therefore necessary to ensure your baby is able to absorb what he needs (see also The Importance of Being Iron Fortified on page 48).

Persistent Problematic Pooping (Hirschsprung Disease)

In order to move on to a discussion of what can cause persistent problems with pooping, it's necessary to take a moment to discuss the involved anatomy of the intestinal tract. When all of a baby's parts are in working order, poop makes its way southward through the gut, or intestines, until it comes to rest in the last part of the digestive tract, called the *colon.* It accumulates there while awaiting its release from the anus. Every now and then, the nerve cells that control the anus (and sometimes those in the lower part of the colon) don't develop properly. As a result, the muscles responsible for letting the poop out can't relax. This condition is known as *Hirschsprung disease* (also called *congenital megacolon*). Only about 1 out of every 5,000 babies will have it. In more serious instances, the anus is unable to open at all, in which case pooping is noticeably absent from birth. Many babies with Hirschsprung disease, however, lack only some of the nerve cells and are still able to relax enough to let some poop out, just not as easily or as often as expected. This milder form of Hirschsprung disease can result in constipation, as characterized by infrequent or difficult poops that may not signal a problem until the parents or a pediatrician begins to notice a chronic pattern over time. While we've taken time to give you only the quick and dirty explanation, it should be enough to give you a sense of what to keep in the back of your mind and what to consider should you find yourself concerned about your newborn's potentially problematic pooping practices.

7

other unmentionables and inconveniences

• • • • • • •

In addition to encountering peeing and pooping, parents of newborns seem to encounter a disproportionate number of other unmentionables and inconveniences—namely, gas, burping, spitting up, and vomiting. The following two chapters will help you sort through what's considered normal, what's considered a nuisance, and what should not be ignored.

Full of Hot Air

With all the gulping some babies do during feedings and crying, it's no surprise they swallow quite a bit of air. Once air makes its way in, there are only two logical ways for it to escape—up and out as a burp or down and out as gas. Air that is destined to be passed as gas must travel through many (as in 8 or more!) feet of intestines—a process that invariably takes longer and is often believed to cause more fussing and discomfort than if that same air manages to come back out in the form of a burp. While we aren't entirely confident that this theory has been proven, it doesn't usually take a lot of convincing to believe that gassy babies tend to be uncomfortable babies. For this reason alone, it's worth taking some simple steps to minimize the amount of air your baby swallows.

- **Feed early and often.** Whenever possible, feed your baby before she is screaming her demands at you. The more she cries before a feeding, the more likely she is to fill up with air.

- **Rise to the challenge.** When feeding your baby, keep her body at somewhat of an upright angle—at least so her head is a little higher than her stomach. Try to do this even if you have already figured out how to breast-feed lying down. This position theoretically allows the liquid to sink to the bottom of a baby's stomach while the air stays on top, making it easier (and less messy) to burp out. Any air bubbles trapped below the milk are more likely to be burped up with liquid (spit-up) or have to pass through the intestinal tract.

- **Bottoms up.** When bottle-feeding your baby, hold the bottle at an angle so there is always milk filling the entire nipple. This position helps keep babies from sucking air. (See also The Model Bottle on page 57.)

- **Let things settle.** Before sitting down for a feeding, consider letting any bubbles in recently mixed and shaken formula settle first. During or after each feeding, keep your baby upright for a few minutes to let things settle and then try to burp her.

Burping

Babies and parents alike seem to get significant relief from getting out whatever gas happens to make its way in—and the sooner, the better. The next best thing to helping your baby avoid sucking in a lot of air in the first place is to get any resulting air bubbles to come out in one or two big, satisfying burps shortly afterward. That said, some babies seem not to be bothered by the presence of stomach gas. As a general rule of thumb, if it doesn't bother them, you don't need to exert too much effort in the following burping endeavors.

Burping Techniques

Given the amount of attention paid in the parenting world to the topic of burping babies, you might be led to believe that nothing short of a class on the subject could properly prepare you. Well, in hopes of bursting your bubble, let us stress that burping is not rocket science by any stretch of the imagination. Burping is actually a relatively natural process that you simply stand to help along. If anything, most parents benefit from just a little guidance on if, when, and how vigorously to do it. We've seen too many a parent frantically try to elicit a burp every few minutes during and after each feeding. The fact of the matter is that some babies just don't swallow as much air or need to burp as much as others. If your baby is going to burp, he will probably do so within a few minutes of having his back patted. Ideally, you simply want to decrease his chances of discomfort by coaxing out whatever air has found its way into his stomach. With that in mind, here are some basic burping techniques.

- **Positioning.** The classic burping technique (and often the most popular) involves holding up your baby so he's up against your chest, facing you with his head resting just over your shoulder. You can also sit your baby upright on your lap, providing necessary support by simply putting one hand across his chest and under his armpits while patting his back with the other. Or you can lay your baby on his belly across your lap or on the floor to help compress his stomach and press the air out.

- **Patting.** Pat or rub your baby's back for a couple of minutes after he drinks. Your patting should be less forceful than an all-out clapping motion but harder than a soft touch. Many parents either burp a little too delicately or, on occasion, with a little too much enthusiasm.

- **Postponing.** If your baby hasn't burped after a couple minutes of coaxing, you can stop trying to elicit the elusive burp and simply lay your baby down for several minutes. If he seems uncomfortable, simply try again later. Sometimes, allowing the air bubbles to settle will make burping easier. Quite honestly, however, when left alone for a few minutes, many babies are able to muster a burp all on their own. If you find your baby spits up a lot, swallows a lot of air, or is uncomfortable during feedings, you can certainly try stopping and burping him in the middle of each feeding. Just be forewarned that in our combined experience, babies often mind being interrupted while they are eating more than they mind any potential gas bubbles.

- **Patience.** Accept that some babies do not need to burp (or be burped) with every feeding—especially when they don't swallow much air, aren't prone to spitting up, or just don't tend to burp much. It's definitely not worth losing sleep over if you're unable to elicit a burp.

Pumping Gas

Despite your best efforts, some air will inevitably make its way past the stomach and into your baby's intestines. If you find that your baby seems uncomfortable as a direct result of gas, try laying her on her back and "bicycling" her legs to help work the air bubbles out. You can also try gently putting her face down along your arm, her legs straddling either side with your hand supporting her belly, chest, and chin. If you're now wondering how to go about coordinating this whole one-arm thing—which hand and facing which direction?—you can instead opt to rest your baby belly down on top of a flat surface. Lifting up slightly on her belly so you can slide your hand under it, use your fingertips to lightly massage or gently apply light pressure to her tummy area for a few minutes. These motions seem to help break up gas bubbles or at least help make gassy babies and their parents more comfortable with their predicament.

Gas Busters?

You may hear that some babies seem to respond well to over-the-counter anti-gas drops containing simethicone—the key ingredient found in Mylicon, Gas-X, Phazyme, Little Remedies, and certain colic drops. To tell the truth, we can't find definitive evidence to show that the effort and expense of anti-gas drops pay off. In fact, with respect to colic, studies suggest that simethicone does not help. It is for this reason that pediatricians are increasingly recommending that you just shouldn't use them. If, however, you still feel your baby's gas may benefit, there's usually no harm in trying them as long as you consult with your pediatrician first (just as we hope you would before introducing any medication). As but one example, one study found that simethicone interferes with a drug used to treat congenital hypothyroidism. In any case, be sure to hang on to your receipt. Should you come to your own conclusion that they are ineffective, we've been told that some companies will reimburse your money.

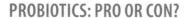

PROBIOTICS: PRO OR CON?

Probiotics, commonly known as "good" or "friendly" bacteria, have been getting positive press for their beneficial effects on digestive health. Thought to help restore "bacterial balance" and generally considered safe, probiotics have been proposed as a possible solution to many bodily disturbances, including (but not limited to) gas and maybe even colic. While probiotics have very quickly grown into a multibillion dollar industry, it's worth pointing out that research confirming their benefits for babies is not yet definitive, with some researchers finding little evidence that supplementing infants provides any health benefits at all. Also of note, for those interested in making sure their babies get probiotic bacteria (as well as prebiotics), breast milk is naturally full of them (and free!). Although probiotic supplements do not require a prescription, we recommend you discuss their use with your pediatrician.

Hiccups

The good news about hiccups is they're not dangerous and are usually more bothersome to parents than they are to babies. At best, your baby won't get any at all or will have only an occasional, cute little run-in with them. At worst, they'll make their presence known at all hours of the day and night and effectively disrupt what may already be a delicate balance in your baby's stomach, giving your baby yet one more excuse to wake up or spit up. Quite simply, newborns have a lot of very active reflexes, and hiccupping can be one of them—sometimes even popping up before birth. Hiccups are thought to occur when a baby's diaphragm is "tickled" for any reason—by sudden swallowing or irregular breathing—or for no apparent reason at all. It is our understanding that any form of breath-holding (which, for a newborn, is pretty much limited to sucking or crying) effectively helps stop them. If you're convinced that your baby is uncomfortable, you can consider offering a pacifier or, if you just can't resist trying it out, you can experiment by giving a little sip of breast milk, formula, or water to see if it stops the process. If you ask us, however, breath-holding doesn't seem to work so well—often even for adult hiccups—and you might be better served by simply ignoring them, knowing they're harmless and likely to be short-lived.

8

spitting up and vomiting

• • • • • •

We have found that many baby books describe spitting up as a harmless nuisance that goes away over time while, at the very same time, cautioning parents that vomiting—sometimes described as *projectile*—is to be taken seriously. You're then given the following definitions:

- **A typical definition of spitting up:** *The easy flow of stomach contents through the mouth that may or may not accompany a burp.*

- **A typical definition of vomiting:** *The expulsion and passage of stomach (gastric) contents through the mouth.*

Now for a little reality check: Does anyone else besides us happen to think the definitions seem somewhat similar? Well, that's because in real life, spitting up and vomiting can at times be difficult to distinguish, especially for those who have never had to give it much thought before. If you've already discovered you've got a "spitty" baby on your hands, you may be wondering just how to determine what qualifies for the upgraded status of vomiting. Don't beat yourself up if you discover you were born without the innate ability to distinguish between the two. The distinction between "happy spitters" and those with bigger issues has been known to elude doctors at times too. In this chapter, we do our best to prepare you for the run-of-the-mill spit-up challenges while familiarizing you with warning signs that can signify something more serious. Take the following descriptions for what they're worth, do what you can to differentiate between the two, and then go with your own gut instinct as to whether you need to involve your pediatrician.

Spitting Up

If you are fortunate, you will be blessed with a baby who, from birth, has the ability to politely keep whatever he drinks to himself and realizes that spitting up does not count as sharing. The information that follows will not be as relevant to you as it will be to those parents who discover that some part of every feeding is likely to come back up and out. If you happen to already be sitting with a spit rag over your shoulder(s) and protective coverings over most of your furniture, you'll undoubtedly be able to relate to this part of the chapter—a section we like to think of as the "what you've worked so hard to put in always seems to come out, even when you don't want it to, despite all your best efforts to keep it in" section.

For most babies, spitting up—also referred to as *normal reflux*—is the result of a not yet fully developed muscle at the top of the stomach that is supposed to serve as a gatekeeper—in general, allowing food (drink, in this case) into the stomach and then *keeping* it there. For those of you who are dying to know the name of the muscle most likely to blame for your spit-up woes, it is called the *lower esophageal sphincter,* or LES for short (**Figure 8-1**). For a clearer picture, take a minute to visualize your baby's stomach as an upright

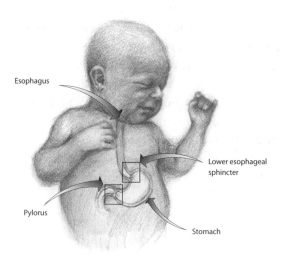

Esophagus

Lower esophageal sphincter

Pylorus

Stomach

Figure 8-1. *The anatomy of spitting up.* Esophagus, pylorus, lower esophageal sphincter, and stomach

water balloon with a narrow opening at the top. For a baby who spits up a lot, picture a water balloon left a little too loosely secured. It's not hard to imagine how any amount of applied pressure—a poke or squeeze on the side—or a change in position could cause its contents to overflow, especially at times when the balloon (ie, stomach) is relatively full. For some newborns, a simple gas bubble or press on the belly may be all it takes to overpower a novice sphincter muscle and cause spit-up and/or reflux to happen. Fortunately, most of the time spitting up doesn't bother babies. For the parents of these so-called happy spitters, a loose sphincter muscle simply means being more diligent about burping, stockpiling a larger supply of burp cloths or spit rags, and investing in a bottle (or three) of stain remover.

THE SHAPE OF THINGS TO COME (UP)

No matter how curdled or "spoiled" your baby's spit-up appears, reassure yourself that it doesn't really matter. The curdled appearance just reveals that your baby's stomach had already started processing the milk before it managed to escape and nothing more. On the flip side, it's also entirely possible to have spit-up that occurs an hour or more after the last feeding that still doesn't look as if it's been digested at all.

Remedies for Spitty Babies

Burping and spitting up often go hand in hand for newborns. The air in a baby's stomach decides to come up, and the stomach contents opt to tag along for the ride—a tendency sometimes referred to as "wet burps" that serves to explain why you'll find a fair bit of overlap between burp prevention (see Burping Techniques on page 84) and spit-up avoidance techniques. If you find that your newborn spits up quite a bit, there are several things you can try to remedy the situation.

- Position your baby's head higher than the rest of her body when she's eating.
- Step up your burping efforts. You can either put a little more effort into eliciting a good burp after each feeding or try burping your baby more frequently during the feeding—after every 5 minutes of breastfeeding or every ounce or so from a bottle. Only you and your baby can decide whether the interruption in feeding is worth the results.
- Feed your baby smaller amounts more frequently.

- Try holding or positioning your baby relatively upright for a good 20 to 30 minutes after meals.
- While some parents find that simply switching brands of formula (see Formula Intolerance on page 47) or eliminating certain foods in a breast-feeding mother's diet can help decrease the amount of spitting up, it's always worth checking with your baby's doctor before considering such changes (see Into the Mouths of Moms on page 39). While on occasion a change might help, for many newborns and their parents it's an unnecessary inconvenience.

THE PATH OF LEAST RESISTANCE

Many parents get alarmed when liquid comes spewing out of their baby's nose. Let us reassure you that this is an anatomically normal (albeit potentially surprising or unpleasant) occurrence. In case you haven't already discovered it for yourself, we all have a direct connection between the backs of our throats and our noses. As stomach contents are expelled, whether from spitting up or vomiting, they generally follow the path of least resistance. Depending on the circumstances—your baby's positioning and the force of the eruption, to name a couple—the exit route may be his mouth, his nose, or, on occasion, both!

Assessing Your Losses

Only rarely do babies spit up enough that it becomes more than a matter of inconvenience and affects their overall nutrition and weight gain. That's not to say that the amount an otherwise healthy baby spits up doesn't seem impressive from a parent's-eye view. When looking at the spit-up stains on your baby's clothes (or your own), it is very easy to overestimate the amount being "tossed." To get a better idea of the true volume, you can try pouring some milk or water in measured increments onto a clean towel or cloth diaper. You'll see that the liquid will spread out quite a bit on the dry fabric. Compare the size of a spot made by 1 teaspoon, 1 tablespoon, or 1 ounce to the size of a spot made by your baby's spit-up or vomit and you may be reassured that all has not been lost. The bottom line: a happy spitter who continues to eat well and gain weight well does not generally need much, if any, intervention. On the other hand, any newborn who isn't eating well, isn't gaining weight as expected, seems generally miserable, or is increasingly spitting up larger amounts more frequently or more forcefully needs to be seen by a doctor.

CHARACTERISTICS OF A HAPPY SPITTER

In attempting to distinguish between normal spit-up (*reflux*) and something more serious, consider these common spit-up characteristics of a "happy spitter."

- Small amounts, often associated with burps, hiccups, or pressure on the belly

- Not associated with crying, pain, or distress

- Starts in the early weeks, is generally associated with feeding, and fortunately tends to resolve during the first year without incident or treatment

Overall, one of the most important characteristics to keep in mind is that a happy spitter shows no adverse (negative) effects as a result of spitting up (no effect on growth, no pain, no problems with the spit-up being aspirated and getting into the lungs, etc).

What Is GERD?

GERD is simply the acronym for gastroesophageal reflux disease. In simpler terms, it's often thought of as the baby equivalent of heartburn—the result of stomach contents making their way back up into the esophagus, sometimes causing discomfort and on rare occasion resulting in more significant intestinal or breathing problems. That said, studies now suggest that the cause of irritability in the great majority of infants is not directly attributable to their reflux. It is the diagnosis typically given to babies who experience choking, sputtering, heartburn, discomfort, and/or poor weight gain associated with their spitting up or vomiting. GERD symptoms occur in less than 1% of infants and warrant a discussion, an evaluation, and potential medical treatment. GERD is not something a book can (or should) diagnose for you but something it can only make you aware of. If in doubt, get it checked out.

Vomiting

More often than not, new parents worry about more serious causes of vomiting when it's more likely harmless spitting up. That said, newborns can and do vomit for a variety of reasons. Your baby may occasionally vomit if, for example, she has a particularly sensitive gag reflex, you have a particularly forceful milk letdown when breastfeeding, or she's a little overly eager and happens to overfeed. Some other causes of what may seem like persistent vomiting include intolerance of whatever it is they are being given to drink, an underlying infection, or a digestive tract problem that doesn't allow things to flow through as directed—all of which should be discussed with and evaluated by a doctor. If you suspect true vomiting, be on the lookout for fever or other signs of illness. Also keep an eye out for blood in the poop, diarrhea, or excessive fussiness and gassiness. These sorts of signs and symptoms are always helpful to report to your pediatrician and can indicate intolerance to formula or breast milk. Regardless of the cause, vomiting can lead to dehydration and electrolyte imbalances much more quickly in newborns than in older children and adults, so don't wait until your baby seems lethargic or dehydrated (as signaled by less pee, a dry mouth, doughy skin, sunken eyes and fontanelle, and weight loss) to contact your pediatrician—just do it right away.

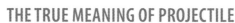

THE TRUE MEANING OF PROJECTILE

Projectile is a word often used in the context of spitting up and vomiting. Some parents graphically describe their baby's vomiting as "shooting across the room." While parents often say moderately forceful spitting up or vomiting can cause liquid to "jump" or "gush" out a few inches from a baby's mouth, true projectile eruptions—more force, longer distances—especially when they occur regularly, may indicate more serious problems. For more information, read on.

How Much Vomiting Is Too Much? When to Consider Pyloric Stenosis

At the point when vomiting seems to be getting progressively worse and becoming more and more out of hand, you or your pediatrician may suspect a condition known as *pyloric stenosis.* The muscle at the far end of the stomach (the pylorus) serves the important role of another gatekeeper, allowing food to pass out of the stomach and into the intestinal tract (see **Figure 8-1**). In contrast to its often too lax counterpart at the top of the stomach, this sphincter muscle can sometimes become a bit too thick and strong for its own good (or anyone else's)—doing *too* good of a job limiting what gets out of the stomach and into the intestinal tract. *Stenosis* refers to any type of narrowing. In the case of pyloric stenosis, the opening at the bottom of the stomach becomes progressively narrower than it should be. The more difficult it becomes for stomach contents to go down and out through this narrow region, the more they head up and out instead.

Pyloric stenosis occurs in about 3 out of every 1,000 babies and is much more common in firstborn boys and those with a family history of the condition. It typically causes babies to start spitting up in the first few weeks, usually around one month. Unlike the frequent but happy spitters or even the occasional and intermittently impressive vomiters, babies with pyloric stenosis vomit with increasing force and frequency—an increase most often building up to the full-fledged projectile vomiting by six to eight weeks of age. If your baby's spitting up or vomiting is persistent and seems to be progressing, it's worth contacting your baby's doctor sooner rather than later. If your baby happens to be diagnosed as having pyloric stenosis, there is a surefire remedy to stop the vomiting. Babies with pyloric stenosis require a straightforward operation to widen the pylorus muscle's opening at the bottom of the stomach. Recovery is usually quick and allows babies to begin feeding normally within a couple of days following surgery.

DOUBLE TROUBLE

If an infant vomits most or all of a feeding for 2 or more feedings in a row, it should be taken as a warning sign of something potentially more serious, and prompt medical evaluation is needed.

Gagging and Sputtering

Some babies have more sensitive gag reflexes than others. On the one hand, this is a good thing because the gag reflex is responsible for keeping food (or in your newborn's case, breast milk or formula) from "going down the wrong way" and getting into the lungs. On the other hand, a gagging or sputtering baby can be very scary for parents. If your baby starts gagging or having trouble breathing while feeding, promptly sit him upright, pat his back, turn his head to the side or slightly face down to let any milk or saliva run out of his mouth, and let him catch his breath. In almost all cases, babies quickly recover from such episodes on their own. If your baby has frequent gagging episodes, or especially if he ever stops breathing, even briefly, or turns blue for a moment during a gagging or coughing spell, seek immediate medical attention.

FOR SAFETY'S SAKE

For safety and peace of mind, we wholeheartedly support the recommendation that you and any of your baby's potential caregivers find the time to take a CPR (cardiopulmonary resuscitation) course in case any emergencies arise regarding your baby. You can start by contacting your pediatrician, local Red Cross, or local hospital for class information.

activities of daily living

introduction

· · · · · · ·

Included in the following chapters are many of the newborn topics we consider to be the bread and butter of parenting. In them are answers to the most commonly asked questions new parents typically have about the activities you are likely to be partaking in day in and day out once you are checked out of the hospital and are heading home. Sandwiched between the ins and outs discussed in the preceding sections and looking ahead toward heading out and about, we now focus our efforts and your attention on the important aspects of everyday life with a newborn. While these are the activities that will initially dominate your thoughts and occupy much of your time, they will soon become second nature: newborn sleep, crying, diapering, bathing, and clothing.

9

sleeping like a baby

• • • • • •

It is for good reason that sleep (and a new parent's relative lack thereof) always seems to top the list of popular parenting topics. There's no doubt about it: heading home with a newborn is quite an eye-opening experience, both literally and figuratively. Even the years we spent on call as pediatric residents didn't prepare us for the interrupted sleep schedule that characterizes life with a newborn. It's safe to say that few things will change more dramatically than your sleep habits, at least for the near future when you suddenly switch roles from expectant parent to new parent. Beyond asking the basic questions of when, where, and how much sleep to expect your baby (and you) to get, you may also find yourself wondering what to do about your newborn's blatant disregard for the "rules." These include but are not limited to the sanctity of nighttime sleep, the importance of "beauty" sleep, and just plain letting everyone in the household get enough. As you head into the first few weeks of what is all but guaranteed to be relative sleep deprivation, we suggest you remind yourself of one thing: this too shall pass.

What a Difference a Day (or Two) Can Make

During the first day or two after you have your baby, you might find yourself impressed with and thankful for how much your baby is sleeping. Many a mother of a newborn gets her best rest in the hospital, only to come to the mistaken conclusion that she is destined to be one of the lucky few whose babies sleep through the night from day 1. Although we really don't enjoy bursting anyone's bubble, we feel obliged to give you a heads-up on the changes that are likely to be right around the corner. In the grand scheme of newborn sleep patterns, the first couple of days are often a honeymoon phase. Many newborns spend their earliest days in the outside world catching up on sleep after the exhausting effort it took to get them there. It's almost as if they are briefly too tired to realize they are now out in the real world where there is so much to see and so much fun to be had. But once they wake up to the fact that they have at their disposal new scenery, parents to "play" with, and a lot of eating, peeing, and pooping to do—not to mention they are no longer being lulled to sleep in the cozy confines of a uterus complete with soothing background noise—well then, all bets are off and the games typically begin. As you first set out to learn the rules of this "can you survive your newborn's sleep habits?" game, you'll find there are, in fact, very few rules. Even for the few rules there are, your baby may not be much for following them. As you brush up on what you can expect from your newborn, rest assured that with time (hopefully, just a few weeks), patience, and a bit of endurance mixed in, you and your baby will catch on and adjust.

Safe to Sleep: Back Sleeping and Beyond

Chances are good that some of you were raised as a "belly baby"—spending all your non-waking hours (as well as many of those when you were awake) lying comfortably on your belly. Since those days, when babies were so commonly laid belly down to rest, new information was brought to light about the potential role sleep position plays in the prevention of sudden infant death syndrome (SIDS)—an occurrence that is admittedly uncommon but nonetheless terrifying to think about. Based on an ever-increasing amount of evidence linking belly sleeping to an increased risk of SIDS, the American Academy of Pediatrics (AAP) first recommended back sleeping in 1992 and then partnered with several national organizations to launch the official Back to Sleep campaign (now called the "Safe to Sleep" campaign) in 1994. After more than two decades of education aimed squarely at getting parents and other caregivers to place infants to sleep on their backs instead of their tummies, the percentage of back sleeping babies increased accordingly, while the SIDS rates decreased impressively. If you're interested in the actual numbers, we are happy to oblige: by 2008, more than 85% of babies were estimated to sleep on their backs, in stark contrast to 25% in 1992. Overall, recent studies show that rates of SIDS and other sleep-related newborn and infant deaths (such as accidental suffocation) declined considerably—from approximately 130 deaths per 100,000 live births in 1990 to approximately 93 deaths per 100,000 live births in 2017.

THE REALITY OF SIDS: CREATING A SAFE SLEEP ENVIRONMENT

Sudden infant death syndrome (SIDS), sometimes called *crib death,* is the sudden, unexplained death of an otherwise healthy baby during the first year. SIDS, along with the other sleep-related infant deaths, is certainly not a topic we, as parents or pediatricians, enjoy bringing up with excited new parents but rather one that we are committed to raising in the hopes of saving babies' lives. While sudden unexplained infant death is always a tragedy for the roughly 3,600 babies and families affected each year in the United States, the odds of it happening to your baby are very low, and it is well within your power to minimize the risk. Although SIDS rarely occurs during the first month after birth (the risk is greatest from two to four months), there are simple things you can do to create a safer sleep environment for your newborn right from the start. We suggest you start by following the most recent safe sleep guidelines from the American Academy of Pediatrics (AAP), which may help prevent SIDS and other sleep-related tragedies.

- **Be safe.** Play it safe by making sure you or anyone else who cares for your baby always places him on his back in a crib or bassinet with nothing other than him and a tight-fitting sheet when it's time to sleep.

- **Be firm.** "Being firm" means making sure your baby always sleeps on a firm surface—and by *firm* we actually mean a surface hard enough that it does not become indented when your baby lies on it. Make sure your crib meets all safety standards and that the crib mattress fits securely in the crib. Being firm also means keeping all soft items out of your baby's crib—including such tempting but potentially dangerous items as fluffy blankets, stuffed animals, and crib bumpers (and yes, this means all crib bumpers, including the thin mesh kind).

- **Stay cool.** Overheating increases the risk for SIDS. Dress your baby in light-weight sleep clothing. Consider using a wearable blanket in lieu of a loose one, and keep the temperature in the room where your baby sleeps set at what would be comfortable for a lightly clothed adult. If you are worried about your baby getting too cold, you can dress her in layers of clothing.

- **Clear the air.** Keep the air your baby breathes smoke-free, not only to reduce the risk of SIDS but also for your baby's overall health. This includes your home, car, and any place your baby spends time awake or asleep.

- **Provide a pacifier.** During your baby's first year, consider offering him a pacifier when he is falling asleep. If you are breastfeeding, we recommend waiting until it is going well (typically by three to four weeks) before introducing the pacifier.

(continues)

THE REALITY OF SIDS (*continued*)

- **Share a room but not a bed.** The American Academy of Pediatrics (AAP) recommends sleeping in the same room but not the same bed as your baby until she turns one or for at least the first six months. This can make breast-feeding easier while at the same time help protect your baby from SIDS.

- **Use trusted sites.** The AAP also cautions against allowing infants to sleep on a couch, armchair, or soft surface, either alone or with anyone else. Instead, it may be helpful to strategically place an additional crib, bassinet, or play yard elsewhere in the house if you want to keep an eye on your napping baby during the day. Also avoid sleep products that hold the baby in a reclined position. They are not safe for infant sleep, and many have been recalled.

Putting Back Sleeping Concerns to Rest

We're willing to bet this isn't the first time you've been introduced to the benefits of raising a back sleeping baby. Most new parents today are well-informed when it comes to safe sleep and why back sleeping is so strongly recommended. We'd be remiss, however, if we didn't acknowledge that you may find yourself with some practical concerns when faced with putting principle into practice. For the most part, the following concerns cause parents to worry unnecessarily:

- **Not sleeping "well."** One of the primary concerns (and observations) parents often have is that their babies don't sleep as well on their backs. While it is true that back sleeping babies are likely to wake more frequently, what's most important to understand is that their easier arousability is actually the reason why back sleeping is safer than belly sleeping. While it is certainly understandable for new parents to dream of sleeping longer, you can rest assured that this will come in good time. For now, just remind yourself that you don't want it to come at the expense of your baby's safety.

- **Spit-up and vomit.** The most common concern we hear is the understand-able but unfounded fear that babies will spit up and choke while on their backs. Fortunately, several reassuring studies, as well as the test of time, have demonstrated that healthy babies laid to sleep on their backs are able to turn their heads and protect their airways if and when they spit up. Additionally (albeit counterintuitively), babies' anatomy actually makes choking *more* likely when lying on their bellies. And finally, back sleeping babies are no more likely to have breathing or digestive-related problems than their belly sleeping counterparts of years past.

- **Flat heads (sometimes referred to as *positional skull deformities* or *positional plagiocephaly*).** While there has been a documented increase in the number of babies "walking" around with flat areas on the backs of their heads since back sleeping came into vogue, the fact of the matter is that this condition doesn't pose much of a problem for most back sleeping babies. In large part, that's because you have a good deal of control over the situation. It's important to understand that the shape of a newborn's head is not set in stone and can be affected by spending a lot of time in any given position. It is therefore important to simply remember to try and alternate the direction your baby faces each time she lies on her back—both while she is asleep and when she is awake. By offering your newborn plenty of tummy time and time spent in positions other than flat on her back while she is awake, you can also help decrease the likelihood of a flat or misshapen head. For more on newborn heads, see The Shape of Things to Come on page 296.

- **Delayed milestones.** Some of you will undoubtedly hear or read that back sleeping has been associated with delayed motor development. In addressing the question of delayed milestones—or, more specifically, a delay in the time when back sleeping babies first begin to roll over—rest assured that this all seems to even out in the end. Even if your baby doesn't take to rolling quite as early as her belly sleeping counterparts of generations past and present, to our knowledge no college application has ever asked applicants how early they mastered the ability to roll over (or, for future reference, sit, crawl, walk, or toilet train). When it comes to strengthening the muscles your baby needs to roll and, at the same time, decreasing your baby's chances of ending up with a flat head, just be aware that both can be easily accomplished by allowing your baby plenty of time on her belly when she's awake.

DON'T TAKE SIDES ON SIDS

In the early days of sudden infant death syndrome (SIDS) prevention, both back sleeping and side sleeping were considered to be acceptably safe sleep options for babies. However, subsequent concerns about the safety of side sleeping—fueled by the finding that it doubles the risk of SIDS as compared to back sleeping—led to the current recommendation for exclusive back sleeping. That said, some parents have turned to wedge-like cushions, often referred to as *sleep positioners*. Whether they have unwarranted concerns about spitting up, are worried about flat heads, or simply think side sleeping is safe, it's simply not a good idea. Unfortunately, devices designed to maintain sleep position have not been sufficiently tested for their safety or effectiveness. In addition, they are often made of soft material or memory foam, both of which have no place inside a baby's crib or near a baby's face. For any devices that made medical claims, the US Food and Drug Administration (FDA) (in 2010) was able to require their removal from the market. Regarding any sleep positioners that remain, both the American Academy of Pediatrics (AAP) and the US FDA recommend that parents never use them.

Good Night, Sleep Tight

We'll be the first to admit that sleeping belly up doesn't always seem to agree with all babies. Although it seems to vary, we've found that quite a few babies are prone to startling themselves awake from peaceful slumber. That's because babies are at the whim of their own reflexes—which, by definition, they cannot control—and are born with one particularly inconvenient reflex (the *Moro* or "startle" reflex). This reflex causes infants to jerk suddenly, flail their arms and legs, and even cry out in response to being startled—hence the name (see Reflexes on page 324). And yes, even when you've gone to great lengths to create a startle-free environment for your sleeping baby, he may just take matters into his own hands (and feet), startle himself awake, and proceed to flail around like a bug stuck on his back until someone comes to his rescue. But don't give up on uninterrupted sleep just yet because there is something quick and easy you can do: a handy little technique we call the "burrito wrap."

The Burrito Wrap

Most commonly referred to as *swaddling*, wrapping your baby up as snug as a bug in a baby blanket before putting him down to sleep can be helpful. While there is no shortage of readily available, commercially made swaddling blankets, it's also possible to bundle your baby at home simply using a regular baby blanket. Hands down, the most talented people we've ever seen at this sleep-saving technique are the nurses in the newborn nursery. These baby-bundling experts take uncomfortably free and exposed newborns and almost effortlessly have them bundled into blissful, no-flailing-allowed slumber in the blink of an eye. If you have an opportunity, we highly recommend watching these professionals in action. For those of you who are already home and either missed out on the hospital demonstration or could use a little refresher course, we've laid out the details for you as best we can without actually being there to demonstrate in person.

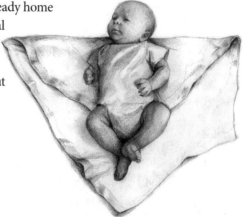

Figure 9-1. *Steps 1–3.* Preparing the swaddle

1. Lay a thin baby blanket out like a diamond in front of you (**Figure 9-1**).

2. Fold the top corner of the blanket down a bit so that the folded corner almost reaches the middle of the blanket.

3. Place your baby on his back, and center him on the blanket with his arms at his sides, his head just above the folded edge, and his shoulders just below it.

4. Take one of the side corners of the blanket and fold it over your baby's shoulder and across his body; make sure to tuck the corner underneath him on the opposite side (**Figure 9-2**).

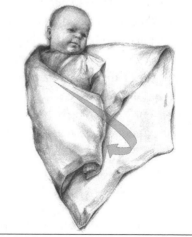

Figure 9-2. *Step 4.* Folding the blanket

5. Then take the bottom corner of the blanket (below your baby's feet) and fold it up over your baby. If the blanket is large enough that the bottom corner reaches up to (or over) your baby's face, you can simply fold it back down until his face is no longer covered or bring it over either shoulder and tuck it under him (**Figure 9-3**).

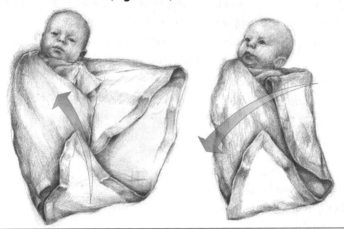

Figure 9-3. *Step 5.* Continuing the swaddle

6. Finally, take the only remaining corner and pull it over your baby's other shoulder and across his body. Again, tuck this corner snugly under your baby's opposite side (**Figure 9-4**).

Once you have the general idea, remember that variations are perfectly acceptable. Feel free to play around with what works best for you and your baby. While the exact details and order in which you do them may not matter too much in the end, we will point out that there is a good reason why we recommend folding the bottom of the blanket up *before* flipping the last corner across (ie, Step 5 always before Step 6) and always tucking corners under your baby; doing so helps keep your handiwork from coming undone quite as easily. However, if you find your swaddling technique to be less than secure, you may want to opt out of the do-it-yourself approach and use a blanket designed specifically to stay in place. Of course, you'll need to always make sure the swaddle is not so snug as to potentially restrict your baby's breathing. As a rough rule of thumb, this means you should be able to fit 2 or 3 fingers between the swaddle and your baby's chest.

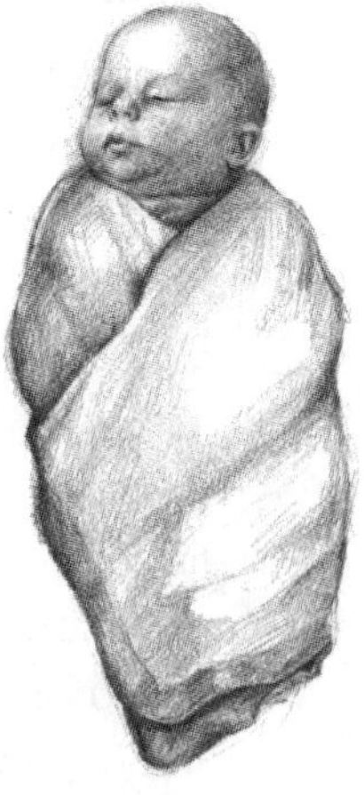

Figure 9-4. *Step 6.* Completing the swaddle

Hands-free Bundling

Some of our esteemed parenting colleagues suggest doing whatever it takes (ie, with regard to bundling) to ensure that your baby's arms and legs stay snugly secured in the blanket. Other equally convincing and respectable experts recommend never restricting your baby's arms—focusing your bundling attention on just your baby's legs while allowing her arms free rein. While there is admittedly no evidence to lend support to either approach, we personally have tried bundling both ways with good results. If you find that your baby seems unhappy having her arms "pinned down" by her sides instead of up next to her head, go ahead and burrito wrap her without placing her arms inside.

Safe Swaddling

According to the AAP, swaddling can be an effective technique to help calm infants and promote sleep when done correctly and so long as babies are always on their backs when swaddled. Most child health experts agree that a baby's hips should not be bundled too tightly. Instead, they should be allowed to relax in their natural frog-leg positions to allow for proper growth and joint development. For safety reasons, you should always be sure that your swaddled baby is on his or her back—never on the side or tummy. Swaddling also has the potential to cause babies to overheat, so be sure to check and make sure your baby isn't showing signs of overheating (sweating, damp hair, rash, and rapid breathing). And finally, for safety and developmental reasons, it is a good idea to stop swaddling by about eight weeks of age, before babies typically start rolling. If your baby is trying to roll earlier than that time (whether swaddled or not), you should stop swaddling sooner.

A NEWBORN'S PERSPECTIVE ON THE COMFORTS OF HOME

In addition to being at the mercy of their own reflexes, babies also tend to take a while to adapt to their new and often less appealing living (and sleeping) quarters. By keeping in mind that your newborn has just spent almost a year inside a continuously warm, dark, snug, and soothing environment, it becomes easier to understand how the sudden transition to lying sprawled out flat on one's back can seem like nothing short of a rude awakening—one that your newborn may take some time adjusting to.

Sleeping by the Book

"Sleeping like a baby" can mean different things to different people—usually depending on whether they've ever had a baby or taken care of one before. For just about all newborns, it fairly predictably means having the ability to sleep at any time and in any place while at the same time being completely unwilling to entertain any "suggestions" as to how, when, or where to put such talent into practice. You may come across those who have ventured down the path of parenthood before you who simply shake their heads sympathetically and wish you luck in getting your newborn to wake up when you want or need him to and even better luck in getting him to go to sleep when you want. Because we're committed to helping you set appropriate expectations for yourself and your baby, we'll help you get into the right frame of mind with some general sleep-related milestones.

- **Daily sleep.** The average newborn spends at least 16 hours a day sleeping, but there can be big differences from one newborn to the next. The total amount of sleep babies need in any given 24-hour day gradually decreases over time but still totals anywhere from 12 to 16 hours between the ages of 4 months and 1 year.

- **Naps.** Sure, many newborns nap in 1- to 2-hour spurts, but before you go planning your schedule around any preconceived idea of nap time, let us add that the length of most newborns' naps is also quite variable, and they tend to be scattered throughout the day (and night) in a completely random and therefore unpredictable manner. The three-nap-a-day schedule with which you may be familiar is a sleep pattern you can aspire to down the road. Most newborns don't settle into this type of nap routine for at least 1 or 2 months. Even then, it can take a few additional weeks or months before you can count on a morning nap, an early afternoon nap, and an early evening nap.

- **Night versus day.** During the first few days and weeks of parenthood, you are likely to find there's not going to be a whole lot that distinguishes your days from your nights. More often than not, they just seem to blend together into one big sleep-deprived blur. That's because it will be almost completely up to your newborn when he chooses to be awake and when he chooses to sleep. Most newborns spend equal amounts of time sleeping during the day and night—a tendency that can be quite challenging for those of us accustomed to more of an awake-by-day, asleep-by-night approach. By the end of their first month, most newborns manage to figure out how to consolidate their sleep into longer stretches and start to get at least one extended stretch of sleep during each 24-hour day. So with any luck, you'll be blessed with a baby who decides to choose nighttime as the right time to do so. And for the real light at the end of the tunnel: by 3 months of age, many babies get approximately two-thirds of their total daily sleep during the night (albeit not yet in a single, uninterrupted stretch).

Reversing the Day-Night Reversal

Some babies settle into a newborn sleep routine dreaded by many expectant parents—the so-called day-night reversal. As the term implies, newborns are known on occasion to mix up their days and nights. These temporarily backward-sleeping babies often begin to increase the amount of sleep they get each time they go to sleep according to plan. They simply do so during the day, while they demand to be fed, changed, *and* entertained throughout the night. As painfully exhausting as this upside-down approach to sleep may be for those of us accustomed to getting most, if not all, our sleep at night, the assurance that this too shall pass once again comes to mind. We can all but guarantee you that hope is not far away. In most instances, that your newborn is learning to replace lots of catnaps with longer stretches of sleep— whether they happen to fall during the day or at night—bodes well for a more "civilized" sleep routine in your not too distant future.

Lights On, Lights Off

If your baby seems determined to play during the night and sleep during the day, there's really no quick fix, but there are some easy things you can do early on to set the stage for more acceptable sleep habits in the future. During your first few weeks at home with your baby, try to establish an atmosphere that clearly differentiates night from day. A good night's rest may not result overnight, but this approach can help get you there sooner.

- **Set your baby's (internal) clock.** After spending nine months in the dark, it's no wonder that newborns seem to have no respect for their parents' sleep schedule preferences. We liken it to being in a casino with the same amount of lighting at all hours and not a clock in sight. You can help sync your baby's body clock with the rest of your world by keeping things bright during the day and dark at night. Taking your baby for a walk in natural light (somewhat shaded of course) can help speed up the syncing process.

- **Allow for active sleep.** During the day, have your baby sleep in more active areas of the house—in rooms with the lights on or perhaps even in the car seat or stroller when you determine that you are ready to make your way out of the house (see also Thinking Outside of the House on page 209). That said, let us be clear in stating that car seats and strollers (and other partially or fully reclined baby products) are okay for when you are on the go with your baby in tow but are *not* recommended for routine sleeping around the house.

- **Create consistent contrast.** While it's a good idea to limit your baby's exposure to background TV from day 1 (see Media Matters on page 205), don't spend too much time worrying about common background noises such as talking, telephones, or music during daylight hours. In contrast, make your nighttime interactions as calm and quiet as possible, limiting any unnecessary light, sounds, or distractions.

- **Maintain focus.** Whenever possible, take a more focused approach to your nighttime interactions—limiting them to feeding, burping, changing, and gentle soothing when necessary.

- **Use a soft-spoken approach.** Get into the habit of taking the aforementioned measures in a dark room and using a soft voice whenever you want to signal to your newborn that it would be a fine time to sleep.

Learning to Sleep, Drink, and Be Merry

Before lying down, closing your eyes, and considering yourself lucky that you have a baby who has precociously caught on to sleeping long stretches at a time, you'll want to first consider whether prolonged periods of sleep could get her into trouble. Some babies—especially those who are born small, who have not yet mastered breastfeeding, or who are just a bit too sleepy for their own good—can be drowsy enough that they don't remember to wake up and eat. Just how long should you let your newborn sleep at any one time, and how often should you feed her? The answer will depend on a variety of factors, not the least of which will be based on your pediatrician's assessment and subsequent recommendation.

Let Sleeping Newborns Lie?

Some pediatricians buy into the idea that full-term, healthy babies do not need to be woken up to eat during the night as long as they are eating and gaining weight well. Others feel very strongly that all babies—at least for the first several weeks—should not be allowed to sleep for more than four or five hours at a time (at most) without being woken up to eat. Our opinion on the matter: wait at least until you are sure your newborn has fully mastered breastfeeding or bottle-feeding, proven himself capable of taking a regular interest in eating, and regained his birth weight according to plan within the first two weeks or so after being born before kicking back and enjoying the luxury of four or more hours of uninterrupted sleep. Whatever you do, be sure you discuss any sleep habits that seem too good to be true (and may, in fact, be falsely reassuring) with your baby's health care provider before reveling in the thought of a good night's sleep.

Waking Up Is (Sometimes) Hard to Do

Now is as good a time as any to discuss briefly the age-old adage "never wake a sleeping baby." Many expectant parents take this advice to heart and prepare themselves and their homes accordingly. In anticipation, they begin by turning the ringer off on their phones and making signs to tape over their doorbells that read, "Please knock quietly—baby sleeping." After bringing home a newborn of your own, however, you're far more likely to discover that most young babies (older babies are a different story) can sleep through just about anything—vacuums, doorbells, and a whole host of ringtones included. Instead of figuring out ways to ensure peaceful slumber, many new parents find themselves wondering if, in fact, their babies would awaken to the sound of a freight train going by or the house being hit by a tornado. You'll find that as your baby gets older, she will probably become a lighter sleeper. For the time being, however, feel free to relax a little on the noise control unless, of course, you need it so you can sleep.

How to Wake a Sleeping Baby

As we mentioned at the outset, newborns have an impressive ability to ignore the world around them when they see fit to sleep. If you find yourself in the position of needing to wake up your baby, here are some simple techniques that sometimes (notice we said *sometimes*) work.

- **The kinder, gentler approach.** You might as well start out with the kinder, gentler approach to baby waking and see what kind of response you get. This can include such basic measures as talking, singing, and gentle stimulation. Pick your baby up, talk to him, move his arms and legs around, and even tickle the bottom of his feet or rub his cheek—whatever works to rouse him.

- **Dressing down.** Whether it's the physical stimulation or the increased exposure to cool air that does it, many newborns absolutely hate to be undressed. Your newborn may find it well worth the time and effort it takes to wake up and voice his opinion.

- **Double-duty diapering.** Even if your baby doesn't technically require a new diaper, going through the motions of a diaper change (even reusing the same diaper, assuming it's still clean) may help if undressing alone doesn't do the trick. This works especially well for babies who have a tendency to fall asleep before finishing their meals. We think of it as dual-purpose diapering because diaper changes not only tend to wake up sleeping babies but are more likely to be needed around feeding times (see The Eating-Pooping Connection on page 79).

- **Cleanliness is next to wakefulness.** Giving sleepy babies a bath certainly takes things a step beyond undressing and changing diapers, but it has been known to work when all else fails. While we certainly don't approve of cruel and unusual punishment in any way, shape, or form, there may be times when some of you may simply have no other choice than to resort to a bath to get your baby to wake up. This more "drastic" measure is most appropriately used sparingly, such as in the event that a newborn is long overdue to eat, and can be modified to accommodate your baby's umbilical cord as needed (see Baby Bath Basics on page 149).

The approaches we have described to you are based on the assumption that your newborn is healthy. While it is true that newborns are known to be challenging to wake up at times, you should also be aware that babies who are not easily aroused or responsive despite their parents' best efforts need medical attention. Do not wait to discuss any questions or concerns you might have about your baby's sleepiness with your baby's doctor. Seek medical help immediately if your newborn seems increasingly sleepy, unresponsive, or hard to arouse.

Now I Lay Me Down to Sleep

Many new baby books matter-of-factly lay out the merits of teaching babies to fall asleep all on their own, without parental assistance. You know: no rocking, no nursing, and no driving circles around the neighborhood in search of sleep. If you have taken heed, you may be wondering to yourself exactly how you are supposed to go about getting your newborn to fall asleep independently without guaranteed screams of protest. Fortunately, the reality is that many babies learn to fall asleep all by themselves within the first four months after birth. And yes, we do mean at nighttime and at nap time. In the early days, however, we suggest you avoid losing sleep over whether you are doing yourself and your newborn a great disservice by occasionally allowing her to start drifting off to sleep cradled in your arms, rocking with you, or snuggled up on your chest before putting her safely into her crib. That said, we suggest taking any opportunity you get right from the start to promote healthy lifelong habits, and that most certainly includes the important life skill of falling asleep without assistance by about four months of age.

TO SLEEP, PERCHANCE TO DREAM

Even though they have shorter sleep cycles than adults, overall an average newborn spends far more time in what is known as active (REM, or rapid eye movement) sleep. This is not only the stage of sleep when dreaming takes place but also the stage when there is likely to be a lot more sucking, kicking, grunting, and moving going on. This is also a good time for you to catch a few of your newborn's first sleepy smiles.

Suitable Sleep Sites

At first, we figured we ought to allot a good bit of time to addressing the various sleep-site options available to you, starting predictably with the crib and then running through everything from bassinets, cradles, and co-sleepers to play yards, car seats, and dresser drawers (the latter of which we feel compelled to point out right from the start aren't recommended as safe sleep settings). Then it occurred to us that most parents we talk with seem to handle this part of new parenthood pretty well on their own and either don't care too much or already have their hearts set on one or the other (or several) of the options. Given that there are plenty of well-respected and informative baby product books and resources around (including *Baby Bargains*, now in its 13th edition, and HealthyChildren.org, to reference but a few), we decided not to take up too much of your time on the subject. Instead, we lay out for you what we consider to be the practical considerations and safety tips most useful in deciding where to safely lay your baby down to sleep.

Sleeping Solo or Filling the Family Bed

Probably since the beginning of time, babies and parents around the world have slept together in what has come to be commonly referred to as "the family bed." However, in recent years, particularly in industrialized nations, including the United States, the trend has been to have children sleep separately starting from birth. Given that this trend is in keeping with what we now know to be safest for babies, we suggest you let common sense and a strong commitment to safety prevail.

- **The family bed.** Whether because of space limitations, cultural norms, or a strong belief that bed-sharing is an integral part of parenting, parents have slept with their babies for thousands of years. In many parts of the world and in a good 60% of US households, many babies still sleep in bed with their parents, at least on occasion, despite increasing concerns about the associated risks. Followers of attachment parenting seem to feel quite strongly that parents and babies benefit most from bonding whenever possible, including during sleep. Proponents also feel that bed-sharing makes breastfeeding easier. We encourage you to read on for some important things to consider before you opt for the family bed.

- **Sleeping solo.** By *sleeping solo,* we don't mean to imply in a different room, just not in the same bed. In the United States, there has been a definite shift toward placing babies down for sleep independently, whether in a crib, cradle, or bassinet. Our country's movement toward independent sleep may well be, in part, attributable to recent and well-founded concerns that bed-sharing in the first year increases the risk of sleep-related infant deaths (see The Reality of SIDS: Creating a Safe Sleep Environment on page 103). Other practical reasons why parents opt for solo sleeping: they find it to be safer, sounder (for their baby and themselves), and less intrusive on their "adult" time.

BEDSIDE SLEEPERS:
THE CONVENIENT ALTERNATIVE TO BED-SHARING

For those of you who find the convenience of having your baby nearby at night appealing but find the prospect of having him in bed with you concerning, a bedside sleeper (often referred to as a *co-sleeper*) may be just the thing for you. If you ask us, these specially designed baby beds are ingenious. Somewhat like play yards, co-sleepers generally rest at the same height as a standard adult bed, have a removable (or absent) rail on the side that fits next to the bed, and can therefore be placed right alongside your bed for easy access, resembling a motorcycle sidecar. While the American Academy of Pediatrics (AAP) does not make any official recommendations for or against the use of bedside sleepers (pending additional research), this sleeping option technically meets the AAP checklist for creating a safe infant sleep environment by having your baby sleep in the same room but not the same bed while facilitating safe and successful breastfeeding. (On the other hand, in-bed co-sleepers are NOT recommended.) Given that they can be pricey and their placement a bit difficult to navigate around for moms just recovering from C-sections, you can alternatively consider use of a play yard with or without a bassinet insert placed next to the bed.

Bed-sharing Safety Concerns

Many new parents are tempted to take their newborn into bed with them—often out of fatigue and convenience, as well as for cultural and philosophical reasons. Whether bed-sharing is safe, however, has been the subject of much debate. Recent studies suggest that bed-sharing may significantly increase the risk of infant suffocation, so you'll find that many experts (including those responsible for writing AAP policy) now strongly advise against it and instead suggest the very practical and safer alternative of sharing the same room but not the same bed during your baby's first year. If you choose to sleep with your baby in your bed, even if only infrequently, here are some extremely important safety considerations.

- **Make your bed like a crib.** The heavy blankets, comforters, pillows, and other accessories typically found on adult beds can suffocate or smother a baby and therefore have no place being in the same location where newborns sleep. (While we're on the subject of simple yet potentially lifesaving measures, we also strongly recommend removing any and all such items that may have already found their way into your baby's crib.)

- **Bed-sharing babies are at risk from falls** or the possibility of being trapped between the mattress and the wall, headboard, or other furniture.

- **Bed-sharing and the use of tobacco, alcohol, or drugs don't mix.** These substances, including over-the-counter or prescription medications, all have the distinct potential to cause excessive drowsiness or impaired judgment, making those who choose to indulge at risk of being less aware of a baby in the bed.

Crib Safety Considerations

Whether you decide to set up a crib for your baby as soon as your pregnancy test turns positive or months after your newborn's much-anticipated arrival, there are a few general safety principles that you'll want to follow to ensure your baby's safety. Some may not seem particularly relevant during your baby's first few months, but given that cribs tend to be big-ticket items and the one you invest in is going to be put to the test for years to come as your baby learns to roll, sit, stand, and climb in it, it's well worth considering present and future safety concerns.

- **Crib slats.** The slats should be no more than 2⅜ inches apart. All new cribs must meet this standard, but older cribs may not. Avoid using any crib that does not meet this 2011 standard.

- **Posts and cutouts.** Steer clear of bedposts taller than ¹⁄₁₆ of an inch (which we realize is almost nothing, but that's the point) and cutouts in the headboard or any other parts of the crib, where a baby's or toddler's body part could get stuck.

- **Bumpers and pillows.** Yes, they're soft and cute. But soft and cute should not be your deciding factor. For safety's sake, keep crib bumpers and pillows out of your baby's crib.

- **Crib toys.** They may seem harmless, entertaining, cute, and cuddly, but it's considered wise to keep all stuffed animals (and most toys) out of your newborn's crib because they can pose a small but nevertheless real safety risk. The exceptions are the types of toys that strap securely to the side of the crib. Some babies like mirrors or toys with parts they can play with (such as spinners, rattles, and music), but your newborn probably won't be terribly interested in them for at least a few weeks.

- **Mobiles.** Mobiles are special hanging toys designed to entertain your baby and can be attached to the crib, ceiling, or wall. Some are even adorned with lights or play music. They are fun but definitely optional. If you choose to use mobiles, make sure they do not hang low enough to entangle your baby, especially once she begins to roll. In fact, once your baby is able to sit up, it will definitely be time for her mobile to come down.

- **Crib placement.** Unless you don't mind a bit of redecorating and rearranging when your baby starts to get around, we suggest you place your baby's crib well away from any windows and no less than an arm's reach away from any nearby dressers or tabletops. Knowing that it won't be long before anything and everything within reach will be fair game, we also recommend limiting your over-the-crib wall decorations to painted walls and wallpaper. Picture frames and mirrors over cribs may be cute, but they are also injuries waiting to happen. Be forewarned that while they may be safe, even paper borders placed within reach of the crib don't often stand up well to prying fingers.

- **Firm-fitting mattress with a fitted sheet.** While they seem to be mostly standardized, cribs and mattresses can and do come in more than one size, so be sure to double-check measurements and read labels to end up with a mattress that fits snugly into your chosen crib. Any extra space between the mattress and crib frame has the potential to trap a baby's arm, leg, or head. Also make sure your fitted sheets are tight enough that they don't slip off easily, thereby posing a serious safety hazard. See the following sections in this chapter for more on bedding for your baby's crib.

- **Tooth-resistant rails.** Some railings are covered by a special plastic to prevent teething babies from gnawing on the paint or wood.

- **Adjustable mattress height.** Many cribs have adjustable heights so you can lower the mattress as your baby gets taller, making it more difficult for him to climb out. You will most likely want to keep it at the highest level while your newborn is relatively immobile and you are coming and going frequently because it will allow you to save a good deal of strain on your back. Remember that by the time your baby is able to sit or stand up, you'll want to lower the level of the crib mattress accordingly.

DROP-SIDE CRIBS: A THING OF THE PAST

In years past, crib railings were almost always *adjustable*, meaning you could raise and lower one or both side railings. While this feature had long been appealing to parents as a convenience factor, in 2009 it became a significant concern. And by *significant*, we mean that numerous injuries from crib side rails resulted in what was the largest crib recall in history (2.1 million cribs!). As a result, the US Consumer Product Safety Commission (also referred to simply as "the CPSC" and the organization that sets voluntary industry safety standards) required all full-sized cribs be manufactured with four immovable sides. Taking an even stronger stand, the government set new federal standards in 2011 that banned the sale (including resale) of drop-side cribs. That's why drop-side cribs are now a thing of the past. The take-home message for all parents: always be sure to check out the latest safety information on the CPSC website (www.cpsc. gov) before dropping your guard.

Bare Is Best

If you come to find that the excitement you feel about having a new baby is wrapped up in the buying of a fancy baby bedding set complete with bumper and quilted blanket, we suggest you work on changing your mindset rather than your nursery decor. Simply remind yourself that the AAP recommends that *nothing* but a snugly fitted sheet be placed with your baby in the crib during the first year.

Monitoring the Situation

Parents now have the option of using the latest in audio and video baby monitoring to listen to and watch their baby from afar. Many parents find that this type of technological surveillance buys them peace of mind, by allowing them to roam freely around the house while they are still keeping tabs on their baby. If you choose to use a monitoring device, camera, and/or app, you may want to keep the following considerations in mind:

- **Nothing beats the real thing.** First and foremost, never let baby-monitoring technology substitute for direct supervision and taking sensible safety measures. Also, be aware there is unfortunately no evidence that using a monitor decreases the chance of SIDS.

- **Range.** Baby monitors themselves are only as good as their technological limitations, so we suggest you take a look at what kind of listening range, clarity of view, and data they each offer. The kind that sync with some of the baby-monitoring apps, of course, have solved what used to be a more common range limitation by making use of cloud-based access.

- **It works both ways.** There are steps you can take to minimize the potential for interference, hacking, or fuzzy reception, starting with simply following the product instructions. This typically includes recommended security precautions such as setting a strong password for the monitor and your home's wireless network, updating software regularly, and keeping other electronic devices away from the monitoring unit as necessary.

- **Disrupting the peace.** Some of you may find that leaving the monitor on at night significantly disturbs whatever limited sleep you stand to get, causing you to be wide awake in response to your slumbering baby's every twitch or snort.

- **Channel surfing.** In this age of modern electronics, there's more than enough to interfere with your monitor, including cordless phones, cell phones, radio stations, and other monitors. Try to find a monitor with good reception and more than one channel to decrease the likelihood of interference. We also suggest holding onto your receipt in case you run into any unforeseen technological conflicts that become apparent only once you put the monitor to use at home.

- **Bells and whistles.** Give some thought to which bells and whistles you really want and which simply serve to raise the price. Some of the available added features include a portable receiver with a belt clip, two-way walkie-talkie radio capability, night vision, a room-temperature sensor, a receiver that vibrates or flashes lights so you can leave the sound turned off, the ability to watch your baby on your computer or other devices using your wireless network, and the possibility of purchasing multiple portable receivers that can accompany a single base station.

- **Safety reminders.** All monitor bases and additional units should be wireless or, if they have a cord, must be well out of baby's reach.

Parental Sleep Priorities

We couldn't end a chapter on newborn sleep without addressing what you can do to get yourself some much-needed rest too. Typically offered by those who've been in the trenches before you, the often-repeated advice to sleep whenever your baby is sleeping actually makes very good sense—regardless of whether you considered yourself the type of person to take naps in your pre-parenting days. After all, if you don't take any and every opportunity that comes your way, we're pretty sure you'll come up quite short when trying to squeeze in your own REM cycles. We encourage you to put sleep high on your own priority list and either delegate or let other activities take a back seat for the first few weeks or months. As a point of practicality, let us also mention that trying to accomplish routine but complex tasks, such as balancing your checkbook, preparing elaborate meals, entertaining, or operating heavy machinery in a sleep-deprived state, is best avoided whenever possible (more on this in Taking Care of Yourself on page 173). And in all seriousness, do not attempt to drive when you're extremely exhausted. Finally, take friends and relatives up on their offers to help out around the house so you can get some much-needed rest. They wouldn't offer if they didn't mean it, right?

CHAPTER

10

crying

· · · · · ·

All newborns are supposed to cry—and most of them do a very good job
of it! In fact, most newborns tackle this important rite of babyhood immediately after being delivered. A newborn's first cries actually serve an important
purpose. By helping fill the lungs with air, crying allows a newborn to make
the momentous shift from depending on the oxygen carried to him in his
mother's blood before birth to breathing it in on his own as soon as he enters
the outside world. Even without an explanation of fetal and newborn circulation, you probably don't need us to tell you that delivery room cries are
worthy of eager anticipation; generally represent the arrival of a happy, healthy
baby; and are almost universally met with tears of joy and relief. What cries
may come in the days that follow can vary considerably from baby to baby.
At least at first, you're more likely to find yourself with a relatively sleepy baby
(see Sleeping Like a Baby on page 101) who only cries to be fed (see Into the
Mouths of Babes on page 1).

Why Cry?

Once newborns have slept off the excitement of delivery and opened their
eyes to the brave new world that lies before them, you can bet that they all
inevitably and intermittently start crying. That said, one of the first and most
helpful lessons to teach yourself is that babies don't always cry for the same
reasons as adults. After all, most of us cry when we are (a) hurt or (b) upset.
We assume it is for this reason that many parents become distressed at the
sound of their baby's cry and feel like absolute failures if they can't stop their
baby's presumed cries for help, much less stop them immediately. Babies,
though, have the uncanny ability to burst into tears (minus the tears, of
course, which don't tend to show up in any noticeable amount for the first
month or so; see No More Tears...Yet? on page 300) if they're startled,
hungry, hot, cold, tired, wet, bored, annoyed, gassy.... You get the picture.

The way we look at it, babies are justified in crying a lot if for no other reason than that they really don't have many other ways of communicating their feelings. By reminding yourself that a newborn's cries aren't always synonymous with pain or upset, you'll be much less likely to find yourself on the verge of tears in the months to come.

LOUD AND TEARLESS

Most babies typically don't seem to shed tears in the first month or so—not for a lack of trying but, as we understand it, simply because their tear glands don't make enough to be very noticeable. While you may not exactly treasure your baby's cries (at least after the first one in the delivery room), you may actually find yourself a little misty when she reaches the teardrop milestone and her cries are accompanied for the first time by overflowing tears.

Tales of a Telltale Cry

Most books tell you that your parenting instincts will quickly take over and you'll be able to identify the reason for each of your baby's unique cries. We definitely don't want to minimize the importance of taking crying seriously, and we wholeheartedly agree that you should try to understand the underlying meaning of each of your baby's cries, but in our experience, this is often easier said than done. When you're not quite sure why your baby is crying, look first for the "obvious" causes—hunger, pee, poop, tiredness. At the same time, reassure yourself that it's not due to something potentially more serious. These can include causes such as fever, illness, a tight diaper or piece of clothing, poking pins, an eyelash or scratch in the eye, or wayward hairs or strings wrapped around fingers or toes (the latter few being universally listed causes we felt obliged to include when, in reality, they're actually pretty rare). Should you ever find yourself unable to pinpoint why your newborn is or was crying and feel hopelessly incompetent as a result, we hope we can convince you to be less critical of yourself. After all, we did not always find cry identification to be a simple task with our own newborns either. We did what we could, and we gave it our all (although sometimes our "all" was a bit limited because of sheer sleep deprivation). If our children could remember their infancies and were allowed to publicly discuss our parental "inadequacies," we're sure they would tell us they were fed when they were wet, put to bed when they were hungry, and overstimulated when they were tired. Sure, there will be times when your baby's needs are obvious, but it's worth keeping in mind that there will also be times when you're just not sure about anything except, perhaps, wanting to pull your hair out.

CALCULATED CRYING

In your first weeks and months of parenthood, remind yourself that it is absolutely normal for babies to cry. A typical newborn will cry for about two hours a day for the first 6 weeks or so. Light at the end of the tunnel: the amount of daily crying that babies do gradually decreases to about 1 hour per day by 12 weeks (and even less after that). Even better, the reason(s) for their crying usually become much easier to figure out as time goes on.

Is It Colic?

Pick up any baby book and you're sure to find mention of what many parents refer to as the dreaded "C word." Even though the rule of thumb for colic is that it doesn't usually settle in until three to six weeks or so after birth, we've included it front and center in our discussion of newborn crying because without any frame of reference, quite a few parents start worrying about it even before their babies are born and then worry that every cry or fussy spell is only one step shy of all-out colic (or might signify the start of it).

Colic Defined

This is the one time when we warn you that turning to the dictionary will not serve you well. That's because the dictionary definition listed, which defines *colic* as "severe, often fluctuating pain in the abdomen caused by intestinal gas or obstruction in the intestines and suffered especially by babies," is simply incorrect given the current pediatric understanding of colic in the context of crying babies. In this much more relevant context, colic is defined as "excessive crying" in an otherwise healthy baby. In other words, it is no longer believed to be related to or explained by simple intestinal causes. The excessive crying that has come to define colic occurs with equal frequency in up to 40% of babies, regardless of whether they are male or female, breastfed or bottle-fed, full-term or premature, or firstborn. For practical purposes, we like to think of colic as a spectrum ranging from repeated crying episodes that last just a few minutes to those that go on for hours at a time. Only time will tell if your newborn will prove to be a colicky baby—one who has regular crying spells that present themselves usually in the evening, for no apparent reason, at least three days a week, and for more than three hours at a time. The good news is that a majority of babies with colic outgrow it by three months of age (60%) or four months of age (90%).

Controlling Colic

While no one knows the true cause of colic, and many parents and experts continue to attribute the crying to stomach pain or something in a baby's diet, a sensible and logical analysis of colic (and what to do about it) has been laid out for all parents to benefit from in a well-written, practical parenting book and related DVD by a fellow pediatrician named Harvey Karp. In *The Happiest Baby on the Block,* Dr Karp takes a close look at previous colic theories and introduces parents to the 5 Ss (swaddling, side/stomach positioning while awake, shushing, swaying, and sucking) that we agree can be very effective in calming crying or colicky babies during the first few months after birth.

DOES SOOTHING EQUAL SPOILING?

You certainly don't need to hold back on responding to your newborn's cries for fear of spoiling her. In fact, for the next several months you can take spoiling off your list of parenting concerns altogether. Each time you try to respond promptly to your newborn's cries, you simply send your baby a message that you're there to tend to her needs.

Soothing the Savage Beast

How, exactly, can you tell what your newborn's needs are so you can more successfully soothe him? Even though we've already told you it's not always simple, after a few days you are likely to notice your baby has a characteristic cry every time he starts to fall asleep. Or maybe he'll have a certain wail that stops as soon as he is fed. Once you start picking up on these cues and responding accordingly, your baby will take comfort in knowing he's able to communicate with you, at least some of the time. If you can't identify the cry, consider the last time your baby ate, slept, or had his diaper changed. If a few hours has passed, it may be time again to tend to each of these needs. Here are some other techniques to try if your baby just won't stop crying.

- **Get professional help.** Most books save the worst-case scenarios for the end of the list. Not us. We want you to know right off the bat that if at any point you feel your baby is simply inconsolable or crying for longer than you're comfortable with, or if he seems sick or has an unusually high-pitched cry, then by all means, put down the book(s) and enlist the expertise of your pediatrician without delay—that's what they're there for!

- **Soothe yourself.** Okay, we're now going to assume that you've evaluated your situation and don't think it warrants a doctor's intervention. The next step is to take a deep breath and try to relax. Babies can pick up on stress around them and may start to cry if they get negative vibes. Sometimes the best first step you can take is to calm down, even if that means putting your crying baby in a safe place and giving yourself a quick break first.

- **Stay snug and secure.** Try swaddling your baby snugly (as described in Good Night, Sleep Tight on page 106). The way we reason it, newborns have all spent nine months (give or take) accustomed to feeling snug and secure in the very close quarters of the uterus. By simulating this cozy feeling of confinement, the swaddling technique often helps with crying, as well as sleeping.

- **Keep things moving.** Any newborn who's spent any amount of time in utero is simply not going to be born accustomed to sitting still. As a result, you may find that yours takes a while to buy into the notion that the absence of movement and activity can be pleasant and peaceful. In the meantime, you can try the time-tested methods of movement such as carrying, rocking, strolling, or driving to appease your crying or restless newborn. The ever-popular vibrating infant seats, rocking cradles, and baby swings also serve the purpose of keeping babies comfortably moving as well. Just keep in mind that you'll want to always secure your baby according to these products' instructions, keep an eye on him while you're using them, and be aware that they are only considered safe and recommended for use when babies are awake. Be sure to look for features designed to safely accommodate newborns such as additional recline options, harnesses that adequately secure small infants, or low settings on automatic swings. Even more importantly, make sure you never use any inclined seat as a sleeper (see The Dangers of Infant Inclined Sleepers on page 129).

- **Supply simple sound effects.** Your baby may also crave the soothing muffled noises similar to amniotic fluid waves or the swishes and pulses of mom's heart and blood vessels. You may find, as many before you undoubtedly have, that the sound of a vacuum cleaner, washing machine, shower running, or human heartbeat (hold him against your chest, or play a recording of heart sounds) works wonders. For some of these efforts, you also have the added bonus of a cleaner house, clothes, or body! Whether you're musical or not, try singing or playing some music. Some parents find that their newborns seem to be particularly soothed by music that was played or sung to them even before they were born!

- **Opposites attract.** Feel your baby's hands and feet. If they are cold, put another layer of clothing on him or wrap him in a blanket. If the back of his head and neck are warm or sweaty, remove a layer (and consider checking his temperature, as discussed in Fever: Trial by Fire on page 325). See if he's interested in a change of scenery. If it's bright, turn off the lights. If it's dark, turn some on. If it's very noisy, turn down the volume. If it's unusually quiet, try out some of the simple sound effects just described. Too still? Move around. Bottom line: no actual science is involved; it's more a matter of finding and fine-tuning your own calming solutions.

- **Resist unfounded cure-alls.** We have yet to meet the parent of a crying baby who wasn't tempted to buy products marketed to help stop the crying. While there may be some that do work, or at least help, there are plenty of others with no proof to back up their claims. As but one example, many parents faced with colic are tempted to try using simethicone-containing drops (you may be more familiar with the brand names Mylicon or Little Remedies) to treat it. Lactase enzyme and herbal remedies are other products that are marketed to treat infantile colic. Unfortunately, last we checked, studies still show that these interventions are not proven to help with colic. Before trying any of these products, be sure to discuss them with your baby's pediatrician to make sure they are not harmful.

- **Hand off.** If others are around, enlist their help until you're ready to try again yourself.

- **Give it time.** If all else fails, just hold your baby and patiently wait for him to settle down. Crying in and of itself won't hurt your baby, so if you're not in a mindset to handle it, it's okay to let your baby cry for a while. If you're at your wit's end and need a break, don't feel guilty about putting him in a safe place (such as a crib) while you compose yourself.

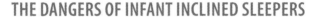

THE DANGERS OF INFANT INCLINED SLEEPERS

In 2019, 4.7 million Fisher-Price Rock'n Play sleepers were recalled following dozens of infant deaths. A subsequent study commissioned by the US Consumer Product Safety Commission (CPSC) found that *no* inclined sleep products that were tested and evaluated were safe for infant sleep. As a result, both the CPSC and the American Academy of Pediatrics have concluded that there is no such thing as a safe infant inclined sleeper and recommended that they should all be taken off the market and no longer be used by parents or other caregivers.

When You Feel Like Crying

While entire books are written on the subject of the so-called baby blues and postpartum depression, we didn't want to finish off this chapter without telling you that if you don't feel like crying in the first few days or weeks after becoming a parent, congratulations! You're definitely in the minority. The "baby blues" are a real thing, and up to an attention-worthy 80% of new moms reportedly experience some form of them. For most of you, we suggest you don't spend too much time trying to explain your tears or wondering whether the hormonal roller coaster, sleep deprivation, or sheer newness of parenthood is to blame. The mild depressive feelings associated with the baby blues, while common, are just that—mild. And they fortunately tend to go away on their own within a week or two.

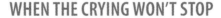

WHEN THE CRYING WON'T STOP

Now that we've tried to give you a better feel for why newborns cry, we want to leave you with a general rule about newborns and crying. Even though inconsolable crying does not always mean there is a serious underlying cause to blame, it always warrants a call to the doctor.

Postpartum Depression: Beyond the Baby Blues

For an estimated 15% of new mothers, the feelings of sadness and anxiety can be much more extreme and persistent, interfering with their ability to care for themselves or their families. These are not the symptoms of the baby blues, and they don't just go away on their own. They represent postpartum depression. Postpartum depression most commonly sets in sometime during the first month after delivery (although it has been known to start even before delivery) and can affect any woman regardless of age, race, ethnicity, or economic status. The symptoms associated with postpartum depression can last anywhere from a month to a year and usually require counseling and treatment. Of note, as many as 1 out of 10 new fathers experiences symptoms associated with the diagnosis of postpartum depression as well. If ever you find yourself overwhelmed, frustrated, anxious, persistently teary, or depressed and unable to explain or shake the feeling, please don't suffer in silence or shame. Talk with your doctor right away, as there are effective treatments readily available. Although you may well feel lonely, you are not alone.

GETTING HELP FOR POSTPARTUM DEPRESSION

Given all that is known about the serious effects of postpartum depression, we wanted to leave you with the following valuable information from the National Institute of Mental Health regarding what to do if you or someone you know has or may be experiencing postpartum depression.

What are the symptoms of postpartum depression?
- Feeling sad, hopeless, empty, or overwhelmed
- Crying more often than usual or for no apparent reason
- Worrying or feeling overly anxious
- Feeling moody, irritable, or restless
- Oversleeping, or being unable to sleep even when her baby is asleep
- Having trouble concentrating, remembering details, and making decisions
- Experiencing anger or rage
- Losing interest in activities that are usually enjoyable
- Experiencing physical aches and pains, including frequent headaches, stomach problems, and muscle pain
- Eating too little or too much
- Withdrawing from or avoiding friends and family
- Having trouble bonding or forming an emotional attachment with her baby
- Persistently doubting her ability to care for her baby
- Thinking about harming herself or her baby

What can happen if postpartum depression is left untreated? Without treatment, postpartum depression can last for months or years. In addition to affecting a mother's health, it can interfere with her ability to connect with and care for her baby and may cause the baby to have problems with sleeping, eating, and behavior as he or she grows.

How can family and friends help? Family members and friends may be the first to recognize symptoms of postpartum depression in a new mother. Encouraging her to talk with a health care provider, offering emotional support, and assisting with daily tasks such as caring for the baby or the home are all important steps to take.

When and how to get help quickly. If you or someone you know is "in crisis" or thinking of suicide, get help quickly.

- Call your doctor.
- Call 911 for emergency services or go to the nearest emergency department.
- Call the toll-free, 24-hour National Suicide Prevention Lifeline at 800-273-TALK (800-273-8255).

Adapted from *Postpartum Depression Facts.* Bethesda, MD: National Institute of Mental Health. Accessed April 27, 2020.

11

the art and science of diapering

• • • • • •

The Facts About Diapers

It's probably not news to you that becoming a parent will inevitably involve changing a lot of diapers—as many as 8 to 12 a day once you get into the swing of things—but who knew there was a whole art and science to the task? The fact is that most parents will go through nearly 3,000 diapers during their baby's first year alone and average six diaper changes a day for an estimated total of 8,000 over the course of a baby's diaper-wearing career. With toilet training not often achieved until children are two to three years or older in the United States (although it may occur much earlier in other cultures), diapering is an unavoidable part of parenthood. Need we say more? Obviously we think so because not everyone (ie, almost no one) is born with an innate mastery of this necessary parenting skill.

DIAPER(LESS) TRIVIA

Did you know that in certain Asian and African cultures, babies are not put into diapers? When a baby awakens or the parent notices certain cues, the parent places the baby over a bush or another designated area to pee or poop. Although you may want to adapt this technique when it comes time to potty train, based on social norms in America, we don't recommend you try this with your newborn at home!

The Debate: Cloth Versus Disposable

As a newcomer to the world of parenting, you may not have heard of the ongoing cloth versus disposable diaper debate, especially because use of disposable diapers has become so accepted as a modern-day convenience that many parents wouldn't dream of using a substitute. In contrast to 1955, when essentially all American babies wore cloth diapers, an estimated 90% (or even 95%) of 21st century American babies are sporting the latest in disposable fashions. While a simple internet search on the subject quickly makes it clear how strongly some people feel about the cloth versus disposable debate, we have no intention of taking sides. Instead, we figure we'd offer you some facts and practical advice related to the use of each type, with the rest of our information weighted toward disposable use only because it is applicable to a majority of parents these days.

DO YOU SEE WHAT I PEE?

Disposable diapers these days are so effective at absorbing whatever pee may come their way, they can actually pose a challenge to parents who are trying to keep close tabs on just how much their newborns are peeing (see also In Search of a Little Pee in a Big Diaper on page 76). Fortunately, some diaper brands now come with a colorfully effective solution: a strip on the diaper that changes color when wet, allowing you to more clearly see when your baby pees.

- **Disposable.** Disposable diapers are very absorbent, a feature that can be good and bad. Using them may mean your baby's skin has less contact with pee and poop and may offer the added convenience of less frequent changing. However, it may also be more difficult to monitor exactly how much your baby is peeing—a task that is especially important during the newborn period, as well as when you're faced with watching for signs of dehydration (see Vomiting on page 93).

  Some cloth diaper advocates argue that babies in disposable diapers have a much higher incidence of diaper rash (presumably due to longer contact with diaper contents resulting from less frequent changing). Interestingly, however, one of the commonly recommended approaches to treating diaper rashes is for cloth diaper users to switch to disposable. Also garnishing a lot of attention is the fact that "disposable" diapers are not biodegradable, and billions (with estimates around 20 billion diapers, or 3.5 million tons) make their way into landfills each year. We have been happy to learn that some communities have begun recycling or responsibly composting used disposable diapers, while some of the country's leading diaper makers seem to be making an effort to be more eco-friendly, improving everything from the materials they use to the amount, transport, and packaging of diapers. We certainly hope that this sustainability-minded approach continues across the entire disposable diaper industry.

- **Cloth.** Cloth diapers are supposedly more comfortable than disposable diapers (we say *supposedly* because neither of us has any personal recollection, and we aren't exactly sure how one would otherwise prove such a claim). Proponents also claim that babies who wear cloth diapers are five times less likely to develop diaper rashes than their disposable diaper-clad counterparts. But unlike disposable diapers, cloth diapers are not as absorbent, need to be changed more frequently, and usually need to be worn with an overlying stay-dry cover. These covers typically come in the form of plastic, cotton, or terry cloth. As for the materials used to make them, cloth diapers have long been made of cotton—a material that is notorious for requiring a lot of water to produce. Those focused on reducing the environmental impact of diapering point to bamboo-based cloth diapers as more eco-friendly, as well as a more readily available alternative to cotton. And because cloth diapers (and their covers) require a lot of washing by either the parents or a diaper service and therefore use a great deal of water and detergent, people in the disposable diaper camp point out that cloth diapers also have a negative effect on the environment—especially when they are washed in small, half-full loads of laundry, put into a dryer instead of line dried, or both washed and dried.

AN ENVIRONMENTALLY SUPERIOR DIAPER?

One of the most significant concerns parents have when it comes to the use of diapers these days is the effect they have on the environment—a concern that is well worth paying attention to. What may come as a surprise, however, is that it's in no way clear that disposable diapers have any greater effect than their cloth counterparts. Both disposable and cloth diapers have an effect on the environment that is determined by taking into account the full "life cycle" of the diaper, from start to final use. This includes how much energy, water, and raw materials are used, as well as how much atmospheric emissions and water-borne and solid wastes are created. While studies suggest that disposable diapers use more raw materials and produce more solid wastes, cloth diaper use potentially consumes significantly more water and produces more waterborne wastes. The conclusion: we wish we had a definitive one for you. When it comes to declaring environmental superiority of cloth versus disposable diapers, it still seems to be a wash.

The Art of Diapering

Yes, believe it or not, there is an art to diapering. After all, who wouldn't be proud of the ability to diaper a moving target, save five cents a diaper, always be prepared for (if not prevent) a blowout, or simply get the darn tabs to stick when and where we want them to? While parenting inherently requires a whole lot of diaper changes, the art of diapering involves doing it better, faster, cheaper, and with less mess or stress.

Choosing a Diaper

Whether you choose cloth or disposable, brand name or generic, or any combination thereof, you and your baby may develop some preferences for the diapers you use. Some babies are "well contained" using a variety of brands and styles of diapers, whereas others may do best with a certain brand. Some require extra absorbency, while others do just fine with the less expensive, not quite as absorbent types. Some babies may be sensitive to particular materials in diapers and may, on occasion, seem more prone to rashes when wearing certain brands. The bottom line: each baby is different. More expensive brands are not always better, but some are worth their absorbency in gold. Finding a suitable diaper for less may take some trial and error, but doing so can clearly be a good way to save money. So don't be afraid to try something new.

Diaper Sizing

The exact numbers vary from brand to brand, but in general, newborn diapers are designed for babies until they reach about 10 pounds. Unless your newborn is particularly small (in which case you might start out with "preemie" diapers for babies weighing less than 6 pounds), you may find yourself jumping up to size 1 diapers fairly quickly. Given that size 1 diapers are designed to fit infants from approximately 8 to 14 pounds, you may find yourself rounding up and bypassing the newborn diapers altogether.

Diapering Around the Umbilical Cord

Until a newborn's umbilical-cord stump fully dries and falls off, it is recommended that you leave it exposed to air as much as possible, as well as limit its exposure to pee- or poop-filled diapers (see The Care and Keeping of the Cord on page 311). While newborn diapers usually have umbilical-cord cutouts, you can also use diapers that don't and simply fold the front of the diaper down below the level of the belly button (**Figure 11-1**).

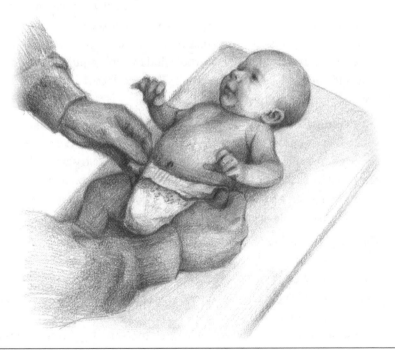

Figure 11-1. *Diaper folded below umbilical cord.* Fold the front of the diaper down below the level of the belly button until the cord falls off

Buying Diapers

At an average of nearly 30 cents a diaper for brand-name disposables and about 3,000 diapers, you can expect to spend around $1,000 during your first year of diapering—and that's not even factoring in wipes, diaper creams, and all the other diapering paraphernalia. With those figures in mind, we thought it would be useful to point out several potential ways you can save yourself some money in the diapering department.

- **Start small.** Start out by buying diapers in smaller quantities. You'll want to make sure you've found a good match, but also, keep in mind that your newborn will be growing very quickly in the months to come. If at first you happen to settle on a more expensive brand, remember that as your baby gets older (ie, potentially has less sensitive skin, less leaky poop, and pees less frequently), you may want to experiment with less expensive brands.

- **Divide and conquer.** Calculate your cost per diaper. This may sound obvious, but by simply dividing the cost of a pack of diapers by the number of diapers in the pack, you can figure out whether what you're getting is really a good deal or is just being advertised as one. Quite often, the retail (and virtual) stores list this price-per-diaper cost for you, if you just remember to look for it. If and when you do, you'll find that mega-jumbo packs aren't always the best bargain, and one store's sale price doesn't always beat the everyday price at another.

- **Cut coupons.** If you're the coupon type, it won't take much convincing for you to find a quick search for diaper coupons well worth your while. If you're not the coupon type, you might want to give it a try anyway. At the rate you'll be using diapers, there's really not a good reason to pass up $1, $2, or even $5 off a pack. While you're at it, consider using your coupons at stores that double manufacturers' coupons.

- **Think big.** When you find a sale or have coupons, buy extra diapers in advance to spare yourself a middle of the night run to the grocery store because you've used your last one. If you're going to take advantage and really stock up, you might just want to consider having your reserve supply be a size up from the one your baby's currently wearing. That way, you don't wind up having a stockpile of leftover, too-small diapers that don't fit as your baby outgrows them faster than you can use them.

- **Join the club.** Take note of frequent buyers' clubs. You know you're going to be in the market for diapers for a long time to come, and by simply collecting proofs of purchase (or "diaper points"), many companies reward you with baby clothes, toys, music, and other products. Similarly, some grocery and drugstore chains now tally up dollars spent on baby items and offer rebates or coupons each time you reach a certain total (eg, a $10 store coupon every time you spend $100 on baby items at that store).

- **Consider your options.** Consider using cloth diapers and washing them yourself. By some estimates, using a diaper service instead of paying for disposable diapers only lets you break even. By others, washing cloth diapers yourself has the potential to cut your diapering costs by as much as half.

Wipes for Newborns?

It's not uncommon for a new or expectant parent to hear through the parenting rumor mill that wipes are not to be used during the newborn period. As with many parenting recommendations, we're not exactly sure why this one exists. So we scoured the pediatric literature (which is not exactly extensive on the subject), and it seems most experts believe wipes are perfectly fine to use on newborn skin, even if there is a rash or break in the skin. In general, they are thought to be as mild as using a wet washcloth.

WIPING AWAY UNFOUNDED FEARS

In this day and age, cautionary parenting media posts—whether well-founded or not—have the potential to go viral before anyone has time to fact-check them. This is what seemed to happen in 2014. A concerning headline about doctors warned parents to never use baby wipes because they contained a harmful chemical. As you can imagine, this caused considerable parenting concern. At the time, an estimated half of all baby wipes sold in the United States reportedly made use of said chemical—a preservative called *methylisothiazolinone*. While it is true that this particular preservative was shown to cause rashes, what the alarmist headline failed to mention was that a total of only six children exhibited an allergic reaction that resolved as soon as the use of baby wipes stopped. The study authors thus concluded that patients with that particular allergy should avoid the preservative-containing baby wipes. This is a far cry from the "no one should use baby wipes under any circumstances" type warning that resulted.

A Word on Wipes

Although we haven't officially counted, there have to be about as many brands and types of wipes as there are tennis shoes—environmentally friendly, all-natural, scented and unscented, with aloe and without it, in round containers, in refillable rectangular containers, and in reusable or disposable travel packs. And while they may cost only a few cents a wipe if you don't go for the top of the line or opt for fancy packaging, the cost can nevertheless add up. While the principles discussed in Buying Diapers on page 138 generally apply to buying wipes as well, here are a few additional things to consider when buying and using wipes.

- **Packaging.** After one look at the shelves, you won't need us to tell you that when it comes to buying wipes, you pay for packaging. However, doing so is not always a bad thing. For example, someone who clearly had firsthand experience in the use of wipes on the go must have come up with the handy little travel-sized packs, and many parents find the added convenience well worth the extra money. That said, it is useful to hang on to reusable plastic travel containers and full-sized refillable plastic containers. By simply buying large refill packs and restocking them yourself, you can save the extra expense.

- **Don't flush 'em.** Enough said—almost. There are very few wipes on the market that don't have the potential to wreak havoc on your plumbing. Be sure to check package labels before buying if you are determined to find wipes that are flushable because most of them are not. Even then, seasoned plumbers will tell you that despite their name, the flushable ones still have the unfortunate tendency to get stuck.

- **The overuse of wipes.** Believe it or not, not every diaper change requires the use of wipes. This is not only because pee is rarely irritating but also because today's superabsorbent disposable diapers effectively limit the amount of pee that comes into contact with your baby's skin. Reserving wipes for cleaning up poop can save you a considerable amount. Also, keep in mind that a moist tissue, a wet washcloth, or even a quick rinse in the tub may be used in place of baby wipes when convenient.

Wipe Warmers

It seems some people are convinced that warm wipes are less shocking to newborns. It sounds reasonable: given that a baby's body temperature is 98.6°F and regular damp wipes are roughly 60°F, we're talking about a 40°F difference. Presumably to address this gap, the number of wipe warmers on the market seems to have multiplied since we last looked. By heating up the wipes to just below body temperature, wipe warmers can lessen the shock, so to speak. There are many options when it comes to choosing a wipe-warming unit—AC power adapter and/or car charger, heat from the top or heat from the sides, a constant 104°F wipe temperature inside the unit, built-in night-lights, and more.

In reality, however, most parents only briefly warm up cold wipes with their own hands, if at all, before using them on their baby. Those who own warmers tend to only use the warmed wipes in the room where the wipe warmer is kept. And we have yet to meet a parent who bothers to take their wipe warmer with them when venturing out of the house. Realistically speaking, most babies are not afforded this luxury and get used to cool wipes right from the start.

TEMPERATURE TRIVIA

While we're on the subject of temperatures and heated wipes, we thought we'd point out, for the sake of comparison, that the US Consumer Product Safety Commission recommends a toasty hot tub never exceed a temperature of 104°F, and indoor swimming pools are generally kept below 85°F. And lest we leave room for misinterpretation, let us emphasize that we are *not* suggesting you take your newborn in either but simply offering you a temperature frame of reference.

Changing Diapers

Location, Location, Location

Wherever you choose to change your baby's diaper—whether it's on your brand-new changing table or next to you on your bed—you'll want to pre-pare the area so everything you need is accessible. At a minimum, this means a diaper and something to wipe with. Changing tables are clearly the norm when it comes to location. Some people, one of us included, even opt to have more than one around the house. As convenient as they may be, you should be aware, if you aren't already, that changing tables aren't inherently necessary. If you decide you don't want your diaper changing to be limited geographically by where your changing table happens to be, or you want to save yourself the expense, simply consider keeping diapers accessible in convenient locations around the house (and in the car, once you start to venture out). That way, you can limit how far you have to go to take care of business. Some people opt to use a simple diaper-changing pad in lieu of the table, and the floor, bed, or couch or even the back seat of your car can easily serve the same purpose once you are comfortable with the routine. That said, some particularly messy episodes might require not only a new diaper but also an extra pair of hands, a new outfit, and even a trip to the tub. On such occasions, you'll be much better off if you choose your changing station in close proximity to all your supplies.

The Technique

Before starting to change your baby's diaper, keep in mind that some babies have a tendency to pee as soon as they are exposed to open air. By keeping them relatively covered as much as you can during the course of a diaper change, you can help keep yourself, your changing surface, and your baby's clothes from getting unnecessarily wet.

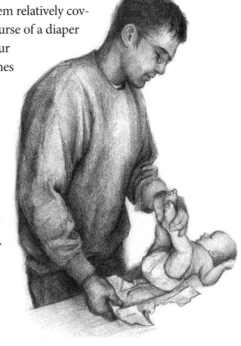

- If your baby is cooperative, which most babies are at least until they learn how to roll (somewhere around four months of age), you can first lift her legs with one hand. Using your other hand, place an opened clean diaper under her still-diapered bottom (**Figure 11-2**). Make sure you have the picture side of the new diaper in front, face down on the changing surface, and the side with the tabs underneath your baby.

Figure 11-2. Clean diaper positioning

- Once you have your clean diaper appropriately positioned, go ahead and unfasten the old diaper. Wipe your baby's bottom with the front (inner side) of it as you remove it. While you clearly don't have to wipe with the old diaper before taking it off, doing so often removes a significant amount of poop before you reach for your first baby wipe.

- If the old diaper isn't overwhelmingly messy, leaving it folded over on itself but still under your baby's bottom can help prevent her still-dirty bottom from getting the new diaper soiled before you've had the chance to clean her up. It can also serve to absorb any new pee that may present itself during the uncovered stage of the diaper change. Next, wipe your baby's bottom and surrounding dirty areas with a baby wipe, moist tissue, or washcloth.

- Then remove the old diaper, along with the wipes, from underneath your baby (**Figure 11-3**) and find a "safe" place to set them so you don't end up with your baby's foot in poop or find yourself with a new mess to clean up after accidentally knocking the diaper and its contents onto the floor.

- Securing the new diaper simply involves making sure that the front of the diaper is centered between the legs and pulled up to at least the same level in the back that it is in the front—usually around the level of the belly button. Check to see that the tabs are evenly secured in the front so there aren't any gaps around the hips.

- Also, to help prevent leakage, make sure the fringe around the legs isn't tucked into the diaper's elastic edges.

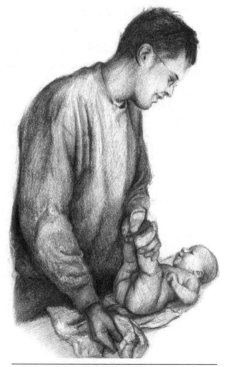

Figure 11-3. Dirty diaper removal

A WORD ON THE PERILS OF LOOSE-FITTING DIAPERS

Many of you will know precisely what we are referring to when we suggest you use caution and not let the back of the diaper sit too low or loose on your baby. This plumber-style method of diapering (no offense to plumbers intended) leaves way too much room for less-than-desirable contents to escape from your baby's diaper. Even if you quickly become a master diaper changer with impeccable technique and flawless fit, be sure to check the work of those well-meaning friends (and pediatricians) who may pay less attention than you do to detail when it comes to the end result of their diaper-changing efforts!

Disposable changing pads, available in most drugstores and sometimes referred to as *bed liners, underpads,* or "chux," can be helpful in protecting your changing table, crib, bed, floor, or wherever else you may choose to set up shop. These are especially good when you're away from home because they can be used first as a changing pad and then to wrap the dirty diaper for a quick and easy disposal. If you're at home and don't mind a bit of extra laundry, a towel can easily serve the same purpose.

A Word on Boys

Baby boys are notorious for indiscriminately spraying their parents, grandparents, and pediatricians. Simply being aware of this inherent hazard can help limit the amount of time you leave yourself vulnerable during a diaper change. So can holding your hand, a diaper, or a tissue over your baby's penis during the process. If you find yourself caught in the line of fire, take comfort in knowing it happens to the best of us. While it may not help you much, those of us in the medical profession who have been peed on more than once find some comfort in reminding ourselves that urine is, after all, a sterile bodily fluid. If you can get the diaper on without being doused but nevertheless find yourself faced with urine sneaking out of your baby boy's diapers, you can also try aiming his penis downward before covering it with the diaper.

DIAPER-CHANGING SAFETY CONSIDERATIONS

Although they may soon seem obvious (if they aren't already), we want to reinforce some of the basic and most relevant diaper-changing safety considerations. They include

- **Never leave your baby unattended.** Keep one hand on him at all times. Even though he may not even be able to lift up his head yet (much less roll over), it's a good habit to establish right from the start.

- **Prevent changing table falls by using the safety straps.** If you use a changing table pad, make sure you use its safety straps to secure your baby. Make sure the pad itself is safely secured to the table as well. These measures are not, however, substitutes for staying within arm's reach.

- **Beware of powder.** When inhaled, powder of any kind (whether it's talcum powder or cornstarch) can cause damage to a baby's lungs. If you choose to use baby powder, be sure to keep it away from your baby's face. First carefully rub a little onto your hands, then apply it to your baby's bottom.

- **Stay safe.** Keep plastic bags, safety pins, and any other potentially harmful tools of the trade out of your baby's reach.

A Word on Girls

Baby girls obviously have more nooks and crannies to deal with in their diaper areas, and as a basic principle, you shouldn't forget to look in them for hidden poop. That said, it is not necessary to wipe vigorously in an attempt to remove all the normal white discharge commonly found between the folds of the labia. In fact, doing so can cause undue irritation.

For many of you, this will be stating the obvious, but in hopes of promoting good hygiene and potentially decreasing the likelihood of urinary tract infections, we also feel compelled to remind you that baby girls should be wiped from front to back to prevent spreading poop into the region around the opening where the pee comes out (called the *urethra*). Sure, the poop may already have made its way there without your help, but at least you won't be adding to the mess.

UDOS: UNIDENTIFIED DIAPER OBJECTS

- Many parents are at a loss when they first find clear or yellowish beaded, gel-like particles in their infant's diapers, but you can rest assured that there is usually a simple (and harmless) explanation. Although we haven't actually seen any in years, diaper manufacturers still mention that the materials used to make the inside portion of the diaper have a tendency to form little gel-like beads when the diaper becomes over-soaked. By simply changing your baby's diaper more frequently, you can stop them from appearing.

- Also common are small harmless crystals made in the kidney that may appear during periods of relative dehydration, when the urine is very concentrated. For this reason, they are occasionally discovered along with pee in the diapers of newborn boys and girls who are not quite up to speed with their drinking and peeing. These *urate crystals,* as they are called, can leave a brick red–, orange–, or pink–tinged stain on the diaper and are usually not cause for concern in the first week or so. You can just mention them to your pediatrician at your baby's next visit.

- And finally, it is not uncommon for newborn girls to have some pink or even bloody spots appear in their diapers during the first few days or weeks. The bleeding, which is caused by exposure to mom's hormones before birth, typically resolves on its own but can really throw new parents for a loop in the meantime.

If you have any concerns about unidentified objects or discolorations appearing in your baby's diaper, be sure to consult your baby's physician.

Disposing of Diapers

Several manufacturers are in the market of selling diaper disposal systems designed to cut down on the odor associated with dirty diapers. These systems generally use built-in deodorizers, plastic bags, and airtight containers to seal off the smell. While many parents swear by them and love to use them, the main concerns some parents have about these systems include inadequate elimination of odor once things start to get smellier and the added expense of buying replacement bags. They also tend to be less useful for parents who choose to change diapers in a variety of locations around the house instead of at the official changing station where the disposal system is typically kept.

It comes down to a matter of personal preference, how sensitive your nose is, and how often you take out the garbage whether a special odor-eliminating diaper disposal system is worth the extra money. Parents who conclude that mildly wet or soiled diapers don't actually smell all that much may choose to use the disposal system for only the truly smelly diapers. Others find it just as easy, if not easier, to toss the smelly diapers into one of the zillions of extra plastic grocery bags (or newspaper bags or bread bags or any other sorts of bags) we all seem to accumulate. Doing so helps minimize the smell of the diaper enough that it can be placed into a regular garbage can in your house or a trash container outside. Once your baby starts having more solid and stinky poops—a milestone that tends to happen when solid foods are introduced, if not sooner—you may find it worthwhile to dump any solid poop into the toilet first.

The Medical Side

A Word on Diaper Rash

Quite simply, anything that appears as an irritation or rash on the skin in the diaper area is a diaper rash. While there are several types and causes of diaper rash, they fortunately don't seem to show up too often during the newborn period. That said, the types you are most likely to become personally familiar with are those caused by contact irritation or yeast. Contact with pee or poop can sometimes be enough to cause irritation of the skin. In other instances, a type of yeast known as *Candida albicans* is responsible for causing considerable redness and irritation. *C albicans* is commonly found in moist, warm areas, which helps explain why it primarily targets the diaper area—one of the most likely spots on a baby's body to be excessively moist. When *C albicans* finds its way into the inside of an infant's mouth, it can also cause white plaque-like spots, a condition referred to as *thrush*. Changing your baby's diaper regularly (every couple of hours during the day) and allowing her skin to air-dry before putting on a new diaper can definitely decrease her likelihood of getting a yeast diaper rash.

IT'S A WRAP

If you haven't figured this one out yet, the simple technique of folding up a dirty diaper before disposing of it is actually quite useful. Simply take the old diaper and lay it flat with the inside facing up and the tabs out to the sides, just as you would if you were spreading out a new diaper to put on your baby. Place any wipes you may have used into the center crotch area. Lift up the front portion of the diaper and roll it up like a sleeping bag. Once it is bundled up into a compact roll, take the side tabs and fold them over the rolled-up part to keep it closed and its contents well contained. This technique not only saves space and decreases odor but also limits your likelihood of spreading poop around.

Treating Diaper Rash

The treatment of diaper rashes depends on the underlying cause. If irritation is to blame, simply getting rid of or limiting your baby's contact with whatever is causing the irritation—whether a particular type of soap, detergent, or baby wipe or even just irritating poop—is often all that is necessary. In addition, the use of zinc oxide creams, ointments, or petroleum jelly–type products that provide a protective barrier over the skin can help limit the amount of contact and severity of the resulting irritation. Last, mild over-the-counter anti-inflammatory steroid creams such as hydrocortisone can often help reduce redness and pain, but parents should always be sure to discuss the use of this type of treatment with their baby's doctor before using it. This is necessary in part because of the possible harm that improper or prolonged use of steroids can cause to the skin but also because of the potential for steroid creams to worsen a rash if it is caused by yeast. Yeast infections require specially medicated antifungal creams—some of which are over-the-counter and others that can only be purchased with a prescription.

12

baby bath basics

• • • • • •

While it is true you are solely responsible for all your newborn's nooks and crannies, you may be relieved to know the task of bathing your baby does not need to be added to your daily routine just yet. The fact that you need to work around your newborn's drying-up umbilical-cord stump actually gives you a bit of a break-in period—giving you a good reason to get used to periodic sponge baths before you try your hand at more frequent and full-fledged immersion baths. After all, it can be daunting and challenging to handle a slippery bundle of body parts that don't follow directions. As you get the hang of giving your baby a bath and no longer have to accommodate a crusty, old umbilical cord, we hope you'll find that bath time becomes a less stressful and more enjoyable activity for everyone involved.

To Bathe or Not to Bathe

Contrary to popular belief, babies do not need to be bathed every day—especially as newborns. As we enter parenthood, we should all consider ourselves fortunate that we are given a few months in which to become comfortable with our baby-bathing duties before our children effectively figure out how to make themselves truly messy. It's really not until babies start crawling around in dirt, in sandboxes, or even just on the kitchen floor (depending on how dirty yours is) and begin exploring baby foods—with more smeared on their faces than in their mouths—that they warrant frequent full-body washes. Until then, you have the practical option of focusing your attention on a relatively limited number of parts. Your primary area of focus will predictably be the diaper area and, of course, the surrounding areas, the size of which will depend on whether your baby has taken to having blowouts (see What Goes In Must Come Out on page 71). Other areas to pay particular attention to include around the mouth and anywhere there are skin folds. While some of you may be looking at your newborn and thinking to yourself that there are few, if any, skin folds to be found, rest assured that they will soon appear. The present-from-birth and all-too-often-neglected armpit and groin folds are likely to be joined in mere weeks by double chins and thigh rolls. By making it a habit to regularly spot-check these hot spots and clean them as needed using a wet washcloth, you shouldn't have to bathe your baby every single day. In fact, bathing a couple of times a week is often enough until your baby becomes more mobile and figures out how to get dirtier. With that as a lead-in, it's high time we move on to the practical details involved in achieving cleanliness for all.

The Bathing Part

The First Bath

Parents of years past may have images of having their brand-new baby being whisked off for their first bath within minutes of birth before being returned for feeding and family bonding. The philosophy was that it was best to remove any residue and possible bacteria that the newborn might have encountered during pregnancy or delivery. In a recent change of routine practice, however, it has become more common to wait until about 24 hours post-birth (or as soon as 6 hours, if cultural norms dictate it), as recommended by the World Health Organization (WHO).

There are multiple reasons behind this shift in first-bath timing. Delaying the first bath can help maintain a normal body temperature and blood sugar levels in newborns. It also allows for quicker bonding and skin-to-skin exposure, and the earlier feedings have proven to increase breastfeeding success in the hospital. Finally, leaving on the protective waxy, white vernix on your baby's skin can act as a moisturizer and possibly prevent infections.

Tub Timing

When it comes to deciding when during the day is best to sit down (or kneel or bend over) and give your baby a bath, it is simply a matter of personal preference and convenience. From a practical viewpoint, we suggest you consider timing your baby's baths around your work schedules, your baby's sleep schedule, your own bathing schedule, or after a feeding. If you opt for after a feeding, you may want to wait a while to let the contents in your baby's belly settle a bit and allow any spitting up, peeing, or pooping to happen preferably beforehand. One time-tested tip we have to offer you is that babies really do respond well to routines. While you don't need to cling to a set schedule at all costs—there's definitely nothing wrong with accommodating a trip out of the house or visiting guests—over time you and your newborn are likely to benefit from a comfortable routine. Our personal favorite, and one we highly recommend you start sooner rather than later, is to offer a breast or bottle first. Follow this with a relaxing warm bath, and finally, share a few moments of cozy time curled up with a good book and your baby on your lap before bedtime (see Books and Babies on page 197).

Conditioning

The title of this section is not a reference to conditioning your baby's hair (if, in fact, he has any) but rather to conditioning your newborn to water in general—the look, sound, and feel of it splashing around. (We cover the hair care part in The Bathing Technique on page 154.)

While there are certainly several bath-time safety measures we address that you'll want to educate yourself about, you need not be timid about occasionally getting water in your baby's eyes or ears. Newborns are fully capable of blinking away splashed or even a bit of poured water. And to tell you the truth, few seem to actually mind it. That is why we have become convinced that there is such a thing as being too careful about splashing around newborns. From what we've seen, babies who grow up without ever being splashed with a few drops here and there, hearing the sound of the shower spraying, or getting a bit of water in their face every now and then are more likely to grow into toddlers who are afraid of water, put up a fight at bath time, and struggle through hair washing.

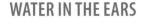

WATER IN THE EARS

As far as ears are concerned, your baby's ear canals dead-end at the eardrum (as do your own). What this means for bathing purposes is that water is conveniently blocked from getting into the middle ear. It also means that having a little water in one's ear canals from time to time doesn't cause middle-ear infections (*otitis media*) and may even help keep them clean of wax.

Stocking the Deck

If you buy into our philosophy of parenting preparedness, a good portion of the thought you put into bath time will be in the form of forethought. Since babies should never be left alone in the bath even for a minute, it's of primary importance that you have anything and everything you think you'll need within arm's reach before getting started. Whether the "deck" is the edge of your bathtub or the counter next to the kitchen or bathroom sink, stock it with all the bath-time supplies you intend to use before, during, and after. Some of the most useful supplies to have on hand include

- **Water.** Seem obvious? Of course you need water, but we suggest you make a habit of filling whatever tub you choose to use *before* putting your baby in it. In general, we've found that a water level in the tub of about 3 or 4 inches is easiest to work with—full enough to get the job done but not so full that you (or your baby) are going to make waves. You may also find that limiting the amount of water you put in the tub will make your number one job of keeping your baby's head above water logistically easier.

- **Soap and shampoo.** Washing your baby with plain water is fine so long as you remember to adequately rub and rinse problem areas (the notorious diaper zone and skin folds). Many parents, however, opt for a foamier form of cleaning, in which case there are plenty of baby soaps, bodywashes, and shampoos from which you can choose. We suggest simply finding a mild one designed for babies that's agreeable (ie, doesn't cause a rash or otherwise bother you or your baby) and sticking with it.

- **One washcloth or two.** We have found that many adults are unaccustomed to using a washcloth in their daily self-hygiene regimen. This is the reason we thought we would state what might otherwise seem obvious: washcloths are quite useful for sponge baths and baths alike. We like to use them both wet for cleaning and dry for wiping off.

- **One towel or two.** We think it's pretty safe to say that no one likes to step out of a warm bath or shower into the cold air. Babies are no exception. In fact, they are often quite vocal about their dislikes. You're likely to be met with considerably more enthusiasm if you plan for your newborn's quick escape from the tub to a warm, dry towel. Feel free to use the cute little hooded baby towels if you are so inclined, or simply opt for a regular bath towel. We should point out that for newborns, many parents find adult-sized towels more difficult to work with than the custom-sized baby towels—just too much towel to work with and considerably more towel than you actually need. Other than that, we suggest you go with your intuition and use towels that are soft, absorbent, and cozy. Remember that if you're going to be laying your baby onto a towel during a sponge bath, you'll definitely want to have a second one designated for drying off.

- **Moisturizer.** Despite that most newborns have dry, peeling skin, most of them, if not all, don't need moisturizers. In fact, some moisturizers may cause rashes when applied to the sensitive skin of a newborn. If it makes you feel better to apply a moisturizing cream, ointment, or lotion to your baby's skin, don't hesitate to discuss with your pediatrician which are best. In general, it's thought to be best to use moisturizers that are hypoallergenic. When it comes to effectiveness, sticky, oil-based moisturizers tend to get the job done better than those that are water based (see also The Drying Effect of Water on page 157).

- **Diapering supplies.** Remember that it is a newborn's prerogative to poop wherever and whenever she feels like it, and you may well be met with a mess just before or after putting your baby into the tub. Coming to the tub prepared means coming with baby wipes, a clean diaper (or two, in case of diapering mishaps), and any diapering supplies you typically use.

- **Change of clothes.** Your newborn is likely to appreciate any extra effort you make to get her out of her damp towel and into a clean diaper and warm, dry clothes because we have yet to find a newborn who likes to lie around naked, especially when wet.

Bathing Around the Cord

Having to avoid getting your baby's umbilical-cord stump wet is going to be a short-lived nuisance because dried-up cords typically fall off within the first two to four weeks. To the best of our knowledge, there's no serious medical reason why you need to keep your newborn's umbilical-cord stump 100% dry at all costs; it doesn't directly connect to anywhere, and there's nothing to panic over if you should accidentally get it wet. What we can tell you, however, is that cords usually need to dry up before they fall off, and wet cord stumps can be a bit messy and gooey (in other words, a general annoyance). With that in mind, most parents find it easiest to stick to sponge baths until the momentous day of cord detachment arrives.

PRELUDE TO A BATH

If your newborn is still the proud owner of a pesky little umbilical-cord stump or has a healing circumcision, or even just for those days when you don't have it left in you to fit a full bath into your routine, you'll find that sponge baths make for a great alternative. With your baby either lying on a towel spread out on a flat surface or placed into a baby bathtub (with or without a little bit of water at the bottom), simply take a warm, damp sponge or washcloth; put a little bath wash on it if you like; and then gently dab or wipe, targeting especially those areas in most need of cleaning. Rinse with a clean, wet sponge or washcloth; follow up with a dry towel or washcloth; and…voilà! Your baby is squeaky clean.

The Bathing Technique

Whether you choose to bathe your baby in an infant tub or a bathtub, shower, or sink, here are some practical principles common to all.

- **Full support.** Once you've gotten yourself and your baby situated and your supplies ready, you'll likely find it easiest to use your non-dominant arm and hand to support your baby's head and back as needed. For example, use your left hand for support if you're right-handed. By reaching behind and under your baby and holding on to his opposite arm throughout the bath, you will help ensure that he has your unwavering support while still leaving your preferred and more functional hand free for cleaning (**Figure 12-1**). Using a plastic cup, washcloth, or tub sprayer or your free hand, you can then wet your baby's body from the head down with clean, warm water.

- **Head down.** When you work from the top down, it helps keep areas that were already rinsed clean from getting soapy again.

- **Focus on the face.** Wipe your baby's face with a clean, wet washcloth, using a corner of it to also clean the outer part of the ear and behind the ear.

- **Hair it is.** If your baby has any hair and you think it actually warrants washing, add a small amount of all-purpose baby wash or shampoo to your palm or a washcloth and gently rub it into your baby's hair. To rinse it off, we recommend either using a wet washcloth or pouring water from a small plastic cup. Then simply tilt your baby's head back slightly to prevent getting water, soap, or shampoo into his eyes or ears.

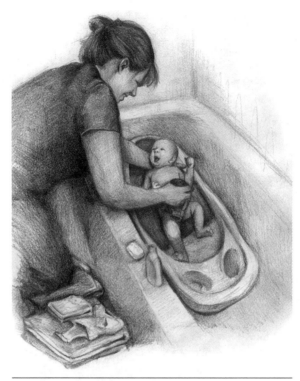

Figure 12-1. Bath-time head support

- **Lift and separate.** Remember to lift and separate as best you can any folds in your baby's neck, armpits, and groin.

- **Soap talk.** If you're going to use a mild soap or baby wash, put a small amount onto the washcloth or your hand and gently rub it onto your baby's body from the neck down. For safety's sake, we highly recommend keeping your holding hand soap-free to prevent a slippery situation. If you get soap on your baby's hands, try to rinse them off fairly quickly before your baby decides to rub his eyes or put them into his mouth.

- **Bend at the knees.** As you finish up, carefully hoist your baby out of the tub or basin without putting too much strain on your back. By bending at your knees and hips, or situating yourself comfortably on a stool or chair (or toilet, depending on the configuration of your bathroom), you can hopefully avoid unnecessary aches and pains.

- **No hands-free options.** For safety's sake, always keep at least one hand and both eyes on your baby (see Undivided Attention on page 159).

It's a (Post-bath) Wrap

Especially if you are bathing your baby solo, you'll definitely want to have a towel set out within arm's reach before you start. While the following technique is sure to seem obvious once you've done it a few times, we hope that by sharing it we can take the stress out of those first few times.

- **The lap wrap.** When you're ready to take your baby out of the tub, lay a towel vertically on your lap or another firm surface (a plastic baby bathtub works well, assuming you didn't use it for the actual bath). Simply grasp your baby under the arms and support her head carefully as you place her onto her back, just enough below the top of the towel that you can cover her head with it. Then flip the remaining (longer) part of the towel up over her legs and body and gently pat her skin dry.

- **The upright wrap.** Try holding your baby's towel vertically against your chest with the top part of it hanging just over your shoulder. Pick up your baby carefully and hold her up against your chest facing toward you. Wrap her by bringing the bottom of the towel up over her feet and legs (**Figure 12-2**). Once you get comfortable with the technique, you can hold your baby against your chest facing outward, bring the towel up under her chin, and use the excess cloth draped over your shoulder as a bath hood. You may find this technique easier to master while sitting down, although standing is also okay if you're comfortable with it. Once you've done the quick wrap and dry, you can move your bundle to a more convenient location to safely finish diapering and dressing.

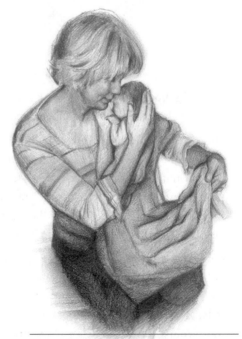

Figure 12-2. The upright wrap

THE DRYING EFFECT OF WATER

The fact that water itself can dry out the skin—yours and your baby's—may come as a surprise, but it's true, at least for some people. The drying effect is thought to take place when wet skin is exposed to air and the moisture subsequently evaporates or is rubbed off. Should you find that your baby errs on the side of dry skin, you can try to counteract this drying effect by simply patting her dry with a towel instead of providing a vigorous post-bath rubdown and applying a moisturizer to her skin while it is still damp—a technique that is thought to help lock moisture in the skin. However, many pediatricians will tell you not to bother with lotions, creams, or ointments for the first month or so. This is not only because newborn skin can be more sensitive but because it is predictably dry and flaky and almost invariably resolves on its own if you simply ignore it and let it run its course. For more on dry skin and rashes, see On the Surface: Your Newborn's Skin on page 320.

Have Tub, Will Travel

Baby bathtubs are quite popular these days, and you will undoubtedly have plenty to choose from—from rigid to inflatable to collapsible and from spongelike to those made of soft or hard plastic. While it is entirely possible to live without a baby bathtub, most parents find them to be quite practical, not to mention relatively inexpensive and multipurpose.

- They allow you to bathe your newborn on a counter, on the floor, in a sink, or in the bathtub (the "tub-within-a-tub" technique)—basically, wherever you are most comfortable.
- Many baby tubs are designed to "grow" with your baby by making use of newborn inserts that can be removed for extended use as your baby gets bigger.
- Even after your baby graduates from baths in the baby bathtub, it can still prove itself useful as a towel-wrapping station or a safe place to temporarily set your wet or towel-wrapped baby after a bath. Some are even specifically designed to convert into other useful toddler tools, such as a sturdy step stool.
- Once you become comfortable with the nuts and bolts of baby bathing, you may decide to take a bath or shower *with* your baby—an activity we consider to be a somewhat risky but admittedly convenient business. If you do decide to try and coordinate your bathing times, baby bathtubs can prove to be very logistically convenient, safe, and waterproof places to set babies before, during, and after.

TUB UPDATE

As of October 2, 2017, it became illegal to sell baby bathtubs in the United States that don't meet updated safety standards. These new mandatory standards, issued by the US Consumer Product Safety Commission (CPSC), were in response to multiple reports of infant deaths and aimed at helping prevent bathtub-related drowning. Among a few other requirements, the regulation thus mandated improved drowning and fall warning statements printed on all tubs to make sure caregivers have easy access to critical information about bath-time hazards. According to the CPSC, the standards not only help ensure safer new bathtubs but, equally important, serve as a reminder that "baby bathtubs are not babysitters."

Caution: Slippery When Wet

It is definitely not our nature to scare new parents. Instead, we want to introduce and reinforce a few simple but extremely important bath-time safety measures that will keep you and your baby from getting in over your heads. It probably goes without saying that the reason bathing a baby can sometimes seem like a daunting prospect is because there are some definite (albeit avoidable) risks involved. It's hard to miss that babies are slippery when wet, much less ignore the occasional news report about a baby or child unintentionally scalded or left unattended and drowning in mere inches of water. The good news is that most childhood injuries in general are preventable, and those related to bathing are no exception. In the committed spirit of tub safety, there are several hard-and-fast rules well worth committing to memory and putting into practice from day 1.

Hot Tubs

- **It's a matter of degree.** The ideal bathwater temperature is thought to be somewhere between 95°F and 100°F. Water warmer than 105°F is considered to be too hot; cooler than 90°F, too cold. In contrast, many water heaters are installed at 140°F to 150°F. At 140°F, it takes *less than 5 seconds* for a child to get a third-degree burn. Before you christen your baby's tub, we suggest you pay a quick visit to your water heater and/or engage your plumber or handyperson to make sure the upper temperature limit is set to no higher than 120°F—a temperature at which you should be able to hold your hand under a running stream of hot water without getting burned. While most parents have heard this advice at least once, very few actually follow through. We suggest you make yourself one who does.

- **Fill 'er up first.** Run the bathwater first. Put your baby in it only *after* you've turned off the water. Having water flowing directly into the tub when your baby is already in it is an unnecessary risk because the temperature of running water can be inconsistent, and hot water controls can be bumped.

- **Know what your baby's getting into.** Make it a habit to always test your baby's bathwater on your own skin (preferably on a more sensitive area, such as your wrist or elbow) *before* putting your baby in it. Testers and bathtub thermometers are also easy to find and use. Either way, be sure to know exactly what you're both getting into.

- **Don't just go with the flow.** Anti-scald devices designed to stop (or slow) the flow of dangerously hot water are recommended as yet one more way to ensure you and your baby can keep your cool at tub time. We're told they're available at plumbing or hardware stores and, of course, can easily be found online.

Undivided Attention

Above all else, committing your undivided parental attention to your child's bath time will serve a particularly important purpose for many years to come. The fact is that a mere inch of water can pose a drowning risk for infants, even as they become more skilled at sitting up. And for children between the ages of one and four years, Safe Kids Worldwide still recognizes drowning as the leading cause of injury-related death. For children younger than one year, drowning is more likely to occur in the home, in a bathroom, or in a bucket. Keep in mind that drowning is often both speedy (in a matter of minutes) and silent. For the foreseeable future, but most especially when it comes to newborns, you'll always need to lend at least one hand of support and keep both eyes focused on the task at hand, regardless of how much or how little water you have in the tub.

13

clothing and accessories

The Big Picture

As parents, we all tend to have one thing in common when it comes to baby clothes, whether you're the type who is looking forward to shopping for baby attire or you happen to have very little interest beyond having your baby's clothes fit properly and adequately serve their purpose: inevitably, we all dole out a sizable amount of money on our children's wardrobes. For a glimpse of the big picture, consider that on average, parents in the United States spend an estimated $15,000 to outfit their children—an amount that equals 6% of the total estimated cost of raising a child to the age of 17.

This chapter is especially meant for those who haven't had much, if any, experience outfitting and dressing infants prior to becoming a parent. Even if you have picked out baby apparel as gifts for other people's children before, let us just say that the approach you take will likely be a bit different once you're faced with choosing (and paying for) your own baby's attire.

Learning the Layette of the Land

We wanted first to include a basic rundown of what's available in the world of baby wear and help you get a sense of what your baby might realistically need in the days and weeks ahead. The term *layette* itself comes from the French word for "drawer" or "trunk." Technically speaking, *layette* describes a newborn's full clothing wardrobe, bedding, and accessories. Nowadays, however, the term is used much more loosely. You'll find that newborn sleeper gowns are sometimes called *layette gowns,* and many manufacturers market coordinated sets of baby clothing—often accompanied by matching accessories (such as hats, booties, and blankets)—as layettes. These conveniently coordinated set versions of layettes are especially useful as quick gifts. While there's no reason you can't buy some for your own baby if they catch your eye, be aware that you could pay a premium for a group of items you might be able to purchase individually for less.

ONESIES DEFINED

As far as we know, credit for the term *onesies* goes to Gerber, the baby product manufacturing company that first used it to describe their baby undershirts that snap at the crotch. Just as many other brand names—Kleenex, Xerox, and Coke, to name a few—seem to have taken on lives of their own, *onesie(s)* is often used generically to describe all brands of snapping undershirts. The name is sometimes even applied to entire one-piece outfits, which personally, we consider to be more accurately called *rompers* (when they are worn in public) or *sleepers* (when they are used for nightwear).

With that in mind, here is a description of some of the more commonly found items in the baby-clothing department and our opinion on their usefulness.

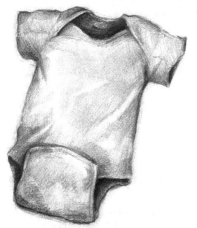

Figure 13-1. The undershirt onesie

- **Undershirt onesies.** These are handy in cooler weather as undershirts during the day and at night and can double as stand-alone outfits in warmer weather. Some look like undershirts (**Figure 13-1**), while others are fancier and come in a variety of colors or complete with patterns and cutesy sayings emblazoned on the front (or rear). We suggest using the same rule of thumb as many adults do when buying themselves underwear: buy enough to last you at least as long as it will take you to do laundry. Then buy a few extra for good measure.

- **Pajamas and sleepers.** While your baby is still young, you may find that you don't venture out of the house all that often. When you do, dressing your baby in sleepwear (as opposed to a fancy outfit) is not only convenient but also socially acceptable. Many parents of newborns don't end up making much of a distinction between their baby's daytime outfits and his nighttime outfits. If you plan on using sleepers as your baby's primary clothing, we again suggest you take into account leaky diapers, spitting up, and other common bodily function mishaps when you are calculating how many to buy.

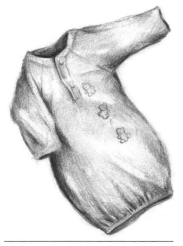

Figure 13-2. Baby nightgown

- **Wearable blankets and baby gowns.**
Wearable blankets typically zip up the middle or side. While they can be long- or short-sleeved, or even sleeveless at the top, they all tend to resemble sleeping bags at the bottom. Baby gowns are not only similar but often come in lighter weight material—sometimes with buttons instead of zippers up the front and often with an open elasticized bottom (**Figure 13-2**). Either type allows for use overtop a onesie or other infant attire and can prove particularly useful in the early weeks for easy access (see Easy Access on page 165 for more information) and for keeping your baby well covered in lieu of a baby blanket (see Bare Is Best on page 120).

- **Socks.** There's not a lot of enlightening information to share with you about baby socks that you wouldn't already know from your own sock experiences, so we'll just point out a few quick considerations: When you go shopping for baby socks, consider how many of your own socks you lose over the course of a few months first. Then picture them smaller and with a much greater tendency to disappear or fall off tiny feet and you'll realize why we suggest buying quite a few. If you find you like using them under (or even over) pajamas and footed outfits in addition to over bare feet, add a few more to your shopping list. You won't need to search for no-skid bottoms until your baby starts walking, but you will want to make sure you buy socks that are well elasticized to maximize the likelihood that they'll stay on.

AN OUTFIT A DAY...

...is rarely enough for most new babies. If you buy baby clothes with the expectation that your newborn will wear only one outfit a day, we predict you will be doing laundry very frequently. With spit-up and diaper breaches alone, you may find yourself going through at least two (if not three or maybe four) outfits on any given day.

Size Matters

After "preemie" and newborn sizes, just about all baby clothes come with relatively age-specific size labels, starting with 0 to 3 months and continuing up in three-month increments throughout the first year. This approach to sizing seems very straightforward—that is, until you actually have a baby of your own and start putting labels to the test. You'll quickly find that one manufacturer's idea of newborn doesn't always match another's, and many newborns don't fit in newborn-sized clothing at all. Some may fit into size 0 to 3 months at birth and grow into size 3 to 6 months within weeks of being born. While it's theoretically possible to take a baby into a fitting room and try clothes on to see whether they fit, we find the thought of actually doing so quite comical and have yet to meet anyone who has done so! If you want to come away with a few practical pieces of sizing advice, rather than reserve a dressing room, we suggest you consider the following tips:

- If a label reads "3 to 6 months," an average-sized infant is more likely to fit into it around three months of age. We definitely don't recommend holding your breath for it to fit at six months.
- Look for tags that offer weight and height guidelines and age ranges, as they can give you a better sense of how the clothing will actually fit your baby.
- Remember that sizing varies by brand. Just as with adult clothing, some brands run big and others run small. Once you become familiar with one or several brands, you'll have an easier time with gauging what size your baby needs relative to the specific brand.
- Leave the price tags on and pay attention to return policies and periods. That way, you can return or exchange an item if and when your baby outgrows it before she gets to wear it.

SUPERSIZING

Right from the start, you'll discover you're able to get longer wear out of your baby's clothes if you supersize them—or, in other words, buy big. Onesies are well suited for being worn big, especially if you use them as undershirts because no law says they have to fit perfectly. Well-elasticized cuffs at the wrists and ankles of rompers, shirts, and leggings help keep longer than necessary sleeves and pant legs from hanging way over your baby's hands or feet. This feature allows him several inches' worth of room to grow, which can translate into extra months' worth of wear. Just make sure they aren't uncomfortably tight or binding. Outfits or pants with attached "footies" can also be worn big if you put socks over the footies—a simple but ingenious way to keep your baby's feet snugly inside them.

Profiles in Color

Before you buy a lot of clothes for your baby, we suggest you give some brief thought to whether you consider yourself color casual or color conforming. If it's all the same to you, you may as well limit the number of outfits you buy in baby blue and pastel pink in favor of more gender-neutral colors (pastel yellows and greens and primary or neutral colors)—especially if you don't know whether you're having a boy or a girl or would like to raise your child gender-neutral. This advice also holds true if you see more children in your future and hope to use your baby clothes more than once. Alternatively, if gender-neutral clothing is unappealing to you and the mere thought of an onlooker mistakenly referring to your yellow-clad baby boy as a beautiful little girl horrifies you, you may be better off opting for more gender-traditional pinks or blues.

Principles of Practicality

Think back to your pre-parenting days and the most recent time (if ever) you purchased a cute little baby outfit as a gift. Did you opt for one adorned with pretty ribbons? Splurge on matching dress shoes or the color-coordinated hair bow (which, as a sidenote, we have decided should more appropriately be called a "head bow" because most babies are significantly lacking in actual hair)? Well, many of these eye-catching features, while they are admittedly appealing, also tend to be impractical. We're not by any means saying that we haven't succumbed to temptation and bought adorable but inconvenient outfits for our own babies or that there's no place for them in your baby's closet. It's just that as you find yourself faced with the reality of day in and day out dressing, not to mention coping with changing weather, frequently changing diapers, and even more frequently washing clothes, you are also likely to find that practicality becomes more of a priority. In the spirit of practicality, here are several fundamental principles to consider.

Easy Access

It's exceedingly easy to disregard the access factor the first couple of times you set out to buy clothes for your baby, but the moment you're faced with dressing and undressing your baby several times a day—including the middle-of-the-night blowouts (you know, the occasional explosions that defy even the most absorbent and well-secured diapers)—you'll instantly gain a new appreciation for easy access.

- **One piece or two.** There are definitely benefits to both one-piece outfits and two-piece outfits. For easy-on, easy-off clothing, many parents find that two-piece outfits are more convenient. This finding is especially true for those late-night diaper changes that end up requiring a full wardrobe change. Once you've tried to remove a soiled one-piece outfit over your baby's head without making more of a mess, you, too, may decide to go for two pieces instead of one. The benefit of a one-piece outfit is that it involves, by definition, fewer pieces to coordinate. A one-piece outfit also generally keeps babies more reliably covered. Bottom line on one or two: personal preference prevails.

- **Zippers, snaps, and Velcro.** All these options are generally easier to do than buttons—especially in the middle of the night or when you're on the go.

ZIP-A-DEE-DOO—OW!

If you think it hurts to zip your own skin, think about how you'd feel if you inadvertently zipped your baby's skin. We suggest you get into the simple but highly effective habit of lifting the fabric and zipper away from the skin and putting your finger underneath the zipper whenever you zip.

Newborn Dressing for the Beginner

If you haven't had any experience holding or otherwise handling babies before, it's quite understandable that figuring out how to get your baby's arms and legs going in the right direction while you are properly supporting your newborn's head and getting everything snapped and secured may take some practice. We've come across enough new parents who are embarrassed to admit they aren't comfortable dressing their new babies that we decided to include this step-by-step tutorial (**Figures 13-3 to 13-5**).

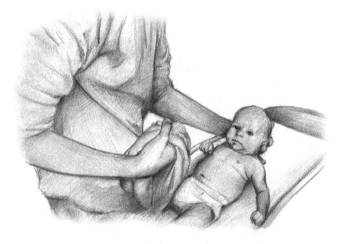

Figure 13-3. Position and head support of a newborn being dressed

1. **Position.** Lay your baby down on her back as if you're going to change her diaper.

2. **Head support.** Gently put one hand behind her head and neck for support.

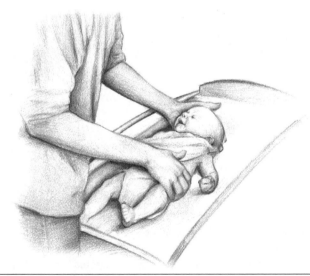

Figure 13-4. Placement of clothing over the head of a newborn being dressed

3. **Over the head.** With your other hand, put the neck opening over your baby's head and gently pull the clothing down over her head and your supporting hand and arm first. Then let her head rest on the changing area while you remove your arm from underneath it.

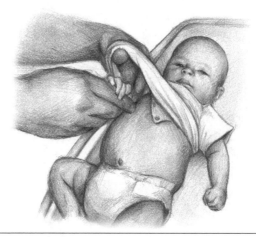

Figure 13-5. Placement of clothing onto the limbs of a newborn being dressed

4. **Limbs.** One by one, guide each arm through the armholes first. For sleepers and rompers with zippers or snaps down one leg, it is generally easiest to put the leg into the side without the zippers or snaps in first because the fit tends to be tighter. Then put the other leg in.

5. **Securing.** Fasten any zippers, snaps, or buttons. If you've chosen an outfit with back snaps or buttons, consider picking your baby up against your chest to access them or simply lay her on her belly to access them.

REMOVING SOILED ONESIES WITHOUT ADDING INSULT TO INJURY

If you find yourself faced with a blowout—the kind where poop is up your baby's back and onto his clothes—we suggest you first place your baby onto a towel, changing table, or disposable pad. Next, put a washcloth, baby wipe, or paper towel against the area of dirty skin and leave it there to prevent further spread. With your baby still in it, roll up the soiled piece of clothing (usually a shirt or onesie) as best you can so that the mess is as well contained as possible. Then carefully remove each of your baby's arms and lift the rolled-up clothing over your baby's head. For some outfits, you may actually find it easier to pull the clothes down past your baby's waist and legs instead of up and over. Having done your best to minimize the mess during the removal process, you can finish cleaning up and redressing your disrobed baby.

Comfort Is Key

It shouldn't come as a surprise to you that your newborn is as likely as you are to appreciate wearing soft fabrics and well-designed clothes that don't scratch, poke, twist, or irritate. On the surface, decorative collars, frills, bows, and lace can definitely add to the appeal of an outfit, but cute isn't always what it's cut out to be. Be sure to consider whether added frills might get in the way or, worse yet, irritate your baby's skin. In addition, the more ornate an outfit is, the more challenging it will probably be to clean.

Keeping Hands Covered

Newborn outfits often have fold-over sleeves that allow parents to keep their babies' hands covered during the newborn period. That's because young infants have a disconcerting tendency to scratch themselves on the face with tiny yet rapidly growing fingernails (a problem we cover in more detail in Nails, Nails Everywhere on page 322). Their usefulness is generally limited, however, to the first couple of months at most. Once your baby begins to try using her hands and gains control of the flailing movements typical of her first few weeks, you'll definitely want to uncover her hands and let her explore.

Safety Considerations

You'll want to always take safety into account when you are choosing baby clothes. Fortunately, there aren't too many hazards lurking out there when it comes to baby clothing if you just put the necessary forethought into your choices. A government organization, the US Consumer Product Safety Commission (CPSC), provides safety standards for clothing, as well as other baby and consumer products, and routinely issues recalls to alert the public about potentially unsafe items. In addition to directing you to its website (www.cpsc.gov or https://saferproducts.gov) for the purpose of identifying specific products as potentially unsafe, we've listed some good general baby-clothing safety considerations.

- **Safe at sleep.** Baby sleepwear should be flame resistant and snug fitting. That said, not all pajamas for babies come with a flame-resistant or flame-retardant finish. After determining that loose-fitting clothing could catch fire more easily, the CPSC required in 2000 that all tags and labels on sleepwear for children nine months and over (who are mobile enough to possibly expose themselves to an open flame) alert potential purchasers if they are not flame resistant and therefore need to be snug fitting. In other words, check the labels.

- **No strings attached.** Simply put, anything in which a baby could potentially become entangled is best left on the rack. While clothing safety standards have made it far less likely to find potentially dangerous outfits in the stores, items with strings or large, loose hoods (as well as any homemade clothing) should be carefully scrutinized before use. The CPSC recommends that no strings whatsoever be used in the neck or hood region and advises shortened drawstrings (measuring no more than 3 extra inches at either end) at the waist.

- **Loose object liability.** Get into the habit of evaluating baby clothes for small and potentially removable objects. The most obvious, of course, are buttons. It's amazing how many small 3-D objects you can find attached to baby clothing in the name of fashion these days. If it isn't securely fastened, be sure to avoid or remove anything your child could choke on should it come loose.

Cleaning Baby Clothes

Washability is definitely something to consider. Be sure to look at the labels not only for size, flame resistance, or snug-fitting information but also for washing instructions. Unless you relish the thought of handwashing a lot of baby clothes and frequently replacing those that don't hold up well, we suggest you give some serious thought to the durability and washability of baby clothes you buy—especially your baby's everyday outfits, onesies, and sleepers.

- **Washing.** Because some newborns may have sensitive skin (and because you don't know who has handled the clothing and with what before it made its way into your possession), it's generally a good idea to wash all clothes prior to using them. An exception might be outerwear, such as coats and jackets, that doesn't have much contact with the skin (and tends not to wash and dry easily). As a helpful hint, consider putting small items such as socks into a mesh bag for washing and drying. Remember to also fasten any Velcro tabs (such as on bibs) before tossing them into the fray to prevent them from snagging other clothes. (See As Good as New on page 171 for more information on washing new clothes.)

- **Detergents.** It is a common recommendation that baby clothes should be washed separately using special "baby" detergents that supposedly leave fewer residues and are therefore less likely to cause skin irritation. In reality, we've found that many parents simply toss their baby's clothes in with the rest of the family's laundry without causing any problems. That said, it is worth paying attention to the fact that detergents in general don't strip away the flame-retardant properties of sleepwear, but soap flakes can. Given that information, you can choose your detergent as we do: buy one that smells good and gets the dirt out, and only feel compelled to invest in a milder baby detergent (or hypoallergenic, fragrance-free "adult" detergent) if your baby has or develops signs of skin irritation.

- **Stain removal.** The best approach to managing stains made by breast milk, formula, spit-up, or poop is to try wiping or rinsing off the offending substance as best you can while it's still relatively fresh. We realize this may be easier said than done—especially if you find yourself in the middle of a diaper change or feeding with a clothing stain that is settling itself in for the long haul—but if you can remove even some of it with a baby wipe or soak the clothes in some water and detergent, you'll be glad you did. We also suggest stocking your laundry room with a good stain remover and designating a place for soaking stained or soiled items.

As Good as New

Having told you it's a good idea to wash your baby's clothes before using them, let us point out one important caveat: instead of washing them all well in advance (which many parents do before their babies are even born), we suggest you wash a couple and leave the tags on the rest until you are ready to use them. By getting into this habit, as well as keeping all your baby-clothing receipts in a convenient place, you can more easily return those you end up not using. Believe us when we tell you that probably not a parent out there hasn't bemoaned the number of outfits that have gone unworn in his or her baby's closet. Even if you're not able to return or exchange an outfit at the store where you bought it, unused clothing that has its tags still on retains a significantly higher value at resale or consignment shops, on eBay, when donating to charity, or—dare we say it (lest we be perceived as publicly admitting to it)—if you are tempted by the thought of re-gifting.

These Shoes Weren't Made for Walking

Because most babies don't walk before their first birthdays, you may be wondering why one might need shoes as an infant. In reality, one really doesn't. Until your baby reaches the point where she's pulling up to a standing position (which probably seems impossible to imagine at this point but will happen before you know it), the only reasons we can come up with for needing shoes are to keep socks in place, to help keep feet warm, or to look good in pictures if you or your family consider bare baby feet to be unacceptable in an otherwise formal portrait. If you decide to buy shoes for your newborn, we suggest soft, roomy ones that are easy to put on and allow for plenty of wiggle room without falling off.

PARENT ATTIRE: NEW MOMS DON'T WEAR SILK

Okay, so maybe some new moms wear silk, but as for us, we sure stuck to sweats and other practical, comfortable, easily washable, no-ironing-or-dry-cleaning-required clothing for several months after our babies were born. We put together a quick list of things to consider and watch for when laying out your own new-parent attire so you, too, will be dressed for success.

- **Dress like your baby.** Especially during this time when you're spending most of your waking (and non-waking) hours tending to your newborn, we highly recommend choosing soft, comfortable clothing over frills and fancy duds. As you make your selections, remember to keep an eye out for inopportunely placed zippers, buckles, snaps, or any other adult clothing accessories that could end up scratching, poking, or irritating your baby. And remember, unless you want to devote extra time, attention, and money to keeping your clothes stain-free and clean, we strongly suggest adding "machine washable and dryable" to your own clothing must-have checklist.

- **Easy access.** Accessibility is going to be especially applicable to you breastfeeding moms. Whether you opt for specially designed (and accordingly priced) breastfeeding attire or simply a loose-fitting shirt and an accommodating bra is up to you (see Breastfeeding on page 5), but it's a safe bet you'll find yourself more at ease with your new role if you aren't wrestling with your own wardrobe at the same time.

- **Comfort.** We can't emphasize this consideration enough: make yourself comfortable. Now is not the time to worry about snapping up pants and zipping up jeans if drawstrings or elastic waistbands feel better.

- **Personal style.** Bottom line advice: don't expend any more time and effort on pulling your outfits together than you need to make yourself feel good. Some of us feel just fine about how we're handling new parenthood even as we lounge around for the first few weeks in ponytails, sweats, and T-shirts. Others, we have found, find themselves feeling further removed from the life they used to lead and more like they aren't rising to the challenge of new parenthood unless they get up and make themselves outwardly presentable. Either way, whatever works for you, wear it!

CHAPTER

14

taking care of yourself

· · · · · ·

Have you ever noticed that flight attendants routinely recommend that adults traveling with small children take a moment to strap on their own oxygen masks before tending to their children if faced with a loss of cabin pressure? Well, not unlike this standard announcement, we make a point of telling all new parents we encounter (which now includes you) that you shouldn't expect to do a perfectly wonderful job of tending to someone else's needs (namely, your newborn's) if you completely neglect your own. We're not suggesting regular days at the spa and weekly pedicures (although we think one of the all-time best presents to receive as a new mother is a gift certificate for a relaxing massage). No, we're talking the basics—as in hygiene, food, and sleep. While we're well aware that many of the take-home messages we've included in this chapter have been said before, including several suggested elsewhere within this very book, we think they're worth drawing your attention to as much more than side comments or afterthoughts in the grand scheme of newborn parenting.

Tending to Your Own Activities of Daily Living

Try to allot time for your own activities of daily living, not the least of which include such seemingly simple tasks as brushing your teeth, bathing or showering, and getting dressed in the morning. Those of you who have yet to have your babies may be laughing at this advice and wondering, "How hard could completing such basic tasks possibly be?" We are confident in telling you that we are not the only ones who found ourselves routinely going on upward of 36 hours with bad breath, wearing the same clothes, and in need of much more than a quick deodorant application. Unless you sincerely don't mind sitting around in pajamas all day with fuzzy teeth, make time to attend to your own basic hygiene each day, get a bit of fresh air, and offer yourself a change of scenery or a little extra time to do some grooming every now and then—in lieu of housekeeping or doing dishes, for example—which often works wonders in helping new parents feel accomplished and in control.

Supplying Yourself With the Strength to Carry On

It's unreasonable for you to expect yourself to keep up with the pace of new parenthood without providing yourself with adequate nourishment, regardless of whether you're asking your body to nourish your newborn as a breastfeeding mom (see Breastfeeding on page 5). Anything you can do in the early weeks (if not months) to make mealtime easier and less effort intensive, the better. If you don't exactly have anyone volunteering to do all your grocery shopping, prepare you gourmet meals, and bring you breakfast in bed, we highly recommend considering the following time- and sanity-savers:

- **Hydrate.** Remembering to sit down and drink can be a bit of a new-mom challenge. We recommend building this necessary habit into your daily routine by simply grabbing a bottle of water or drinking a glass of whatever healthy fluid you choose each time you sit down to feed your baby. Now, we're not saying you can't indulge in your caffeinated or alcoholic drink of choice every now and then, but when it comes to keeping well hydrated (especially as a breastfeeding mom), you'll be better served by keeping a good stock of water, milk, and 100% juices close at hand.

- **Splurge.** Whether splurging means buying more prepared foods (fresh or frozen) or indulging in take-out (better yet, home-delivered) meals, it's entirely possible to do so without overindulging in a lot of fried and/or overly processed fast foods. You most likely will pay a bit more, but you may also find the added expense seems like a small price to pay for the convenience of getting the tasks of food shopping and preparation off your plate.

- **Stock up.** Accept and even suggest the gift of freeze-and-heat casseroles or other premade meals from friends and well-wishers. If no one is offering and you have not yet had your baby, now is the ideal time for you to prepare a few (dozen) of your own. It's also useful to keep plenty of relatively healthy "adult" snacks around the house, as well as have them available to take with you if and when you find yourself on the go (see Thinking Outside of the House on page 209).

- **Streamline.** Consider using disposable (or easy-to-clean) plates and utensils for a while if keeping up with doing dishes is not your strong suit. Try to enlist the help of others to take over any preparation and cleanup involved, regardless of how much or little there is to do to get meals on and off the table.

In Search of Sleep

Getting rest is a great way to help your outlook on life, not to mention your physical condition and general sense of well-being. It is therefore an unfortunate and sometimes even painful fact of new parenthood that getting an eight-hour stretch of sleep quickly becomes a distant memory, and your nights will undoubtedly be interrupted for the next few months. Nevertheless, we want to reassure you that it is possible to compensate, at least to a certain extent.

- **Get your priorities straight.** Start by making sleep a priority on your to-do list—ranking well above entertaining, checking email, posting on social media, and doing dishes or housework.

- **Be partners in sleep.** Make every attempt to follow the age-old adage to sleep when your baby sleeps. Granted, it's not going to be eight hours at a time, but that just makes whatever stretches of sleep you can get all the more important to prioritize. It's amazing how good it can feel to get an extra hour or two of sleep when you're functioning under conditions of relative sleep deprivation.

- **Set the mood.** If you're the type of person who can sleep anytime, anywhere, if you're tired enough, you can skip this tip. For the rest of us who need peace and quiet to fall (and stay) asleep, do whatever you can to create a sleep-conducive setting for yourself, whether it's simply finding a quiet room with a door you can shut while someone else takes over baby duty for a while or investing in light-blocking shades.

- **Outsource.** If you have the means to do so, consider enlisting a relative or hiring a night nurse to help with nighttime feedings so you can get a little rest.

Find New Friends

In no way are we saying you need to forsake the friends you've already got for new ones now that you are (or are about to become) a parent. It's just that we find new parents aren't always aware of just how big and broad the parenting world is. The support you stand to find if you simply look around in your neighborhood, in your community, or even on the internet can work wonders for giving you an almost-instant and understanding support group. These are people who, like you, are quite likely to benefit from sharing the joys, as well as the newness and occasional rude awakenings, of parenthood. Regardless of where you find your support, the bottom line is that having a supportive social network of friends who can relate is an invaluable part of parenthood.

More Than a Feeling

We've said it before (see When You Feel Like Crying on page 129), but it's so important that we're going to say it again: postpartum depression is more than just feeling the "baby blues," and new moms and dads are at risk in the months following a baby's arrival. Unlike the baby blues, which typically get better within a few days, postpartum depression can last for weeks or months. In addition to having your obstetrician and your baby's pediatrician screen you, a new parent, for signs and symptoms of depression (as well as for anxiety, which can also cause problems in the postpartum period), we encourage you to be on the lookout as well and to seek help immediately if needed. Once you are familiar with the warning signs, you can also keep an eye on other new parents to see whether they might be struggling and need support.

A common two-question patient health questionnaire (known as the PHQ-2) asks, "Over the past two weeks, how often have you been bothered by the following problems?"

- Little interest or pleasure in doing things
- Feeling down, depressed or hopeless

More specifically, there is another questionnaire tailored to the postpartum period, called the *Edinburgh Postnatal Depression Scale,* that screens for the presence of ten different symptoms over the past seven days. You can also check out online "calculators" such as the one at Perinatology.com to see whether depression might be present. No matter the results, however, if you have had *any* thoughts of harming yourself, your baby, or anyone else, or if you are having hallucinations, be sure to seek medical attention *immediately.*

SECTION

activities of daily learning

introduction

· · · · · · · ·

We now know that the early learning experiences you offer your newborn can literally connect neurons, influence brain structure, and ultimately have a lifelong impact on your baby's potential. Sound like a big responsibility? Well, it is. But before you scramble to find the latest and greatest baby video (also see Media Matters on page 205) or put the classical music playlist on continuous play, read the following few chapters to gain a better understanding of which learning experiences really make the most difference. While we address some of the more-formal learning activities parents often ask about—including books for babies, classical music, sign language, and baby videos—we are true believers in the notion that just about every seemingly routine interaction you share with your newborn over the next several weeks and months will qualify as an activity of daily learning for your baby. By sharing what we know about how babies think, learn, and communicate, we hope you learn something new and valuable as well.

THE 5 RS OF EARLY EDUCATION

We now know with increasing certainty that babies' brains are very sensitive to early experiences and relationships—particularly those that occur within the first 1,000 days (or roughly 3 years). This period of early brain and child development (EBCD for short) is thought to be so important that it has become the focus of national attention, and the American Academy of Pediatrics has officially deemed it a strategic priority in their overarching agenda for children.

What has also become clear is that the 5 Rs (listed at the end of this box), as fundamentally simple as they may seem, are some of the most effective ways we know to ensure a healthy start and build a solid foundation for your baby's future school success and lifelong productivity. While some admittedly don't apply in the immediate newborn period, they all will prove to be valuable during the months and years to follow.

- **Read** together every day.

- **Rhyme,** play, and cuddle every day.

- Develop **Routines,** particularly around meals, sleep, and family fun.

- **Reward** your child with praise for successes to build self-esteem and promote positive behavior.

- The strong and nurturing **Relationship** you establish with your baby now will serve as the foundation for your child's future healthy development.

CHAPTER

15

baby brain basics

● ● ● ● ● ●

We are parenting realists, and as such, we are well aware of the day-to-day realities of new parenthood. But just as we plan on reminding you to take time to preserve some of the guaranteed-to-be-priceless memories of the next few months (see Thanks for the Memories on page 355), we also want to make sure you take a few moments to look past the piles of diapers, onesies, and wipes and marvel at the potential of your newborn's brain power.

Making the Connections

What modern-day neuroscience now reveals about the way the baby brain works and develops is truly remarkable. By the time you find yourself heading home with your newborn, most if not all of his actual brain cells (*neurons*) will have already been formed. Yet despite being born with a lifetime supply of neurons, his brain will still be the most immature organ in his body and weigh only a third of what it will at age two and only 25% of what it will by the time he reaches adulthood. As your baby grows and develops, the cells in his brain busily make lots and lots of new connections (called *synapses*)—on the order of up to a million new neural connections per second. So many, in fact, that by the time he is eight months of age, it is estimated he will be the proud (and now babbling) owner of hundreds of *trillions* of synapses—a number that's hard to even comprehend. Infancy isn't just about building connections, however. The baby brain also becomes more efficient over time by strengthening those connections that are used frequently while pruning away others that aren't. What do all these neurons and synapses mean to you in what we realize may be a very sleep-deprived state? Let us summarize the extensive literature as best and concisely as we can by simply saying that you will play a very influential role in your baby's brain development. How newborns develop—right down to their trillions of neurons and synapses—is known to be fundamentally and significantly shaped by all their day-to-day activities, experiences, and interactions. In other words, as the Harvard Center on the Developing Child so compellingly summarizes, early experiences literally affect the development of brain architecture and provide the foundation for all future learning, behavior, and health. Before you take that summary to be more intimidating than it should be, let us make it a bit clearer. When we're talking about the critical importance of early experiences, what we're really talking about are such eagerly anticipated and enjoyable everyday activities as talking, cooing, singing, playing, and reading books to your baby. Nothing more, nothing less.

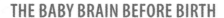

THE BABY BRAIN BEFORE BIRTH

The first brain cells, or *neurons,* are thought to develop very early in pregnancy, forming at a mind-boggling rate of 250,000 per minute as early as the fourth week. A baby's basic senses begin to develop early in the last trimester, which accounts for the ability to respond to a clap, tap, sound, or friendly nudge from the outside. It isn't until right before birth that babies are thought to begin feeling, thinking, and remembering. When it comes to influencing your unborn baby's brain development, the most important takeaway message is that nutrition, certain infections, drugs, alcohol, and stress during pregnancy all can have a significant effect.

The Secret to a Smarter Baby

As parents, we all want happy, healthy babies. Not only that, we want them to be smart. For anyone entering parenthood today, this desire seems to translate into a trip to the toy store and a significant blow to the baby budget. The difference between what we're now going to share with you, however, and all of the claims you're guaranteed to find on every make-your-baby-brilliant product lining today's store shelves is that we aren't selling anything other than this book, which you've presumably already bought. You don't need to spend a penny to accomplish the noble goal of making your baby smarter. That's right, despite all the hype and marketing, we're not buying it and neither should you. Simply put, there just isn't convincing scientific evidence that any of these expertly marketed, highly sophisticated forms of baby brain stimulation, with all of its bells, whistles, and on/off switches, leads to any more advanced brain development. As you approach your own baby's activities of daily learning, we suggest you start by remembering that the real baby Mozart never had CDs, DVDs, *or* iTunes playlists! What, then, is the secret to a smarter baby? We're happy to report that the gold standard is, above all else, the loving interactions that you and other caring responsive adults will share with your baby over the upcoming days, weeks, and months.

BRAIN GAMES: SERVE AND RETURN

"Serve and return" interactions are the driving force behind what is now recommended for fostering healthy brain development in the early weeks, months, and years after birth. As Harvard Center on the Developing Child so clearly explains in its summary of the most up-to-date early brain research, it's the everyday, back-and-forth interactions—all of the babbling, facial expressions, and gestures shared between young children and the caring responsive adults in their lives—that are now considered to be some of the most essential experiences of all when it comes to shaping the architecture of the developing brain.

The Best Learning Activities for Babies

Perhaps the most important message we hope to get across is that you don't need to put undue pressure on yourself when considering what to do with your baby. The types of activities we're talking about are simple, but to help make sure we're all on the same page, we've put together a quick list to get you started.

- **Time for a talk.** Sound simple? That's because it is. While some new parents feel a bit funny about talking to babies who can't talk back, this isn't the same as talking to yourself. Take time to talk to your baby while changing his diaper, telling him about your plans for the day or commenting on whatever comes to mind. The nuances may be lost on him for a while, but he'll definitely be listening and learning.

- **Take a walk.** Not only does taking a walk get you both some fresh air and you some exercise, it gives you plenty more interesting things to talk about and describe to your baby. We're both fans of front-pouch carriers, wraps, or slings, as they offer you the close contact that is even more conducive for carrying on a conversation. (For more on taking your first trip out of the house, see Thinking Outside of the House on page 209.)

- **Sing, sing a song.** One of the classic Sesame Street songs says it perfectly: don't worry if you're not good enough for anyone else to hear; just sing, sing a song! Your newborn not only will cut you some slack if you happen to sing off key but will instantly become your biggest fan.

- **Imitate.** Start by sticking your tongue out and you may be surprised to find that your newborn copies you. Move on to making some exaggerated facial expressions and repeating sounds your baby makes, and before long, you'll find that she'll imitate you as well. While imitation has been said to be the greatest form of flattery, it also happens to be how babies learn about the world and how to make their way in it starting with one coo, raised eyebrow, or smile at a time.

- **Stay in touch.** Massage is a great way to stay in touch with your baby. Beyond just relaxation, touch is a particularly important part of how young babies experience the world, and massage can be a true bonding experience—whether you make it up as you go along or buy a book on the art of baby massage.

- **Read a book.** The entire reading-with-your-baby experience is custom designed to foster both fun and learning, from the close contact of being held to hearing the sound of your voice to watching the pictures and pages go by. In your baby's first months, however, don't worry too much about pictures because it's the time you share and the sound of your voice that your baby will care about most. In fact, we suggest you take this opportunity to read aloud whatever *you* find to be the most interesting (within reason)—whether that's a childhood favorite of your own, *The New York Times,* or even the daily weather. It will only be a matter of months before your baby expects to have more of a say in what you read together. As enthusiastic supporters of books for babies, we've also included an additional chapter on the subject for your reading pleasure (see Books and Babies on page 197).

OVEREXPOSED

In your quest to be the best parent you can be, it's important to remember that you don't need to (ie, shouldn't) set up a jam-packed schedule of constant singing, reading, walking, and talking. The fact is that simple activities of daily living—right down to the diapering, feeding, bathing, and changing of clothes—expose babies to lots of exciting and "educational" sights, sounds, and smells. All this new and interesting stimulation can really add up, so remember to give yourself, as well as your baby, a break. You both will need time each day to relax.

CHAPTER

16

do you understand me now?

· · · · · · ·

Forgive us for stating the obvious, but one of the most noticeable characteristics of all newborns is the simple fact that they don't talk—a lack of words that can easily leave them misunderstood and you scratching your head asking them, "What, exactly, do you want?" As the proud but potentially perplexed parent of a newborn, it's safe to say you'll need to adopt a somewhat different approach to communicating with your newborn. Sure, you'll still be able to use *your* words from day 1, but establishing a mutual understanding is going to take some time and some new parental powers of observation. We hope this chapter helps you understand what your baby is trying to tell you and helps you appreciate each coo and babble that gets you one endearing step closer to an ongoing conversation.

TALK ABOUT AN OPPORTUNITY!

What's all the talk about regarding language development in the earliest months? Well, when it comes to babies' brain development, we now know there are critical windows of opportunity. One of the very first comes early, as infants are believed to be born with the impressive ability to recognize the sounds of *all* languages. By about one year of age, however, they're only able to recognize sounds found in the language(s) they've heard spoken to them. This finding further reinforces what early childhood experts have long recognized: all of the talking, singing, and reading we do with our babies has an impressive effect on their language abilities.

Look Who's Talking

"Mama" and "dada"—these are two words guaranteed to sound like music to your ears. After all, they represent not only one of the most memorable steps babies make toward talking but a two-syllable recognition of all your devoted love and attention. While many months will pass before your baby is able to master this particular milestone, it certainly won't be your baby's first when it comes to language development. Here are some of the significant stepping stones that lead up to the day when your child is actually able to talk (and talk back to) you.

- **As a newborn.** Crying is going to be your newborn's primary form of vocalization. While crying is admittedly less than perfect in conveying what babies want or need, it's definitely a vocal start.

- **Around 8 weeks.** Cooing and babbling begin. These crowd-pleasing skills symbolize your baby's first more-formal attempts to vocalize, soon to be followed by actual consonants and vowels.

- **Around 6 to 8 months.** Your baby will happily use his voice for making sounds and even some more elaborate streams of babble, but no words yet. The much-anticipated "mama" and "dada" are sure to surface—albeit arbitrarily mixed in with other sounds and, we should note, with "dada" typically being uttered first if only because it's easier for babies to say (ie, with no implications of parental preference).

- **Around 1 year.** By a year, be prepared to celebrate not only your child's first birthday but also the long-awaited "mama" and "dada," now being used intentionally to refer to you. You can also anticipate hearing some simple exclamations, such as "Uh-oh," as well as a few single words. And while there's sure to be plenty of animated babbling and attempts to imitate words, don't expect your toddler's self-expression to string together into full sentences just yet.

- **Around 18 months.** Your ears will likely be graced with the sounds of at least several stand-alone words. Your toddler may even be able to put two words together—such as "all done"—to more meaningfully convey his wishes. Rest assured, however, that your toddler understands far more words than he can speak.

- **Around 2 years.** Now we're talking…as in 2- to 4-word sentences and the start of real conversation along with a whole lot of repetition. Before long, you'll have a hard time remembering the sounds of your newborn's silence.

To sum it up, while it may take well into toddlerhood before your baby is able to put her thoughts, feelings, and demands into words you can understand, she'll be communicating with you long before then.

CAN YOU HEAR ME NOW?

It's important to note that hearing plays a critical role in language development and learning. As a parent, you can look for simple but meaningful signs that your baby is hearing okay as you talk, laugh, and play together. Watch to see whether your baby startles with loud noises and starts turning her head toward the sound of your voice. Also, be aware that in addition to your observations, universal newborn hearing screening is recommended for all infants. For more on this important subject, see Sound Advice for All Newborns on page 303.

17

these hands were made for talking

· · · · · ·

While you may not have come across it just yet, baby sign language seems to have become a mainstay of mainstream parenting these days, at least among a significant handful of proactive parents and child care professionals. As a trend that seems to have real staying power, signing with babies is based on the simple observation that children can be taught to use their hands to "talk" long before their mouths catch up. Sure, you've got a ways to go (ie, 8 or 9 months) before your newborn's dexterity will let her fingers do the talking. But that doesn't mean you can't start learning some basic baby signs in the meantime. Here are a few reasons why we approve.

- **Breaking the language barrier.** From what we've seen in our own children and others (including in Laura's educational child care center), baby sign language really delivers on its promise of improved communication. This is a particularly appealing promise for new parents, given that there's a well-recognized gap between what babies and toddlers *want* to say and what they are capable of saying. It only makes sense that young children who lack the verbal skills necessary to say what they want, feel, or need experience frustration—especially in the period from 8 to 9 months, when babies start to know what they want, and 18 to 24 months, when they typically start to speak their mind. In other words, if basic sign language can help babies use their hands to better express themselves as early as 8 or 9 months, it can mean the bridging of this otherwise months-long communication gap.

- **Bonding fun.** Signing with babies can also offer an opportunity for plenty of positive interaction, and anything that increases parent-baby bonding is a good thing in our book. One creative idea we love: start learning and adding signs to your musical repertoire of popular baby songs such as "Twinkle, Twinkle Little Star" and "Old MacDonald Had a Farm." Long story short: if you approach signing with your baby as an interactive and rewarding activity, then it's guaranteed to be all for fun and fun for all. In fact, if it's not fun, you shouldn't be doing it.

Signs of the Times

There's nothing wrong with teaching young children to "recite" the ABCs of sign language, but the most useful signs—especially for infants and toddlers— are going to be those that convey more than just the letters of the alphabet. Signs you'll want to start with are those that are most meaningful or serve to describe things your baby most often sees, does, or wants.

Here is a list of favorites we've put together to give you a better feel for some commonly used signs during early childhood. Start by learning these, and you're sure to get the conversation going: *airplane, baby, ball, bird, blanket, book, cat, cold, cup, daddy, diaper, dog, done, drink, eat, go, good night, happy, help, hot, hurt, I love you, milk, mommy, more, nap, no, outside, please, sit, sleep, star, thank you, up, water.*

Tips for Getting Started

While signing isn't exactly a must for new parents, it isn't all that difficult to learn either. Books, videos, websites, and apps that handily address the basics of baby signing abound, and it's easy to see why so many parents swear by it, why child care centers include it in their infant and toddler classrooms, and why it has become so commonplace as an activity of daily learning. Here are some big picture tips to get you started.

- **Be patient.** The baby-signing trend is based on the observation that infants taught simple signs at six or seven months of age can begin using them to communicate as early as eight or nine months. While there's no reason you have to wait until your baby turns six months to get started, we encourage you to be realistic in your expectations for any true signs of success.

- **Speak up.** Be sure you don't cut back on the amount of time you spend talking with your baby. As long as signing does not take the place of speaking, it won't get in the way of your baby's learning to talk with her words, as well as her hands.

- **Make it a habit.** As with much of the learning your baby will be doing, repetition is key. For a better shot at success, make signing a daily habit, not a onetime lesson.

- **Sign what you see.** Use signs to describe routine activities and common objects that make up your baby's world.

- **Don't be heavy-handed.** Don't worry if your baby doesn't get the signs quite right or doesn't pick them up right away. Remember, the goal here is to have fun communicating and *lessen* frustration, not add to it.

- **Share your signs.** Be sure you share your signs with your baby's other caregivers so everyone can join in on and understand the conversation once your baby begins to sign. And if your baby's child care provider is going to be the one teaching your baby sign language, be sure to ask for a quick tutorial so you understand what your baby wants when she starts signing to you.

THE ABCs OF AMERICAN SIGN LANGUAGE

While parents choosing to sign with babies who don't have any hearing problems started to gain in popularity in the 1990s, the use of sign language itself has been around for much longer. American Sign Language (ASL) has been developed and used predominantly in the deaf community for hundreds of years. It is estimated that about a million people use ASL, and interpreters can be seen in everyday life, from signing the national anthem at sporting events to translating spoken words on the stages of rock concerts and political events.

18

fun and games

• • • • • •

Parents often ask us questions regarding what toys are best for their babies.

- Can my newborn even see them yet? (The quick answer is yes, but for the more detailed answer, see The Eyes Have It on page 299.)
- Do they have to be red, white, and black?
- Should they play music and flash lots of colorful lights?

We believe the best way to answer questions about baby toys is to help you first understand play itself. After all, play is often said to be the "work" of children, which by definition makes their toys some of the fundamental tools of their trade. However, nothing beats human interaction, especially when it comes to newborns.

For babies (and perhaps for adults as well), playing is essentially the same thing as learning, and we've already given you our two cents on what the best learning activities are for babies: lots of language, books, singing, and other serve-and-return interactions (see Brain Games: Serve and Return on page 183). With that in mind, what makes a toy truly educational is not how much it costs or its color but its ability to entertain and encourage your baby to explore, engage, and interact. This principle is well worth taking to heart now and reminding yourself of over the next several years when you are faced with countless toy temptations.

Safety First

According to the US Consumer Product Safety Commission, bigger is better when it comes to safety and baby toys. While bigger toys can be just as enjoyable, they don't pose the choking hazard that small toys or toy parts do to babies and children under three. One of the simplest yet most important things you can do is to pay close attention and adhere to the age recommendations clearly included on the product packaging. These recommendations are not just based on developmental and educational levels. Rather, they are based on what is and isn't deemed safe for young children at specific ages. To further address the safety of baby toys, specific products or "testers" on the market with carefully standardized diameters can help you determine which toys and other little objects that may be strewn around your house stand to pose a choking hazard. Anything small enough to fit through one of these tube-shaped testers is simply too small for your baby to play with because it could all too easily make its way into her mouth and cause choking or block the airway.

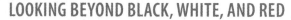

LOOKING BEYOND BLACK, WHITE, AND RED

Newborns are not thought to be very skilled when it comes to color vision and are probably unable to see subtle differences in color until two or three months of age. Young infants, however, are thought to be able to see bright colors and high contrasts fairly well. We imagine that's why manufacturers of baby toys often include lots of black and white (for contrast), mixed with a splash or two of bright red color, in many of their "educational" toys for babies. While this makes good sense, and we've seen everything from mobiles, balls, and toys to bed sets and floor mats in this cute and popular baby motif, in reality you don't need to limit your baby's color palette for the purposes of meaningful play.

What to Look for in a Toy

Babies rely primarily on their five senses (seeing, smelling, hearing, touching, and—yes—tasting) to play and explore. If you keep in mind this concept, along with the following characteristics, it will serve you well when selecting toys for your baby. Just remember, not all toys have to have all of the following characteristics, and some of the "best" toys are the simplest (including those you don't even have to go out and buy):

- **Is eye-catching.** Babies typically prefer objects with bright colors, high contrast, simple designs, and clear lines.

- **Shakes, rattles, and rolls.** Your baby's exploratory efforts will be rewarded with both sounds and movement.

- **Is touchy-feely.** Remember to let your baby explore various textures. Think soft, smooth, fluffy, and fuzzy.

- **Holds its own.** Look for toys that will be easy to hold so that your baby can get a good grasp.

- **Is drool resistant.** As soon as they're able, babies use their mouths to explore their world. Fortunately, plenty of baby toys today are designed with this in mind and are therefore drool resistant and/or washable.

- **Stands up under pressure…**not to mention all of the pushing, pulling, dropping, and squeezing that baby toys are inevitably subjected to.

BOOKS AS TOYS

Whoever invented board books was, in our opinion, brilliant. By making books durable, colorful, and designed to stand up under the scrutiny of inquiring minds (not to mention curious hands and mouths), board books clearly fit the bill as ideal baby toys that are both readily available and relatively inexpensive. Newer to the baby book scene are baby books that not only look and feel more like paper pages but are made out of a drool-proof, tear-proof material that puts them into the same category. For more about books for babies, see Books and Babies on page 197.

Be Proactive

When it comes to toys (and, ultimately, learning), active play always wins out over passive entertainment such as watching TV (see Media Matters on page 205). Although your newborn certainly won't be getting a full-fledged workout just yet, she'll move more in a mere matter of months. As she does, offer her toys she can reach for and hold, look at, listen to, wave, shake, chew on, make noise with, and more. An activity mat that you put on the floor can make an excellent fitness center for your new baby as she learns about the textures and sounds of different objects, as well as works on her depth perception skills by trying to grab such items as hanging rings and plastic mirrors.

The Perfect Fit

Finally, be sure to offer your baby toys that are at an appropriate level for her development. While you may love the idea of building Legos together, it will be a few years before she has the required dexterity to make them a good fit, much less the self-control required to avoid eating (or choking on) the pieces. If a toy is too advanced (or, for future reference, too simplistic), children tend to quickly lose interest or get frustrated.

DON'T JUST THINK INSIDE THE BOX

There's a poignant truth to the observation that children are often more entertained by something as simple as a box than the expensive, sophisticated, well-researched toy or game that came inside of it. That's because a box can offer open-ended opportunities for creative play. We certainly don't recommend giving your baby a box to play with just yet (wait a couple of years for that), but it will serve you well throughout parenthood if you simply remember that a toy can be anything that safely engages and entertains your child. Sometimes the best toys in life really are free!

19

books and babies

. . . . . .

No good parenting book—even one written expressly for the parents of newborns—should be without its own chapter addressing the subject of books for babies. Maybe you're already acquainted with the kinds of picture and board books we're referring to: the classics *Goodnight Moon; Mama, Do You Love Me?; The Very Hungry Caterpillar;* and *Good Night, Gorilla.* If not, we're here to tell you that you're in for a good time. That's not to say you have to sit down and start reading to your baby the first night you get home from the hospital, nor do you have to choose certain books just because they are board-book best sellers, considered classics, or happen to be our personal favorites. Rather, we encourage you to start sharing the joy of reading with your baby as soon as you start to settle into your new parenthood routine. Ultimately, we hope you come away with a deep appreciation for the fact that when loving parents share stories with their babies, babies develop an early and positive attachment to books, as well as to their parents, that can last a lifetime.

Reasons to Read

It is often said that children spend the first years learning to read and the rest of their lives reading to learn. We wholeheartedly agree with this statement but find that it is likely to be lost on new parents who have yet to crack open *Brown Bear, Brown Bear* much less plot out their children's future course to academic success. That said, there is more to reading than what you may recall from your elementary school days when reading was wedged in with 'riting and 'rithmetic. Especially when it comes to reading books with babies and young children, there are some pretty inspiring reasons to read aloud, all of which we hope help you realize it's not just about the book.

- **Instilling a healthy habit.** Just about all parents we know want their children to be able to read well and, more important, grow up with a love of reading. We are also big believers in the notion that healthy habits are more easily introduced sooner rather than later. Put these two observations together and you'll discover that introducing books early and often helps ensure they become both integral to and one of the most enjoyable parts of your baby's daily life (and yours).

- **Bonding through books.** Reading with your baby offers you both the perfect bonding experience. The process of reading aloud is an important part of early learning and literacy by exposing babies to new words, pictures, and even the taste and feel of the board books they'll soon grow to know and love. Add yourself to the experience, however, and what you'll end up with is something much bigger than the sum of the parts. That's because your warmth, voice, and undivided attention are exactly what your baby needs to grow up feeling safe and secure. The time you spend each day setting aside everything else and cradling your baby in your arms to read a good book or two (or three) will be invaluable.

- **Making memories.** Reading books with your baby inevitably involves plenty of the silly sounds, exaggerated voices, and funny faces we encourage you to make to enhance your storytelling adventures, all of which add up to some very memorable moments. Sure, those moments from your baby's first months will undoubtedly be recalled in much greater detail by you than your baby, but over time, the stories you share, as well as the time spent reading them, are sure to hold a place of prominence in both your memories.

- **Books at bedtime.** Whether a child is 4 months, 4 years, or a full 14 years of age, we routinely prescribe books at bedtime. That's because we've often discussed with parents that short of drugging children (which, for the record, we don't condone!), you really can't force a toddler—or teenager, for that matter—to fall asleep any more than you can convince a newborn to sleep through the night (see Sleeping Like a Baby on page 101). We are convinced, however, that one of the best things you can do is establish a predictable bedtime routine that includes books. It's one that will serve you and your child well for years, if not decades, to come.

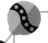

SHOWERED BY BOOKS

If you ask us, there's no better way to decorate a nursery than by lining your baby's bookshelf with a new collection of favorite children's books. Reach out to friends, family, and anyone else you can think of and ask them to share the name(s) of their favorite children's books. Start collecting a few just for fun in anticipation, and remember to put them on your baby registry. If you're fortunate enough to have someone offer, you can even suggest a book-themed baby shower.

The Developmental Milestones of Early Literacy

Some parents choose to read to their newborns even before they can hold their heads up or focus their eyes on the pages. We occasionally hear of those who start even sooner—reading to their unborn children through uterine walls. Our take on this head start? Although babies are thought to be able to hear well before they are born (see Sound Advice for All Newborns on page 303), we wouldn't count on it making your baby significantly smarter or more well-read. If you enjoy it, though, by all means, read away in anticipation of the day when your baby will be able to join in on the fun more actively. The good news is you won't have to wait too long. Just as there are well-defined and eagerly anticipated "motor" milestones that include rolling (4 to 6 months), sitting (7 to 9 months), and walking (anywhere from 9 to 15 months), there are equally well-defined and important milestones of early literacy. For the sake of making this short and sweet, we listed some of the book-related behaviors of early childhood, many of which have been developed by one of the country's most widely respected early literacy programs, Reach Out and Read (see Reaching Out to Read on page 201). That way, you can recognize and celebrate each book-based milestone in the months to come.

- **Around 3 months: Let the games begin.** Your baby will begin to babble and imitate sounds and smile at the sound of your voice. With his head held higher than in months past, he should now be developing a better grasp not only of what you're reading to him (or at least the expressions on your face) but also the books themselves as he learns to swipe at objects and attempts to bring them to his mouth.

- **Around 6 to 12 months: Taking an active interest.** Between the ages of 6 and 12 months, your baby will develop many new skills, including the ability to sit up tall with his head steady and grab at pages. Don't be surprised if books end up in your baby's mouth, as this is not only to be expected but a good sign that he is interested in books and wants to explore them further. This is the time to invest in some durable board and bath books, if you haven't already, as they stand up the best to new teeth and drool and also contain plenty of color, simple objects, and photographs of faces that babies seem to prefer.

- **Around 12 to 18 months: A hands-on experience.** Not only should your baby be able to sit without support, allowing him both hands free for holding books and turning board pages (albeit several at a time), but he's likely to demonstrate his already well-developed love of reading by carrying his books around, eagerly handing them to you to read, and answering your questions of "Where is the…?" by pointing to pictures with one finger. At this age, toddlers also learn to recognize when a book is upside down. If you've never thought about it before, this is actually a fundamentally important step toward reading!

- **Around 18 to 24 months: Taking charge.** By now your baby will not only have turned into a toddler but also a true book connoisseur adept at turning his own board-book pages. Paper pages may still take a while to fully master. Ask "What's that?" and your toddler is sure to respond by naming familiar pictures. Pause before completing the sentence in a favorite book, and your toddler will finish it for you. Listen in and you'll even hear him taking over your role as storyteller as he starts to recite the stories he knows best to his own loyal listeners (ie, dolls or stuffed animals).

REACHING OUT TO READ

As one of the country's leading nonprofit early literacy organizations, Reach Out and Read is committed to reaching families with children from the ages of 6 months to 5 years, especially those living in poverty. Reach Out and Read medical professionals promote early literacy and school readiness by distributing books to children at each well-child (health supervision) visit in more than 6,000 hospitals and health centers across all 50 states. After more than 30 years and with more than 32,000 trained pediatric health care providers, this program now serves nearly 5 million children each year who, as a result, are more likely to be read to and enter kindergarten with larger vocabularies, stronger language skills, and, hopefully, a love of reading that will last a lifetime. You can find out more information about the organization, early literacy, and the importance of reading aloud and a list of doctor-recommended books for babies at www.reachoutandread.org.

The Best Books for Babies

You may be expecting us to share with you our own favorite baby books, but we decided it would be far more useful to tell you that the best books for babies are quite simply those that you and your baby enjoy most. Early on it won't really matter what you read. That's right, feel free to read aloud the Sunday paper, the latest issue of your favorite magazine, or a book club selection you will otherwise never find the time to finish whenever you find yourself without a good children's book handy. Either way, your baby is sure to enjoy the sound of your voice and share in your enthusiastic narration. As your baby starts to develop some interests of her own, make sure you stock up on plenty of durable books designed to hold their own in the face of plenty of touching, tasting, teething, and drooling. You'll find plenty to choose from in the board-book section, but feel free to look for tear-proof books and water-proof bath books that also fit the bill. As for what's inside, young babies seem to be particularly partial to photographs of faces. Continue to add books with colorful pictures of recognizable objects and animals, as well as books with fanciful rhythm and rhyme, to your baby's growing collection.

CHAPTER

20

the sounds of music

· · · · · ·

In recent years, everyone from hopeful parents to well-meaning politicians seems to have jumped on the classical music bandwagon, embracing the notion that something as easy as listening to classical music can make babies smarter. Understandably an intriguing concept that almost certainly contributes to the fact that everything from mobiles and music boxes to crib toys and teddy bears plays favorites from classical composers such as Mozart, Bach, and Beethoven, the relationship between these musical maestros and your baby's brain may not be exactly what it was billed to be when the "Mozart Effect" was first "discovered." That said, we still have good reason to believe that music (classical music included) can and should be an enjoyable part of your baby's early experiences.

A CLOSER LOOK AT THE MOZART EFFECT

Much of the parenting lore about classical music's ability to build a better baby brain—most commonly referred to as the "Mozart Effect"—seems to stem from a single study published in *Nature* in the early 1990s. This study found that college students who listened to Mozart scored better on an intelligence test than those who didn't. After the publication of this short paper, the popularity of classical composers seemed to skyrocket in the popular press and the parenting world. Within a matter of years, scores of classical CDs had found themselves a permanent home in nurseries and on baby registries all over the United States. In 1998, the governor of Georgia even started distributing them to every newborn in his state. Was classical music the secret to success for making babies smarter? Not exactly. While modern-day research involving babies and music is compelling, a closer look at the original study reveals that the so-called Mozart Effect showed only a very short-lived (on the order of 10 to 15 minutes) improvement of a very specific type of intelligence (spatial reasoning) in very few college students. Furthermore, the improvements weren't reproducible (in humans or in monkeys, for that matter) and were never tested for in babies.

The Case for Classical Music

Just because the Mozart Effect may not be what it was originally thought to be, that's not to say you need to replace your best classical music for babies and kids playlist with the sounds of silence. What does seem to be the case for classical music is that

- It has a more complex musical structure than most contemporary pop, rock, or country music.
- Its increased complexity is believed to stimulate areas of the brain responsible for spatial reasoning.
- There seems to be crossover learning between the rhythms associated with music and the recognition of similar rhythms in spoken language (based on studies involving the waltz).

Given what we know about how repeated exposure can lead to new and more well-developed connections in babies' brains, it seems there are still plenty of reasons to believe that music makes a difference.

Music for Your Baby's Ears

When picking music for your baby, don't choose classical (or any other musical selections, for that matter) solely because of its anticipated ability to boost your baby's intelligence but rather for enjoyment. The reality is that you can play just about any type of music for your baby as long as she seems to enjoy it and you keep the following tips in mind:

- **Turn down the volume.** Babies' ears are sensitive to sound, and loud music can cause damage.

- **Sing along.** Even if your pitch is off and you can't remember all the words, the enjoyable interaction you share with your baby each and every time you sing with her is sure to overcome any lack of musical talent.

- **Set the tone.** Music can set the stage for routine daily activities. Put on some upbeat music and your baby will soon learn that it's play and "dance" time. Many parents also find that consistently playing certain soothing tunes at bedtime can go a long way toward calming babies down and getting them in the mood to fall asleep.

- **Listen to the lyrics.** As catchy, calming, or upbeat as a song may be, make sure you pay particular attention to the lyrics. While music written specifically for babies is generally a safe bet, a closer listen to many of today's pop tunes will likely leave you convinced they're not suitable for young ears.

CHAPTER

21

media matters

· · · · · ·

In this day and age of high-tech, multimedia everything, we feel obliged to
at least briefly direct your attention toward a few media matters of particular
parenting importance. While you may not need to look up how to lock your
iPad or use your computer or TV set's parental controls just yet, controlling
how much time your baby spends in front of a screen is a responsibility you
should assume right from the start. iPads, smartphones, TVs, DVDs, video
games, and hi-tech toys have all made their way into early childhood in a
big (and potentially concerning) way. In fact, with today's mobile-enabled
24-hour access, the amount of time young children spend on entertainment
media continues to increase dramatically, with children under the age of two
reportedly engaging with screens an average of 3 hours a day despite clear
recommendations to the contrary. We strongly believe there's no time like the
present for new parents to tune in to the situation so you can make sure your
baby ends up benefiting from a healthy media diet right from the start.

New parenthood is also a good time for you to do a quick assessment of
your own media diet. Given all we know about the critical importance of
human interaction on the developing brain (plus the statistics on how much
media adults consume), we suggest you make a concerted effort to set aside
your own screens whenever you can and offer your newborn the most meaningful gift of all—your undivided attention.

Getting Poor Reception

We imagine that your baby's screen time may seem like a topic of less immediate importance to you as the parent of a newborn than, say, watching your
baby's umbilical cord in anticipation of it falling off. But we assure you that
watching (and limiting) your baby's exposure to screen time is a topic well
worth tuning in to sooner rather than later. While the jury is still out when it

comes to whether TV or any of the many other forms of electronic media for children are fundamentally "good" or "bad" or somewhere in between, there are many valid reasons why tech-enabled babies and toddlers are causing considerable concern—not the least of which are the sheer numbers we're talking about. It has been estimated that almost all infants and toddlers are exposed to TV or videos every day. At the same time, research suggests that for children younger than two years, none of this exposure is actually beneficial to learning. In fact, it may be harmful. As researchers, pediatricians, and parents alike tune in to these numbers, questions are raised about the negative effect of TV and screen time on everything from play and behavior to IQ and language skills. To be fair, we should point out that the news about TV isn't all bad. High-quality educational programs for children over two, along the lines of *Sesame Street,* have shown some benefit—especially in fostering improved language skills.

No TV for the Under-2 Set

The fact that so many babies and toddlers are watching TV is somewhat surprising given that the American Academy of Pediatrics (AAP) has long and decisively discouraged *any* media use or screen time for children younger than 2. This includes TV, computers, tablets, and all the numerous viewing activities touted as educational for babies and toddlers. Although this recommendation has been met with understandable resistance in the parenting world (along the lines of asking devoted football fans to forgo watching the televised Super Bowl), it is important to note that it is based on real concerns. Most notably, we know that what infants and young children need most are positive interactions *with real, live humans.* Unfortunately, there's little way to look past the fact that for the most part, screen time is a 2-D and passive pastime. Until about 15 months, children are unable to translate what they see on a screen to their 3-D, real-life world. The one exception to this screen-time limitation in the under-2 age group is video chatting, such as using FaceTime or Skype to communicate with others in real time.

THE BABY EINSTEIN CONTROVERSY

Exceedingly popular in the 2000s, Disney's Baby Einstein videos catered to very young viewers—playing classical music (*Baby Mozart*), making reference to world literature (*Baby Shakespeare*), and alluding to acclaimed art (*Baby Van Gogh*)—all to a reported tune of hundreds of millions of dollars in annual sales. The problem? In 2009, presumably in response to considerable pressure concerning their potentially misleading claims of educational benefits, not to mention a target audience most definitely younger than two years, the Walt Disney Company offered a full refund to anyone who purchased the videos under the false assumption that the videos would make their baby smarter.

TV (and Screen-Time) Guide

In order to help you figure out your own strategy for how the likes of Doc McStuffins, PAW Patrol, Daniel Tiger, and Elmo will fit most appropriately into your baby's future schedule, we want to leave you with the following TV and screen-time guidelines from the AAP:

- Avoid screen time for children under 18 months other than video chatting.
- Set media limits. According to the AAP, some media programs can be educational for children around the age of 18 months, as long as they are considered *quality* programming. That means age appropriate, informational, and nonviolent.
- For those aged 2 to 5 years, limit screen time to no more than 1 hour per day of high-quality programs, and help them understand what they are watching.
- Turn off the TV and other digital media and screens during meals.
- Monitor what your child watches, and discuss the content with her.
- Keep your child's room screen-free.
- Make sure you ask about (and similarly limit) your child's screen time while she is in child care, as well as at home.

It All "Ads" Up

On a final note, remember that when your child does start to watch TV, it's not just the show's content you'll need to keep an eye on. With advertisements taking up nearly a third of an entire program's time, a discouraging majority of them are for fast food, candy, cereal, and toys. In addition, marketing to preschoolers mostly entails commercials on TV (or some streaming services) because TV is still the dominant medium for young children. Being able to skip this sort of unwanted marketing to children is one particularly compelling reason to opt for pre-recorded shows (during which you can skip over the commercials) and DVDs, in which there aren't any. Or choose online platforms that are ad-free for a fee.

thinking outside of the house

introduction

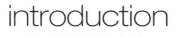

Looking for a Way Out

Having a new baby around the house tends to make even the most routine of pre-parenthood tasks require a bit more forethought. Many of you will find yourselves perfectly content to head home and remain there until you feel you've mastered the primary new-parent challenges of feeding (both your newborn and yourself), sleeping, diapering, clothing, and maintaining a healthy state of household hygiene, to name but a few. Don't be surprised, however, if "homeward bound" starts to feel just that—a bit binding. Looking at the same four walls has a way of making some new parents start to get a little stir-crazy and may understandably leave you longing to get out of the house— somewhere, anywhere, just out. Whether you decide to venture out of the comfort zone of your own home early on or weeks down the road, of your own free will or out of necessity, and with or without your newborn in tow, we wanted to put together a set of basic considerations to help you feel properly prepared.

Dressing for the Occasion

Yes, a newborn's relatively large head is a surefire source for heat loss. No, you shouldn't take your baby out of the house without bundling him appropriately. And no, you won't want to venture out and expose your newborn to direct sunlight. But before you spend any time trying to memorize the seemingly endless don'ts involved in stepping out, we suggest you first focus your attention on a few general wardrobe issues and pieces of advice. By becoming familiar with and applying them, you can significantly reduce the number of don'ts you need to commit to memory before safely and comfortably exposing your newborn to the outside world.

- **At a loss.** Whether you're headed outdoors or in, your newborn is going to benefit from a covered head for several weeks to come. That's because relative to the rest of their bodies, newborns have impressively large heads. This characteristic not only makes them completely dependent on parental head support but also leaves them prone to significant loss of body heat from their uncovered heads.

- **Anticipation.** It's next to impossible to go anywhere and be able to rely on predictable climate control. Regardless of how much faith you have in weather forecasting or the person in charge of the thermostat, your best bet will be to come prepared with several layers of easy-on, easy-off clothing.

- **Overshadowing.** Ideally, you'll want to keep your newborn out of direct sunlight to prevent sunburn. Additionally, we suggest you provide some guaranteed shade by dressing your baby in a thin layer of clothing and a wide-brimmed hat even in warm weather. If you cannot avoid the sun, be sure to apply sunscreen (at least 15 SPF) to any small areas of exposed skin, such as your baby's face and the backs of her hands.

SEEING THE LIGHT OF DAY: SUNSCREEN

While it's best to keep babies younger than 6 months out of the sun, we know from a practical standpoint this is not always possible. Because babies have thinner and more delicate skin than adults, they're more prone to sunburns. This makes the following recommendations particularly important anytime your baby must be out in the light of day:

- Try to avoid the peak hours from 10:00 am to 4:00 pm, when the sun's rays are strongest. This applies on cloudy days, as well as sunny ones, as up to 80% of the sun's UV rays can get through the clouds.

- Keep your baby under a large umbrella, a stroller canopy, or other shade. The next best thing is to keep her covered with a brimmed hat, lightweight long pants, and a long-sleeved shirt.

- The goal is to use sunscreen on your baby only if and when protective clothing and shade are not available. When you do, apply sunscreen with an SPF of 15 or higher to all exposed areas such as the face, neck, tips of the ears, backs of the hands, and tops of the feet. Even though most sunscreen labels state that the product is intended for babies older than 6 months, it is generally accepted that it's better for young infants to risk getting a potential rash from early use of sunscreen than to get sunburned without it.

- Be sure to apply sunscreen at least 15 to 30 minutes before going out and reapply at least every 2 hours.

- Check sunscreen labels to make sure the product protects against both UVA and UVB rays. Products that contain titanium dioxide or zinc oxide are thought to be the best at physically blocking the sun's rays.

- Finally, avoid oxybenzone-containing sunscreen whenever possible. There is concern that this ingredient may affect hormones in the body.

All Dressed Up but Now Where to Go?

You're certain to find a lot of advice regarding taking your newborn out of the house with you. In reality, there are only a few basic principles in action here, with the rest tending to be a matter of opinion as opposed to expertise.

- **Less is more.** You will be better off if you choose to go to places with fewer people around. Close contact with a lot of people tends to be one of the most predictable hazards when it comes to the spread of germs. Enough said, at least until you read Fever: Trial by Fire on page 325.

- **An easy way out.** Consider starting small when you first leave home. A walk around the block is a great example of a doable first choice (weather and neighborhood permitting). Not only does it tend to be a relaxing way to get back on your feet gradually, but new babies often like the soothing motion. You're also less likely to find yourself in close quarters fending off unwanted well-wishers, and it leaves you an easy way out, should you need to cut the outing short and retreat back home for any reason— diaper blowout, fatigue (your own), or a hungry, crying, or otherwise unenthusiastic baby.

- **Overwhelming success.** Heading out of the house can be quite an adventure for a newborn. And, depending on your newborn's temperament and tolerance of stimulation in general, you may find yourself with a crankier-than-usual baby at the end of the day. For some newborns, even a quick trip to the grocery store can feel like a day spent at the amusement park. Any routine you may be working toward stands a chance of being thrown off a bit by overstimulation. We by no means want to imply that heading out of the house is the wrong thing to do. Instead, we want you to set your expectations appropriately, test the waters, and plan your approach accordingly. It is entirely possible to end up with an overwhelmed baby but still feel the outing has been a success.

- **Timing your travels.** This is a subject we address specifically as it relates to airplane travel in Timing Your Ticketed Travels on page 243, but it is a concept you'll want to apply whenever you choose to leave the house— with or without your newborn. Have faith that what now seems like orchestrating a grand production will become a routine you soon fall into.

VENTURING OUT: IT'S ABOUT TIME

You may increase your odds of being met with success when you head out by taking into account a few time-tested recommendations.

- **Just after a feeding.** Given that we've spent many pages addressing how unpredictably and frequently newborns tend to eat, planning your day around your newborn's anticipated feeding schedule may not always go as planned. Nevertheless, it's worth a shot.

- **Off-hours.** Go where the crowds aren't or at least to places at off-peak times when they're less likely to be crowded.

- **When you're well rested.** You're probably now thinking this means we recommend no outings in the foreseeable future. To clarify, we don't mean well rested in the pre-parenthood sense of the phrase but rather in a relative sense. You're bound to have good days/nights and bad ones. We simply suggest giving yourself time to catch up if you've just finished a rough one.

- **You've got coverage.** Venture out when someone can cover for you at home or go along with you and lend a hand with logistics.

Don't Leave Home Without Them

Despite the catchy heading, technically speaking, there aren't many items we consider must-haves before taking your baby out of the house, especially if you're not planning on strolling far from home. There are, however, some useful items we've found best to have on hand. Others may not be essential but rather have earned their characterization as on-the-go conveniences. Here are a few thoughts and suggestions for when you're ready to get on the go again.

- **Diapering supplies.** We consider it Murphy's Law of Newborns that if you don't have a diaper within arm's reach at all times, babies are all but guaranteed to poop the first chance they get.

- **Accommodating change (of clothing).** Expect to need at least one complete change of clothing—definitely for your newborn but quite possibly for yourself as well. Blowouts, leaks, and spills are far less stressful if you've planned ahead.

- **Food for thought.** Newborns don't care how recently they've been fed before setting out on an adventure. The minute you and your newborn step out the door, any semblance of a feeding schedule you may have achieved within the confines of your home has the distinct possibility of flying right out the window. In short, you'll never regret being prepared to feed your baby on the go. With that in mind, we suggest you flip to Into the Mouths of Babes on page 1 for a more in-depth look at what supplies you might want or need for either feeding option—be it breast or bottle.

- **Baby carriers.** We love baby carriers! They offer new parents a comfy, cozy, baby-friendly, hands-free option. While there are many, many options readily available, including carriers that go in front of you, backpacks that go behind you, and slings that drape across you, we narrow our discussion to issues that apply specifically to newborns and include some practical economics-versus-ergonomics considerations.

  - *Weight limits.* Some baby carriers aren't designed for use by small infants. If you plan on using one early on, be very sure to double-check and abide by the lower weight limit.

  - *Safety.* As we've mentioned elsewhere in this book (see Taking It From the Top on page 294), babies are born with minimal head control and neck support. Be sure to choose an appropriate carrier for your baby's development that provides the necessary head support and also provides proper positioning for unobstructed breathing. Soft/fabric carriers should be labeled as meeting ASTM F2236. The carrier should hold your baby in a position that allows the head and neck to be straight and not curled into a letter C shape since a chin-to-chest position can block the baby's airway. The baby's face should always be visible, uncovered, and not pressed into the carrier or the adult's body.

  - *Comfort level.* Not all baby carriers are created equal when it comes to comfort—for you and for your baby. You'll want to consider ease of use—how comfortable you are strapping it on and putting your baby into it—as well as how comfortable you find the carrier to be. Remember to factor in how much you plan on using the carrier because some are perfectly comfortable at first but quickly become less so when put to the test by increasingly heavy passengers.

  - *Price points.* Factor in cost to determine whether you're getting what you pay for. This really is a personal preference. Some parents consider the more expensive, Cadillac-equivalent baby carriers to be well worth the price they must pay for them—especially if they are easier to use and, as a result, end up being put to more use. Others find that the more economical models serve their purposes just as well.

- **Strollers.** From the basic umbrella stroller to a top-of-the-line double jogging stroller, parents these days have nearly unlimited options to meet their needs—whether it's transporting their baby through a shopping center, going on a daily jog, or strolling a colicky baby down the hallways of their home (a "remedy" that, in some parents' minds, justifies the purchase of an extra stroller specifically for use indoors). You may ultimately find that having a few different strollers is worthwhile—a lightweight umbrella stroller for quick trips or to use when traveling, a sturdier stroller for outdoor errands, and a jogging stroller if you're the athletic type (or want to look or feel the part). But for the time being, you'll want to narrow your scope a bit and look for strollers that are appropriate for newborns. First and foremost, this means checking each stroller's instruction manual and following the minimum age requirement and size requirements.

  - *Recline.* In general, newborns need strollers that offer a fair degree of recline because their development does not yet allow them to sit upright and hold their heads high. Some stroller seat backs even recline completely to aid with napping—a feature whose usefulness extends well beyond the first few weeks and months. Most jogging strollers, though, aren't recommended for use during the first five or six months because they typically aren't designed to recline, and babies younger than that age do not have the head or neck strength to withstand the jostling from jogging—reclined position or not.

  - *Canopies and covers.* Whether it's windy, rainy, or sunny out, some type of stroller canopy is guaranteed to prove useful in protecting your baby from the elements both now and for years to come. Some cover more than others, so consider the weather variations in your area. These may also help your baby sleep while in the stroller and keep well-intentioned but nevertheless germ-covered hands from reaching in and touching your baby. Just be sure that any cover-ups have adequate ventilation, and remember to remove them when the weather allows so your baby gets good airflow.

- *Travel systems.* A car seat and stroller may come as a matching set, or a special attachment can allow car seats of various makes to hook on securely to a stroller. Each of these options allows for easy transfer of your baby from car to stroller and back without requiring you to remove her from her seat. If you don't plan on keeping your baby in her car seat while strolling, this option is unnecessary. If you plan on taking advantage of the convenience of (potentially) uninterrupted slumber in the car seat, just be aware that for safety's sake, the American Academy of Pediatrics recommends that infant car seats be used only for travel, not for sleeping, feeding, or any other use outside the vehicle.

TIME TO ADJUST

You may find it interesting to know that traditional Chinese and Indian cultures actually dictate that new moms not leave the house for about a month after childbirth. This gives mothers time to slow down and recuperate from childbirth—something that can be healthy for mom and baby (but, in our opinion, would lead us to develop a serious case of cabin fever).

Taking Your Own Sweet Time

Now that you've read about the preparation that can help with venturing outside the home, we suspect some of you may decide you're not quite ready to do so. That's okay too. In fact, if experience tells us anything, there may well be days when you don't even feel like showering or changing out of sweatpants or pajamas. If you have the luxury of being able to hang out at home (and perhaps let others come to you), enjoy it while you can.

Leaving Home Alone

Want to know where I (Laura) went the first time I left home without my newborn when she was only about a week old? Target. Want to know what I needed to get there? Nothing. I, like many new parents, just started to feel a gradually increasing need to get out of the house and get some time to myself—if only for a brief while. Whether you're enticed by the thought of a walk in the park or a visit to a nearby retail establishment, we strongly recommend seeing what you can do to make it happen if and when the urge strikes you. Start by finding and enlisting trusted help to take over baby duty and give you a chance to do whatever it is (within reason, of course) that you think will help make you feel less like you're trapped or missing out. You may well find that getting some occasional alone time out of the house is invaluable in refreshing your perspective and outlook on your new life.

CHAPTER

22

car safety

· · · · · ·

Buckling Up So You Can Enjoy the Ride

Buying a car seat (more accurately referred to as a *car safety seat*) has become an integral part of the official entry into parenthood—ranking right up there with getting a prenatal ultrasound and picking out nursery furniture. Knowledge about how to keep our children safe in cars has improved dramatically since our own parents were faced with the same task. After all, we've come a long way from the days when new babies were brought home inadequately secured in nothing more than a well-intentioned parent's loving arms. Only a generation or two ago, parents had to be convinced to buy a car seat, much less use one. Today, none of us would dare leave home without one. As you join the ranks of proud parents, you will inevitably become well acquainted with car seats. Not only are they guaranteed to be part of your everyday parenting routine for many years—long after teething, colic, strollers, and diapers have all come and gone—but making sure your child is always secured properly in one constitutes one of the single most important measures you can take to help ensure your child's safety. You may notice we have temporarily put aside our joking tone a bit in this chapter on car seats—something we're doing intentionally for the sake of offering you a serious, useful, and hands-on look at how to get it right.

HOW TIMES HAVE CHANGED

A quick historical look at the evolution of automobile safety may help you understand why a generation of grandparents (and even parents) out there still need to be convinced to buckle up!

1965	Lap belts first required in passenger vehicles
1971	First federal standards for child restraints (car seats)
1973	Lap-shoulder belts required in front seats
1978	First car seat law passed (in Tennessee)
1985	Some type of child restraint law in effect in all states
1989	Lap-shoulder belts required in both outer positions of the back seat
1996	Phasing in of airbags and requirement that all seat belts come with a locking mechanism
2002	Nearly all new vehicles and child seats equipped with universal tethers and anchors—a system referred to as *LATCH* (more on LATCH on page 233)
2008	Significant changes in school bus seating standards such that all small buses (less than 10,000 pounds) required to have lap-shoulder belts
2013	Inflatable seat belts offered in rear seat of select Ford models and designed to provide added protection in the event of a crash. Note that some car seat manufacturers still prohibit their use for securing child restraints pending further safety testing.

Before Leaving the Hospital

Buying a car seat for your baby is certainly one of the most important purchases you'll make and one that you will need to make before your big day arrives—or at least before you leave the hospital. All 50 states now have laws requiring the use of infant safety seats in the car, and it has become standard hospital policy that parents must always have one in their possession before taking their new babies home. Showing up with a car safety seat, however, is not the same as knowing how to use and install it correctly. We strongly recommend that you plan ahead, take time to educate yourself, practice installing the seat in your car(s), and, if possible, schedule a time before your due date, or as soon as you can after your baby is born, to have the seat checked by a certified Child Passenger Safety Technician (CPST) (more on this in Going Pro on page 238).

Selecting the Perfect Seat

Although you may be hoping this is the part of the chapter where we tell you exactly which make and model of car seat to buy, we thought it best to tell you what your options are and then give you the information you'll need to make the choice best suited to your needs. As you read the following information, you'll find that we've included a big picture view of car seats that extends beyond just what you'll need for your newborn. That's not simply because we want to overload you with more information. Rather, we are well aware that new parenthood is the time (and sometimes the only time) when parents pay close attention to the details of car seat selection and use.

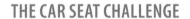

THE CAR SEAT CHALLENGE

The American Academy of Pediatrics (AAP) recommends that all newborns and infants born more than 3 weeks prematurely (less than 37 weeks) be monitored in a car seat—preferably their own—for at least 1½ to 2 hours (or for the anticipated travel time if longer than 2 hours) before leaving the hospital. Taking this simple precaution helps determine whether the semi-reclined position of correctly installed infant car seats puts the baby at risk for breathing problems or slowing of the heartbeat. If this car seat tolerance test results in any such concerning problems, doctors will likely recommend such interventions as supplemental oxygen, further assessment, or a temporary alternative such as an infant car bed, as described in Car Beds on page 227.

Your take-home message in a four-criteria nutshell: the car seat you should buy is the one that

1. Meets all current US federal motor vehicle safety standards
2. Is the right size for your child
3. Can be securely installed in your vehicle
4. Will be used every time your child rides in the car

While manufacturers work hard to appeal to parents' sense of convenience and style, safety should always be your number one priority when choosing a car seat. All child safety seats sold in the United States must be certified for use in motor vehicles—a requirement that must be met and referenced on each car seat label. If only ensuring your baby's safety were as easy as reading the label, but there's clearly more to it than that. Your next step is to determine whether the seat you select is the right one for your baby and if it can be installed properly in your particular car, as correct fit is of paramount importance. Of course, it would be nice if all car seats fit well in all vehicles, but incompatibility is unfortunately not uncommon. And while we've found that some stores—both locally and online—gladly accept returns or allow exchanges, others may not be so accommodating. That means you'll want to carefully explore your options (not to mention the store's return policy) before purchasing.

BUYER BEWARE:
STEERING CLEAR OF COUNTERFEIT CAR SAFETY SEATS

In recent years, fake car safety seats that closely resemble genuine ones have hit the market, and unsuspecting parents have buckled their babies into seats that may not protect them in a crash and may also expose them to flammable or harmful chemical-containing fabrics. Be wary of buying a car safety seat from an unfamiliar seller and deals that seem too good to be true.

Signs that a car seat may not be genuine include

- Labels or parts are missing.

- Seat seems too lightweight, or the plastic is flexible.

- The packaging or online listing has spelling/grammar errors.

- The brand name is unfamiliar.

Fortunately, there are some simple steps you can take to avoid purchasing counterfeit products. These include

- Purchasing from a familiar retail store or directly from a known online retailer, not from a resale shop or third-party marketplace seller.

- Buying a familiar brand. If you are not yet familiar with car safety seat brands or don't recognize a particular brand name, check out the manufacturer's website and, when possible, ask someone who is more familiar/informed (see Going Pro on page 238).

- Looking for the make and model on the American Academy of Pediatrics (AAP) car seat product listing at www.healthychildren.org/carseatlist.

- Registering the car safety seat with the manufacturer either online or using the attached postcard.

- Having your seat (as well as its installation) checked by a Child Passenger Safety Technician (CPST) before using it.

An Overview of Your Rear-Facing Options

Rear-Facing–Only

Rear-facing–only seats (sometimes called *infant-only seats*) are designed for use *only* in the rear-facing position and *only* until your baby reaches the seat's upper height or weight limits. These generally range from 22 to 35 pounds, depending on the seat, and can be used until your baby reaches the top height allowed by the manufacturer, often when the head is within 1 inch from the top of the seat.

Advantages

- The seat is designed specifically for newborns and infants, so it may offer a better fit.
- Adjustable carrying handles allow you to carry your baby around in the seat conveniently.
- Once installed, the detachable base remains in the car so that you don't have to reinstall the seat each time you take it out; simply click it back onto its base. Many car seat manufacturers offer the option of purchasing additional bases if you want one in other cars (**Figure 22-1**).
- In many cases, the rear-facing–only seat can be installed and used without a base. While the seat is not as easy to install correctly when it is used alone, it is helpful to familiarize yourself with how to do so. Having this option can be quite useful when traveling so that you don't have to lug the base around, but be sure to follow the installation instructions carefully.
- Many come with stroller travel systems, where the car seat fits interchangeably with the base and with a stroller (which can also be used alone). While this allows for the much less disruptive transfer of a sleeping baby from stroller to car and into the house (see Travel systems on page 217), be aware that you should not make a habit of leaving your baby strapped in a car seat for extended periods of time when not riding in the car because leaving babies in a semi-reclined position for long durations is not recommended. In addition, the American Academy of Pediatrics (AAP) now recommends that car seats not be used for sleeping or other purposes outside their intended use for safe car travel.

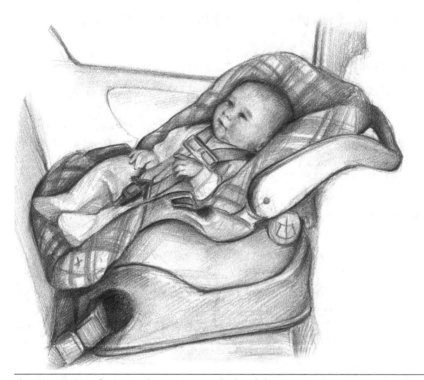

Figure 22-1. Rear-facing–only car seat installed with base

Practical Considerations

- Be sure to consider the lower weight limit for any rear-facing–only seat you're considering. Most standard rear-facing–only seats are only rated for use for babies weighing at least 4 or 5 pounds, which isn't low enough for some low birth weight or premature babies.
- Most babies reach the upper weight or height limits of infant-only seats before their first birthdays but still need to ride rear facing. This means they must be moved to another type of seat that has higher rear-facing capabilities (see Convertible Seats: Rear- and Forward-Facing Use on page 225) to allow them to remain rear facing for as long as possible.
- As your child gets heavier, carrying her around in a rear-facing–only car seat is likely to become less of a convenience and more of a physical challenge.

CARRYING HANDLES

One common mistake parents with infant-only seats make is not putting the carrying handle in the correct position when the seat is being used in the car. While some manufacturers require that the carrying handles on their infant-only seats be put down behind the head of the car seat, other manufacturers allow or even require their handles to remain up while in use in the car. As is true for everything to do with car seat installation and use, this variability reinforces the need for you to actually read your seat's instruction manual.

Convertible Seats (Rear- and Forward-Facing Use)

Convertible seats are so called because they can be used not only as rear-facing infant seats but also turned around, or "converted," to forward-facing toddler seats later on. Perhaps one of the most important things to consider when purchasing a convertible seat (in addition to what it offers in safety and compatibility) is its rear-facing upper weight limit. Most now offer the advantage of significantly higher rear-facing limits than some of the infant-only seats.

Advantages

- Higher rear-facing weight (often up to 40 pounds and some up to 50 pounds) and height limits allow for longer use rear facing.
- They have greater potential longevity because they can later be used forward facing (uppermost weight limits can vary from 40 to 90 pounds when the seat is used with the internal harness), after the child outgrows the rear-facing height or weight limits.
- Come with a 5-point harness that more securely fastens children in their seat (offering harness attachments on either side of the hips, as well as above each shoulder and between the legs).

Practical Considerations

- Most notable, parents often find that their newborns or small infants don't fit quite as well, presumably because convertible seats are designed to accommodate a wider range of sizes.
- They lack the convenience of a carrying handle, detachable base, or stroller attachment.
- They are generally bigger, bulkier, and more expensive than infant seats. They also tend to be taller, a feature making it even more important to check that they fit when installed rear facing in the back of smaller cars.

THE AMERICAN ACADEMY OF PEDIATRICS WEIGHS IN

The American Academy of Pediatrics (AAP) continually updates its important car seat safety recommendations. As we write this, the current recommendation from the AAP is that all children should remain rear facing as long as they haven't outgrown the height or weight limits of the seat. These upper limits will be determined either by the upper weight limit of the seat or when the top of your child's head comes within an inch of the top of the seat (or to the level listed by the manufacturer). These important manufacturer-determined height and weight limits can be found on labels located on the sides of car seats. Fortunately, current limits allow for virtually all children up until the age of 2, as well as most children up to age 4, to be able to safely ride rear facing.

Bottom line: the longer your child can remain rear facing, the better, and be sure to refer to the AAP for the most current car seat safety recommendations.

All-in-One or 3-in-1 Seats
(Rear-Facing, Forward-Facing With Harness, and Booster)

The one-size-fits-all type of seat can theoretically be used from birth (rear facing with the built-in harness, usually 5 to 35, 40, or even 50 pounds) through toddlerhood (forward facing with the built-in harness from 20 or 22 up to 40, 65, or even 90 pounds) and all the way through booster seat age (when used with the vehicle's lap-shoulder belt as a belt-positioning booster seat from 40 or 50 up to 120 pounds). Forward-facing–only combination toddler-booster seats (two seats in one) are also available but should not be used until the child's height or weight exceeds the limits of a rear-facing seat.

Advantages

- Longevity, because one seat fits all.

Practical Considerations

- Longevity. While it may seem convenient at first, some parents come to see little to no benefit in being stuck with the same seat for more than 1 or 2 years—especially those who have witnessed the wear and tear that milk, spit-up, and worse can cause to a car seat over the years. In addition, as improvements are made in children's car seat safety and engineering, you may find yourself wanting the latest state-of-the-art seat long before your child outgrows this one. Expiration dates can range from 6 to 10 years, depending

on the car seat and manufacturer recommendations, so be sure to pay attention to the label over time to make sure your child's seat is still safe to use.

- Fit challenges. Some all-in-one seats are designed to fit newborns weighing as little as 4 pounds by using the supplied inserts and harness length
  adjustments. Just be sure to look for low harness slots designed to fit
  a baby's short torso, and then remember to follow the manufacturer's
  instructions carefully regarding the need to readjust the seat and straps
  as your child grows.
- They lack the convenience of a carrying handle, detachable base, or stroller
  attachment.
- They are generally bigger, bulkier, and more expensive than infant seats.
  They also tend to be taller, a feature making it even more important to
  check that they fit when installed rear facing in the back of smaller cars.

Car Beds

We have intentionally chosen to mention the car bed as a particular type of
child safety restraint not because it is an acceptable option for routine use but
because some of you may come across one. Fortunately, far fewer of you will
actually find yourself needing one. It's most important to be aware that "regular" infant car seats are the preferred method of transportation, and car beds
are *not* recommended for general use. Rather, they are meant to be used only
when recommended by a health care provider for babies who must be transported in a lying down position. Most commonly, this requirement applies to
very small or premature babies or babies who have special medical needs. Car
beds should never be bought secondhand or reused unless you are advised to
by a child passenger safety professional or provided one by a hospital loaner
program. Unlike car seats, most car beds are designed for one-baby use—even
if used for only a few days or weeks.

Used Car Seats: Considerations and Common Pitfalls

We'll admit it, buying a car seat secondhand seems at first glance like a very
good way to get a great deal at a fraction of the cost. Before you decide to use
one, though, we offer you some compelling reasons why we and our child
passenger safety colleagues strongly discourage it. Unless you get a used car
seat from someone you know and trust, you will have no way of determining whether it has been involved in a crash. Fact is, not all seats show outward signs of damage from a crash, but any seat that has been involved in a
moderate or significant crash is considered to be unsafe for use. And if you

don't send in the original registration card, register your seat on the manufacturer's website, or later call or write with your contact information, the manufacturer of the seat will have no way of notifying you if there is (or has been) a recall. In addition, used seats are often expired, missing parts, or without their instruction manuals. The take-home message when it comes to used seats? We strongly recommend "out with the old, in with the new." The money saved by buying used may not be worth the potential price you'll pay.

Proper Use: The Key to Keeping Safe

The key to keeping your baby safe in the car lies not just in buying an appropriate car seat but also in using it properly. Properly installed infant car seats have been shown to dramatically reduce the number of deaths of children younger than one year—by some estimates, more than 70%. Yet some studies suggest that more than 80% of car seats are not installed or used correctly. If you've already tried your hand at the task of installing one, you may have discovered that mastering this necessary task of modern-day parenthood is not exactly easy.

4 Rs of Installation

Just as with the 3 Rs (of reading, 'riting, and 'rithmetic), our 4 Rs of maximizing your infant's safety in the car are not all there is for you to know—as is obvious by the rest of the information we've included in this chapter. That said, *reading, rear facing, recline,* and *recalls* are definitely as good a place as any to start.

Reading

Federal guidelines require that all car seats, unlike babies, come with an owner's manual. Yes, we realize that sitting down and reading an instruction manual is not exactly human nature (we plead guilty as well), but becoming a parent inevitably involves many changes, so just consider this one of them. There are so many different car seats and cars available these days that it is virtually impossible to give you all the information you need to install your own seat properly. While we intend to help you become well-informed on basic safety principles, it is still essential that you take time to read through your car seat instruction manual and your vehicle manual for the exact details that apply to you. If you happen to lose either, call the manufacturer's 800 number required to be on every child restraint or go to their website to download a new one.

REPLACING CAR SEATS AFTER A CRASH[a]

No one plans to get in a crash; it just happens. That's why your baby needs to be in a correctly installed car seat every time you set out on the road. We've found, however, that many parents are unaware that car seats involved in a crash may need to be replaced, regardless of whether a child is in the seat at the time of the crash or whether insurance is likely to cover the expense of replacing any car seats deemed unsafe for use. So which seats are considered unsafe for use? This is not a question you can or should answer alone. The National Highway Traffic Safety Administration guidelines suggest that seats involved in minor crashes may be safe for use if they meet *all* the following criteria:

- No visible evidence of damage to the car seat is found with careful inspection. This includes uninstalling the seat and taking the padding off to look for any cracks or otherwise hidden damage because it's not always outwardly visible at first glance.

- The vehicle is in good enough condition to be driven away from the scene of the crash.

- The vehicle door nearest to where the child safety seat was installed at the time of the crash is undamaged.

- None of the vehicle's occupants were injured.

- No airbags deployed in the vehicle containing the child safety seat.

That said, it is very important to note that not all experts agree with these criteria. The bottom line: car seat manufacturers should always be given the final say, and some recommend replacing the seat after any crash, no matter how minor. In the event that you ever find yourself in a crash, call the manufacturer. Be sure to have any involved car seats in front of you when you call so you can provide the make, model number, and date of manufacture (all found on the car seat label), along with information about the crash. The manufacturer may decide to exchange the seat for you directly or can provide you a written statement saying that replacement is deemed necessary for you to submit to the insurance company.

[a] Derived from Car seat use after a crash. National Highway Traffic Safety Administration website. Accessed April 27, 2020.

Rear Facing for the Long Haul

One of the most important concepts relating to car seats is the recommendation that all children should be kept rear facing until they reach the highest weight or height allowed by their car seat manufacturer and at least two years of age. The fact is that if we could all ride around rear facing in the middle of the back seat in a 5-point harness, we'd be a lot safer. While this situation is obviously not realistic for adults, fortunately, manufacturers of car seats have risen to the occasion. Some convertible seats now on the market have rear-facing size limits of up to 65 pounds and as high as 49 inches, affording children the opportunity to safely remain rear facing well past their second birthdays.

The reason for the rear-facing position is as follows: We know that most crashes involve frontal collisions. During a frontal collision, the crash forces are spread over a rear-facing child's entire body as she is pressed into the back of her car seat. This effect is in contrast to the effect on a forward-facing child, whose head and body are thrust forward with the full force of the crash. Recall that newborns and infants have large heads in proportion to the rest of their bodies. They lack the neck strength and the reflexes that allow older children and adults to resist whiplash-type forces, so the rear-facing position is crucial in preventing brain and spinal cord injuries. Bottom line: instead of asking, "When can I turn my baby face forward?" all parents of rear-facing infants should be asking, "When do I *have* to?"

BUT HER FEET TOUCH THE SEAT

It may seem a long way off right now, but one of the most common qualms that parents seem to have about keeping their newborns and infants rear facing is that their legs eventually grow long enough that their feet press up against the back seat. While this situation may seem somewhat uncomfortable, it should not take precedence over your goal of protecting your baby's brain and spinal cord—a goal that is best achieved rear facing. Luckily, babies and even toddlers also happen to be much more accustomed to and comfortable with keeping their legs bent than adults tend to be!

Recline

All rear-facing car seats need to be installed in a reclined position to keep babies safe. How far back, however, will depend on what your car seat manufacturer specifically recommends. Getting the seat installed at exactly the right angle (which typically ranges from 30° to 45°) can pose a bit of an installation challenge, if for no other reason than the fact that many vehicle seats aren't level themselves. Fortunately, all rear-facing seats now come with a built-in mechanism (in such a form as a dial, a ball, a fluid level, or even a horizontal line on the side of the seat) that can help guide your efforts. Many (but not all) infant-only seat bases also come with an adjustable reclining platform that can make securing the seat at the appropriate angle much easier. As a quick shopping tip, this platform is a feature we suggest you look for when deciding which seat to buy. If your baby's head still seems to flop forward, or you can't get the angle quite right despite your best efforts, be sure to contact a trained CPST for additional assistance (see Going Pro on page 238 for contact information). And remember, more of a good thing is not always better; too much recline, as well as too little, puts babies at serious risk.

BUT I CAN'T SEE HER FACE

Even though it is clearly safest to keep your baby rear facing for as long as you can, we empathize with parents who find it difficult to do so. Nevertheless, we want to stress that there really aren't many, if any, activities related to tending to your child that you can safely undertake while driving. Many safety advocates even discourage the use of back seat mirrors that allow parents to see their baby's face while driving because they inherently require drivers to take their eyes and attention off the road. Our best recommendation: if you are so inclined, sit in the back seat next to your infant while someone else drives. Otherwise, take comfort in knowing that your baby's car seat is properly installed, focus your attention on what lies ahead, and commit to pulling over to a safe spot if and when you feel that your baby's demands warrant an immediate response.

Recalls

If you are like most of the population, you rarely (if ever) fill out manufacturers' product registration cards. Once you buy a car seat, however, it is very important that you do so because supplying the manufacturer with your seat's make and model number, along with your contact information, allows them to notify you in the event of a recall. And despite manufacturers' best efforts, recalls occur. If you've already misplaced your registration card, be aware there are other reliable ways to find out about recalls as long as you remember to look: You can refer to websites or phone numbers for the National Highway Traffic Safety Administration (www.nhtsa.gov/recalls or 888-327-4236). You can also call in your car seat details and contact information to the manufacturer or submit them online, as most manufacturers also have registration capabilities on their websites.

Making Your Efforts Last

We want to emphasize that an important determining factor in keeping your baby safe is not just how secure you are able to make your car seat at installation but how secure the seat is *at the time of a crash.* All too often, well-installed seats are able to work themselves loose because they are not properly locked into place. To prevent this situation, take a look in your own car and ask yourself how you're going to get the seat belt to secure the car seat. The following advice is meant to help you figure out the answer to this lifesaving question.

And You Thought You Knew Seat Belts

Buckling your own seat belt is a task we hope you do without much thought and one that requires little effort or understanding. When installing a car seat, however, a little more thought is generally required—hence our primer on vehicle seat belts.

Lap-Shoulder Belts

If you're using a lap-shoulder belt, you'll notice it can be easily pulled out and spooled back in again on what is called a *retractor.* When lap-shoulder belts were first introduced, they could be pulled out; however, once slack was allowed to spool in, the retractor automatically locked the lap-shoulder belts in so that they could not be pulled back out again. Consumers did not like the inconvenience of these automatically locking retractors, and, as a result, we now have lap-shoulder belts that can be pulled in and out freely—that lock up only when a sudden force is put onto the seat belt. While most adults enjoy the comfort, there's a potential problem with installing car seats by using these freewheeling seat belts that have only emergency-locking retractors: they allow car seats to move just as freely as they do adults until the event of a crash.

Fortunately, two locking mechanisms have since emerged to address this problem. The first is a *switchable retractor*—one that not only affords an adult the comfort of a free-sliding seat belt but can easily be switched into the automatic-locking mode by pulling the seat belt all the way out to the end. Once this seat belt is fully tightened and set to lock, it can't be pulled back out until the seat belt is allowed to spool in completely.

The second mechanism is a locking latch plate (the metal and plastic part of the seat belt where the lap belt threads through and becomes the shoulder belt), which has the ability to lock the seat belt in place. If you have a relatively new car, it should come with either a switchable retractor or some type of locking latch plate. In the event that your car does not have either feature or you are simply unable to get them to work properly, get help from a CPST.

Getting It Right Means Getting It Relatively Tight

Once your baby's car seat is installed, you should not be able to move your baby's car seat more than an inch from side to side at the path of the seat belt or away from the back of the vehicle seat. The trick to getting seat belts appropriately but not unnecessarily tight is to first put some weight onto the car seat base (if you're using one for a rear-facing–only seat) or the car seat itself (while your baby is not in it, of course) and then give the already buckled seat belt an extra pull to remove slack. As you take your weight off the seat, it should be sufficiently secure.

LATCH

Ever since September of 2002, all new child safety seats and vehicles are required to be LATCH compatible. What does this compatibility mean? Well, LATCH stands for **L**ower **A**nchors and **T**ethers for **CH**ildren, and the driving force behind its creation was a desire to standardize the installation of all child safety seats to make it simpler and quicker and to leave less room for error. LATCH involves the use of a top tether for forward-facing seats for older children and two lower attachments that can be used to secure rear- or forward-facing car seats to universal anchor points located in the car (**Figure 22-2**). While it was initially believed that LATCH would ultimately make the use of seat belts to install car seats (and most of the preceding information in this chapter, for that matter) unnecessary, this end goal hasn't exactly been the case. In some instances, LATCH makes installation easier, but in others, correctly using the vehicle's seat belt works just as well (or sometimes even better). Either method is fine as long as you choose just one (because more is definitely not better in this case), and the end result is a well-secured seat. While a handful of manufacturers allow for both the seat belt and LATCH to be used together, at the same time, most do not, so be sure to refer to the instructions that came with your seat to make sure you get installation right. Also, check the car seat label and vehicle owner's manual for any weight limits for use of the LATCH system.

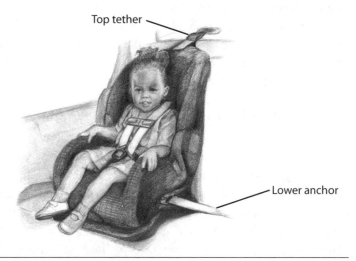

Top tether

Lower anchor

Figure 22-2. Installed seat using LATCH

Securing Your Infant

After you have put time and effort into installing your infant's car seat, it is equally important to make sure you know how to secure your infant in it. All rear-facing–only car seats come with harness straps. There are small variations between brands, but the basic principles are the same: While harness straps should be threaded through the lowest level of harness slots for all newborns, you'll notice that most rear-facing–only car seats have more than one pair of these slit-like openings. Because the harness straps must be at *or below* your baby's shoulders when she is in a rear-facing car seat, you'll want to remember to adjust the straps as her shoulders reach the level of the next opening. Some seats allow for easier adjustment of harness straps by using an adjuster that eliminates the need for harness rethreading.

Getting to the Points

All rear-facing–only car seats now come with 5-point harnesses. This feature means the straps used to secure your baby safely in the seat attach to the seat over both shoulders (2 points), over both hips (2 points), and between the legs (1 point).

Once your baby is placed into the car seat and buckled in, the harness straps should not be twisted and should be snug enough that you can't pinch any slack in the straps at the level of your baby's collarbone. Any extra slack leaves your infant more room in which to move and therefore more susceptible to injury in the event of a crash. The fastener that holds the two harness straps together is called a *harness clip* and should rest across your baby's chest at armpit level (**Figure 22-3**).

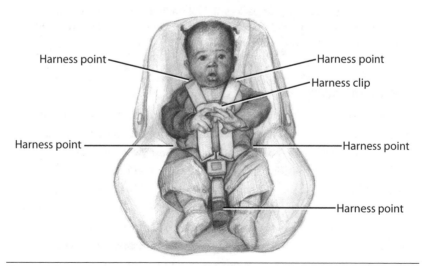

Harness point
Harness point
Harness clip
Harness point
Harness point
Harness point

Figure 22-3. 5-point harness

A Word on Accessorizing

If you look in any baby store, you'll find an impressive array of products with which to "adorn" your infant's car seat. Before you find yourself lured into buying any, there are a few safety considerations to keep in mind. Whether you've got your eye on a cute little car toy or a suction cup mirror, any items that are hard, rigid, and can't be secured well are best left on the shelf of the store or reserved for use outside the car. The reason is simple: the potential for objects to become dangerous projectiles in the event of a crash far outweighs their possible usefulness or entertainment value. In addition, some of these "adornments" can cause choking hazards. All car safety seat manufacturers do not allow use of such objects on the seat during travel, as they may reduce the safety of the seat.

UFOS: UNRESTRAINED FLYING OBJECTS

At the risk of causing you to have a flashback to high school physics, it is worth refreshing your memory about Newton's first law of motion. Quite simply, it states that things in motion stay in motion until acted on by an opposing force. Applying this concept to the context of car safety means that any and all loose objects in your car can easily become projectiles. It's well worth glancing around at what you have lying around and asking yourself what it would feel like to be hit with it at 60, 40, or even 20 miles per hour. You're likely to find that even the tissue box on your back dash looks a little more threatening in this context, and be convinced that it is well worth your time and effort to either restrain them or tuck them safely into your trunk.

Padding the Seats

Specially designed baby headrest cushions that come with a car seat may help prevent young babies' heads from flopping around in their seats and are therefore especially popular among parents of newborns. That said, you shouldn't place any additional padding (including blankets, a bunting, or winter clothing) between your baby and the back of the seat or his harness straps unless it came with the car seat, lest it interfere with the seat's ability to protect your baby. You'll be able to determine recommended use by simply reading the seat's instruction manual. If your baby's head seems to be flopping forward, see whether the instructions say to remove the head cushion. And if you feel that your baby needs another layer of warmth and your choice of clothing seems insufficient, you can secure him in his car seat first and then tuck a blanket or coat over him. If you choose to use a car seat cover that is specifically designed to fit over a car seat like a shower cap, be sure to leave your baby's face uncovered and take care to avoid overheating.

Location, Location, Location

Young Children and Front Seat Airbags

You're probably familiar with the golden rule that *rear-facing car seats should never be placed in front of front seat airbags.* As a point of future reference, neither should young children. That's because airbags deploy at such great force that they can cause serious harm, if not death, to newborns, infants, and toddlers whose car seats are placed in front of them. Granted, there are a few exceptions—such as trucks with airbag turnoff switches—but we want you to think long and hard and enlist the expertise of someone trained in child passenger safety before deciding that you qualify as an exception to this lifesaving rule.

Children and the Back Seat

It is recommended that all children younger than 13 years sit in the back seat. The reason is quite simple: because it is almost always safer than the front. While the middle of the back seat is generally felt to be the safest and most protected location in the car, not all car safety seats can or should be installed there. If the center back seat does not work, the next question many concerned parents ask is which side of the back seat is considered safer: the driver's or the passenger's? While there isn't thought to be a difference in relative safety, the passenger side often ends up being the side of choice for reasons of convenience. It's not uncommon for a rear-facing car safety seat to get in the way of the vehicle seat in front of it, and most parents would rather have the inconvenience of having to scoot the front passenger seat farther forward than the driver's. When the car is parallel parked, removing a baby from it also tends to be easier (and safer) if she's on the same side as the curb.

The Effect of Side-Impact Crash Protection

While most crashes occur at the front of the car, it's well worth noting that close to 1 in 4 crashes is a side-impact crash. Despite being less common than frontal crashes, side-impact crashes are worthy of more attention because of their increased risk of serious or even fatal injuries. While uniform, mandatory standards are not yet in place for car safety seat manufacturers to meet when it comes to testing how well their seats protect children in side-impact crashes, manufacturers and the National Highway Traffic Safety Administration are actively working to come up with them. In addition to keeping an eye out for new safety features and requirements, it's as important as ever that you focus on properly securing your baby rear facing in the back seat and check your vehicle owner's manual and car safety seat manual to determine whether the middle of the back seat is suitable, as this position is the farthest away from any potential point of side impact.

GOING PRO

As you near the end of this chapter, we hope you feel a bit more knowledgeable and confident in your abilities to keep your child safe in the car. But don't feel as if you are on your own. Now more than 43,000 certified technicians across the country are trained in child passenger safety. You can locate one in your area by simply contacting your state department of transportation, local fire or emergency personnel, or a nearby children's hospital or by looking for listings by ZIP code on the National Highway Traffic Safety Administration website (www.nhtsa.gov), SeatCheck.org, or the Safe Kids Worldwide website (https://cert.safekids.org and click on "Find a Tech"). Toll-free numbers such as the National Highway Traffic Administration Vehicle Safety Hotline (888-327-4236) and 866-SEAT-CHECK (866-732-8243) are also useful sources of information. You can also watch for local car seat checkup events advertised in your community. These services are usually offered at no cost, and just about all parents who take the time to have the techniques we've discussed presented in a hands-on setting find the experience to be invaluable.

A Little About Lots

What you, as a parent, consider to be the most convenient spot in the parking lot may no longer be determined purely by the distance from car door to store door but by what lies between. Unless you are one of the lucky few who consider valet parking or a chauffeur as viable options, here are some thoughts to ponder when parking as a parent.

- **Curbside check-in.** Whenever possible, park along the curb so you won't have to cross a busy parking lot. You'll also be able to load and unload without another car pulling up beside you.

- **Last in line.** For those of you who have never considered the option before, parking at the end of the row and away from the crowds can offer you more space for unloading and loading babies, bags, and strollers. However, be aware that others may follow suit or cut across the parking lot from any direction while you attempt to manage your goods.

- **New-parent parking.** Take advantage of new-parent parking if any of your local area merchants have been so kind as to designate special parking spaces for new parents along with their disability access and "stork" (expectant mother) parking.

- **Out of harm's way.** If you can find a spot between two parked cars that has more than squeezing room on either side, you'll be better able to keep yourself, your bags, and, most important, your baby tucked relatively safely out of the way of traffic.

- **Corralled.** Parking next to the cart corral not only allows for quick transfer of baby and goods from car to cart and back but also lets you return your cart without leaving your infant unattended or in harm's way. However, we feel obliged to add that our husbands do not like this choice of parking spots—if only because it puts the cars at risk of being bumped, dented, or otherwise damaged by stray and misplaced carts.

JUST SAY, "YES!"

In some parts of the country, "Do you want help out with that?" is a commonly asked question in grocery stores these days, second only to "Paper or plastic?" Before you selflessly decline the offer, take into account that an extra pair of hands to unload groceries will allow you to focus on securing your child in the car, and you'll undoubtedly be offered the luxury of having someone else put your shopping cart away. The safest place in the parking lot for your baby is buckled into her car seat in your car, away from other moving vehicles, so load your car in order of importance: baby and other children first, purse second, and groceries last.

Mr Carr's Words of Wisdom

Believe it or not, I (Laura) had a driver's education teacher whose real name was Mr Carr. Of all his "take home and remember until parenthood" messages, one stood out above the rest: always, without exception, walk all the way around your car before getting in and driving off. Even before children are able to crawl or walk themselves into precarious positions, the potential tragedy of an infant left in a car seat on top of or behind a car is unfortunately not hypothetical. As a rule to live by, never set your baby in front of, on top of, or behind your car. Also, look into some of the now-available vehicle safety features, including rearview cameras and sensors, that help alert you to potential danger. And if you have to set aside a stroller momentarily while getting your baby into or out of the car, consider placing it next to an open door, which will hopefully serve to keep it out of the path of any oncoming cars.

Keeping Your Wits and Keys About You

Believe us, having experienced it firsthand, when we tell you that getting locked out of your car with a hungry, crying infant can be quite a traumatic experience—one that's even more traumatic if the baby is inside the car along with the keys! Acknowledging that parenthood often makes it harder to keep one's wits about oneself, much less stick to a routine, we strongly suggest you make it a habit to always check for your keys before shutting the car door rather than randomly toss them into a purse, into a diaper bag, or onto the seat of the car.

Maintaining a Perfect Attendance Record

As parents, we've gained a new appreciation of drive-thrus (such as pharmacies, banks, and fast-food restaurants) and drive-up pickup spots (such as Target) in addition to home deliveries of groceries (such as Instacart) or meal delivery boxes, take-out food, and anything else under the sun. Sure, some of these options were convenient before we had children, but we never fully appreciated them until we were faced with all the loading and unloading involved in even the simplest—and what used to be quick—errands. It's no wonder that parents are tempted to quickly run into a store, post office, or gas station without taking their babies along with them. Before you do, stop and ask yourself whether you'd consider leaving a million dollars in the back seat of your car in plain view, even if the windows were cracked for air. Also, consider that in some states, doing so is legally considered a form of child neglect.

IN THE HEAT OF A FEW MOMENTS

The inside of a closed car on a 72°F day can reach temperatures well above 100°F in less than half an hour. In direct sunlight on a day when the temperature is in the mid-80s, it takes less than five minutes. Combined with the fact that a baby's body temperature increases three to five times as fast as an adult's, the heat of a few moments shut inside a car can lead to devastating, if not lethal, consequences.

While we don't need to tell you (although we've found all parents like to hear it) that your child is priceless, we feel obliged to reinforce for you that carjackings turned kidnappings, heat stroke, and even worse calamities can and do happen in cars where children are left unattended. It is for these reasons that we urge you never to get into the habit of leaving your baby alone in the car, however briefly. Bringing your child with you is as much a part of keeping your child safe as having a properly installed car seat!

BACK SEAT REMINDERS

As much as every parent would like to think it could never happen to them, we've all heard of infants being forgotten and left behind strapped into their car seats in the back of the car—sometimes with devastating consequences. More often than not, this nightmare scenario involves a change in routine, sleep deprivation, stress, or any of a host of other factors all too common to new parenthood. Given that it's all too easy to imagine how this out-of-sight, out-of-mind situation could occur, we strongly suggest you make use of any of the tried-and-true ways that parents remind themselves whenever they have precious back seat passengers in tow. Examples of such reminders from KidsAndCars.org, the advocacy group dedicated to keeping children safe in and around cars, include

- Keep a large teddy bear in your baby's car seat and move it to the front passenger seat whenever your baby is in the back seat as a (big) visual reminder.

- Put something you'll need for work, such as your purse, cell phone, or employee badge, on the floor of the back seat whenever you strap your baby in so that you won't ever leave the car with one but not the other.

- Make sure to coordinate with your baby's caregiver(s) and let them know whether your child won't be coming on any given day so they will call you if your baby is ever unexpectedly late or absent.

Your vehicle manufacturer or car seat itself may have other reminder or alarm features, or check out cell phone safety apps that alert you if a baby is in the back seat.

23

flying the family-friendly skies

• • • • • • •

In this age of upward mobility, a large number of new and expectant parents find themselves faced with what we consider to be an altogether new form of travel: airplane travel with a baby. As with just about every other aspect of parenting, this undertaking inevitably involves a lot more advance planning than the trips you used to take alone. In this chapter, we've included insights that apply specifically to flying with your baby—a topic we've found to be especially useful during the early weeks of parenthood when you're laden down with diapers, strollers, and car seats and still settling into sleep and feeding routines.

Timing Your Ticketed Travels

Most parents who find themselves planning airplane travel with their newborns wonder about the age at which it's safe and easiest (relatively speaking) to fly with a baby, not to mention which time of day generally works best with a newborn's "schedule." First, let us say that planning flight times around a young infant's sleeping and eating schedule is a noble idea and one worth pursuing. It's also one that does not always proceed according to plan. Even for those babies who settle into predictable routines conveniently early in life, the phrase "even the best laid plans…" comes to mind. While we have found from personal and professional experience that there isn't one right answer to the question of when it's safest and easiest to travel, newborns and young infants generally adapt fairly well to changes in sleep and eating schedules, including those necessitated by travel.

First in Flight

We have found no wiser advice than for you to take it easy on yourself after having a baby and devote your time and energy to establishing a comfortable routine. In this regard, airplane travel is not exactly conducive to rest and recuperation. Yet it is surprisingly common how often new parents end up faced with taking their newborns or young infants on an airplane. Whether you find yourself traveling by choice or because of hard-to-cancel and faraway obligations, it should be reassuring to know that healthy, full-term babies generally do just fine flying at any time after the first few weeks. Parents, however, don't always fare so well. We recommend you think through your travel plans carefully before embarking on yet another journey because setting out on your journey through parenthood is likely to require a great deal of planning and adjustment in and of itself. Especially during the time when your baby is younger than about four months old, it's worth stopping and asking yourself whether the trip you are contemplating is optional. If not, then jump right into the rest of the chapter for practical advice on how to go about flying the family-friendly skies successfully. If you're unsure, then it is up to you to decide how fatigued you are from your recent and ongoing induction into parenthood, how much you like (or dislike) to travel, what seasonal germs you stand a good chance of running into along the way, and whether your baby is likely to be accommodating. For young infants, their level of "accommodation" often depends on whether they have become relatively skilled at eating and sleeping in unfamiliar surroundings, as well as how sensitive they tend to be in response to stimulation.

FLYING PREMATURELY

While commercial airliners are pressurized and the oxygen level in the cabin is carefully controlled during flight, premature babies whose lungs are not fully developed may be more sensitive to the effects of high-altitude travel. An individual's oxygen saturation level can drop by a few percentage points during commercial air travel, so we strongly recommend you double-check with your baby's doctor before flying (or going to the mountains, for that matter), especially if your baby was born prematurely.

Unwanted Parting Gifts

Even if you're ready to take on the challenges of air travel, consider that airplanes are notorious for their close quarters—a factor that makes the spread of germs all the more likely. Even a good many adults find themselves with the parting gift of fresh colds soon after flying. As discussed in the chapter we devote to the subject (Fever: Trial by Fire on page 325), fever in newborns is more than just an inconvenience and needs to be taken seriously, requiring not only the involvement of health care providers but also the possibility of tests and treatment. In general, avoiding closed-in spaces—especially those filled with people who have the sniffles—is definitely in your baby's and your

best interest. If you fly with your baby, remember that taking extra precautionary measures such as stepping up your handwashing or hand sanitizing and
shielding your baby from any direct contact with coughing or otherwise obviously ill travelers can help minimize your baby's (as well as your own) chances
of catching whatever seasonal viruses happen to be out and about.

Sleeping En Route

Over the years, we've been asked or told about many home remedies rumored
to be effective in getting babies to sleep on planes. As nice as it would be to
have a calm, quiet, and sleeping baby throughout an entire flight, we unfortunately haven't found any ingestible remedy that we can bring ourselves to
recommend. Common sense, never mind our medical training, tells us that
giving babies even a tiny spoonful of an alcoholic beverage or a sampling of
a sedative—while often referenced in parenting humor—is a very bad idea in
real life, however tempting it may seem under duress. Use of sedating over-
the-counter children's medications (most notably antihistamines such as
Benadryl, which is more appropriately used to treat allergies and itchiness) in
hopes of inducing sleep is also not recommended for young infants because
the potential risk of serious side effects outweighs any possible benefits. For
those of you who are still tempted as your child gets older, let us also forewarn you that some children actually have the opposite response and become
hyperactive and irritable instead. If you are determined to use something to
get your child to sleep on the plane—during infancy or in the years to come—
be very sure to talk with your child's doctor about it first to confirm whether
it's safe and, if so, that you have the correct dose. Then do a trial run at home
so that you can determine ahead of time how your child will respond.

Late-night Flights

Once babies master the overall concept of sleeping in the first few months, we
have found they tend to sleep more reliably at nighttime than they do during
nap time travel. That said, before you book a cross-country red-eye, give it your
best guess as to whether your baby will actually sleep through the night if he's
on a plane instead of in a crib. Be sure to factor in whether you'll be able to
sleep as well. If you determine that both you and your baby are up for it, a late-
night flight may be the way to go. Just remember to allow for some extra time
to get yourself *and* your baby settled in safe and sound once you arrive at your
destination because the additional parenting tasks—not the least of which may
include installing a car seat and setting up a crib—can add a fair bit to your

overall travel time and resulting level of fatigue. If nothing else, having a baby along all but ensures you won't have time to sleep in after a late-night or early morning arrival, especially if your baby is well rested and raring to go.

Booking Your Flights

To Buy or Not to Buy

Yes, it's true…. The Federal Aviation Administration (FAA) still does not require the purchase of an airline ticket for any child younger than two years. We openly acknowledge that from a budgetary standpoint, this option of traveling with a "lap child" or "infant in arms" (as the airline industry calls unticketed infants and toddlers) can be financially appealing. You should know, however, that safety experts across the country unanimously agree that forgoing the purchase of a seat for your baby is not an ideal way to save money, and the FAA strongly urges parents to secure all children in an appropriate restraint—a recommendation that inherently requires they have a seat of their own on the plane. Even if it continues to remain optional for parents to purchase infants their own seats on airplanes, we strongly encourage you to save up and pay for the extra seat anyway, if at all possible. Believe us when we say we wish there was a good alternative. But knowing what we do about safety and airplane travel, we can't come up with one. Instead, we recommend getting into the habit if you aren't already of signing yourself *and* your baby up for the airlines' frequent flier mileage programs. Even though it may take a while to get to the level of a free ticket, your baby's accumulated miles (as well as your own) can ultimately help soften the blow to your budget.

Safety First

Securing your infant into a seat of her own in an FAA-approved car seat is an important step in committing yourself from day 1 to the idea that your baby's safety comes first. We're not saying you can't unbuckle to change a diaper or take care of other baby business while in flight, but be aware that turbulence—which poses the greatest safety risk to passengers of all ages—can be unpredictable. Before you set out, keep in mind that not all car seats are FAA approved for use in aircraft, and those that are may still not fit in the airplane seat if they are wider than about 16 inches. Check for an FAA-approved label on your car seat that says, "This restraint is certified for use in motor vehicles and aircraft," and check with the airline if you're concerned about whether the seat will fit. You can also go to the FAA website (www.faa.gov/travelers/fly_children) for more details.

Sitting in the Lap of Luxury

Even if you love to hold and cuddle with your baby when you're at home, you may find that doing it for an entire airplane flight is somewhat uncomfortable. Also, many babies who would otherwise be content to sit in their car seats and entertain themselves or sleep tend to have much greater expectations when they are held.

WHAT THE FAA HAS TO SAY: AN OVERVIEW OF SEAT ASSIGNMENTS

For any infant or child who is going to travel in a child restraint seat on an airplane, the following seat assignments should be considered a must:

- All car seats must be secured in a window seat.
- The exit row is not an option for anyone who has a baby as a travel companion.
- Check the width of your car seat before flying. If it is no wider than 16 inches, it should fit in most airplane seats.
- Use only a Federal Aviation Administration (FAA)–approved car seat, as indicated by a label on the seat that verifies it is FAA approved.
- Be aware that the FAA strongly recommends all infants weighing less than 20 pounds be restrained in a rear-facing car seat during airplane travel.

For future reference,

- Children who weigh 20 to 40 pounds should be restrained in a car seat and not be switched to using just the airplane's lap belt until they reach at least 40 pounds.
- There is an alternative airplane safety harness, called *CARES,* that has been approved by the FAA, but it is not meant to be used for infants. Designed for use by toddlers (22 to 44 pounds) and only on airplanes, the CARES Child Aviation Restraint System provides an alternative to a car seat, but be aware that the back part of the securing strap can sometimes interfere with the tray table of the person sitting behind the child.
- Booster seats are not approved for use during taxi, takeoff, or landing and should therefore be checked or stored overhead.

If You Don't Opt for the Extra Seat

There are those out there who would matter-of-factly tell you that if you can't afford to pay for an extra seat for your infant, you shouldn't be traveling. We, too, feel strongly about keeping children safe, but we also intend to live up to our claim that this is a book about the realities of parenting, and we know full well that not all of you are going to buy your babies airline tickets. While doing so is the only way to guarantee that your baby will be safely secured during a flight, we want to provide some tips about traveling with an infant if you haven't purchased your baby a seat.

- **It never hurts to ask.** While we're not sure about the success rate, the FAA still suggests asking your airline for a discounted infant fare. Given that purchasing a separate seat for your child is the only way to guarantee that she will have one and that you'll be able to secure her into her car seat, it's at least worth a shot. You will most likely need to contact the carrier by phone instead of trying to book a discounted ticket for your baby online.

- **Playing the odds.** Even if you haven't purchased your infant a seat, it is possible on occasion to get one. Some regularly scheduled flight times are notoriously less popular than others, leaving the potential for unfilled seats. If you will be traveling with a lap child, consider booking yourself in a window seat on one of these typically less than full flights and take your chances that there will be open seats left. When you check in at the gate, simply ask the ticketing agent whether any empty seats are still available. If so, chances are good that they will be middle seats, and you may be allowed to secure your infant's car seat in the window seat you had reserved for yourself. Then you can sit in the adjacent middle seat without paying extra. If your flight ends up being full, however, you'll be asked to check your baby's car seat and proceed with your original plan.

- **Picking a seat on a full flight.** If finding an open seat is out of the question, you'll want to decide which you think is going to be the lesser of two evils— a window seat that is out of the way but with less easy access to the aisle or an aisle seat where you'll need to pay attention to a second set of body parts (ie, your baby's) to make sure that head, feet, and limbs don't get bumped by service carts or passersby. In the aisle seat, you may also have to accommodate your middle- and window-seat neighbors' need to access the aisle.

- **Strategic adult ticketing for two.** When traveling with your baby and another ticket-purchasing companion, we suggest booking an aisle seat and a window seat in the same row. Chances are better that the middle seat between will remain unoccupied, potentially allowing you to claim it for yourself and secure your baby's car seat in the window seat as just described. If someone else gets assigned to the middle seat, you can virtually guarantee that person won't mind switching from the middle seat to an aisle or window seat, allowing you and your ticketed travel companion to sit next to each other with your baby on your lap.

- **Baby carriers.** Baby carriers (including slings) are very popular among flying parents, but they by no means offer the same degree of protection as placing your baby in a secured car seat during the flight. Besides, the FAA does not approve them for use during takeoff or landing.

Other Seating Rules, Regulations, and Recommendations

Before your days of flying with your baby, your seat preference was probably based on proximity to the front of the plane, a desire for extra legroom, or an interest in seeing the sights out the window. Not so anymore, at least for most flying parents. If nothing else, you will now be required to install your infant's car seat in a window seat so as not to block passengers from exiting the row, and opting for the exit row will no longer be a possibility. It only makes sense that families traveling with small children aren't exactly the ideal people to perform the necessary exit-row duties in the event of an emergency.

As for the choices you have when it comes to seat assignments, many parents vie for the opportunity to sit in the bulkhead row located at the front of each section of the aircraft, typically right after first or business class. These seats usually offer more room than is found between the rest of the rows and ensure that rear-facing infant car seats won't be in a position to interfere with the ability of the passenger in front of your baby to recline his or her seat. As an added benefit, you also don't have to make your way far down the aisle to reach these seats. Now that we've extolled the virtues of bulkhead seating, let us point out that the odds of getting assigned to bulkhead seats are not that great, and you will most likely have to sacrifice the convenience of stowing your diaper bag under the seat in front of you (because there's often no allotted space) and store it in the less-accessible overhead compartment instead.

If you find yourself in the likely position of considering your second choice in seat selection, you may find that there are benefits to the front and the back. Sitting toward the front of the plane is particularly useful if you're loaded down, whereas the back of the plane will get you tucked out of everyone's way once you make your way back there. That and it is often just loud enough at the back of the plane from the sound of the engines to soothe your baby with background noise or to drown out any crying for all but those sitting closest to you.

Navigating the Airport

Arrivals

As the rules of 21st century air travel changed and airport security heightened, so did the challenges of navigating the airport with an infant. Figuring out how to get everyone and everything checked in and to the gate on time takes a little more forethought these days. We've found that the easiest solution to this problem is to avoid the prospect of parking altogether and get dropped off whenever possible.

Divide and Conquer

If you end up driving yourselves to the airport, you might want to consider the "divide and conquer" approach (assuming you are not traveling solo). Drop off one adult with a photo ID and ticket in hand at curbside check-in with all the bags, including the carry-ons. This leaves the parking parent less encumbered and more easily able to park the car expeditiously and hurry back with the baby to check-in. If your parking prospects look particularly grim, you may want to consider dropping off your baby as well—especially if you don't have a stroller or baby carrier. That way, if you find yourself parking in the remote corners of the economy lot, you'll avoid the frustrating dilemma of how to secure your baby safely on the shuttle because most often, you just plain can't. The final key to success with the divide and conquer approach is to be sure to set a clearly defined meeting place in the airport before parting ways.

STATISTICALLY SPEAKING

We advise you to buckle up your baby on the way to and from the airport, as well as on the plane. The chance of injury from an automobile crash is much higher than that from airplane crashes or in-flight turbulence. Yet in some states, babies are not required to be secured in car seats when riding in the back of taxis, limos, or shuttle buses. It makes us cringe when we hear about parents taking less-than-adequate safety measures in these common travel scenarios based on the misguided reasoning that "it's just a short ride to the airport."

Checking Everybody In

Many airlines now require that infants, even those without a paid ticket, receive a boarding pass. This requirement helps with the inventory of passengers, weight estimates, and age-appropriate emergency equipment for each airplane load. Be sure to let the airline know at the time of booking and when checking in that your infant is traveling with you. You can also take advantage of membership-based time-savers: TSA PreCheck allows children 12 years and younger to accompany a parent or guardian who has the indicator on their boarding pass. Children younger than 18 may use the CLEAR lane for free when accompanied by a CLEAR member. Frequent international travelers may want to explore programs such as Global Entry or Mobile Passport for faster clearance on arrival into the United States at participating airports.

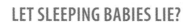

LET SLEEPING BABIES LIE?

As inconvenient as they may seem, safety regulations require that you lift your baby out of her car seat when going through security so that the seat and your baby can be properly inspected—even if your baby is sleeping contentedly. When walking through the metal detector, you may even be asked to carry your baby at arm's length in front of you to prove you are not concealing any objects between your bodies.

Leave the Pointy Parenting Objects Behind

Most adults have become quite accustomed to leaving potentially dangerous objects (tools, weapons, flammables, and even butter knives) at home. Don't forget, however, that this "absolutely no sharp objects on board the airplane" principle may apply to your baby's nail scissors and other grooming supplies as well. By substituting a cardboard emery board for a pair of sharp-pointed metal nail scissors, for example, you'll avoid having them confiscated. Fortunately, most baby supplies are not considered to be security risks. Just be aware that all carry-on baggage, including diaper bags, strollers, car seats, and any other baby items, must go through the x-ray machine, be inspected by a security officer, or undergo both measures. Check the Transportation Security Administration (TSA) website at www.tsa.gov for full details.

Ease on Down the Terminal

When making the seemingly endless trek through airport terminals with an infant in tow, it's best to make the most of modern-day conveniences such as rolling luggage, baggage carts, and your baby stroller or baby carrier. Airport luggage carts may be rented for just a few dollars by using cash or a credit card. That said, some are now conveniently available at no cost. Just be aware that in many airports, luggage carts are allowed only up to the security checkpoints, at which point parents are left to their own devices to find ways to get their belongings gracefully to the gate. In a bind, we've been allowed to use a spare wheelchair to hold carry-on bags and free our hands to hold our babies, tickets, and IDs. Just make sure to ask permission first and then leave the wheelchair at an acceptable location. If you have a long way to go to reach the gate or are really heavily loaded or especially if you have a lightning-fast layover, then by all means request to be transported by one of the airport's indoor electric carts.

Gate Checking Baby Gear

Gate checking is an option well worth knowing about as a parent. If nothing else, it allows you to use your stroller to make your way from the parking lot all the way through the airport and right up until the time you're about to set foot onto the plane. Just be prepared to collapse it or fold it up (after making sure nothing will fall out of its pockets, trays, or baskets) when you reach the security checkpoint. At the gate, you will be given a claim ticket for your tagged stroller and asked to leave it at the end of the Jetway as you board. If everything works the way it is supposed to—which it usually, but not always, does—your stroller should be waiting for you immediately outside the plane as you get off or shortly thereafter. The same holds true for car seats, should you find yourself unable to use yours on the plane, with the added benefit that the risk of damage is apparently a bit lower than if you check your car seat with your luggage at the ticket counter. We've found gate checking to be so convenient that we made a habit of checking even the small umbrella strollers that theoretically could fit into the overhead compartments for the simple reason that doing so gave us one less item (or, in Laura's case, three) to lug on board. As for the "deluxe" strollers that allow the infant car seat to attach, we found them invaluable.

GETTING THINGS ROLLING

Rolling backpacks make for a perfect example of a relatively simple but well–thought-out design that we can only assume was invented by a parent. Even if it wasn't, we recommend that you consider investing in one for use during travel. Many are big enough to hold the same amount of stuff as a rolling carry-on suitcase, but the added hands-free feature of the shoulder straps can be convenient—especially if you're going it alone.

All Aboard

Walking up to the gate with a baby and all your travel accessories should be enough to cause everyone but those we consider to be truly coldhearted to offer sympathetic glances; in some cases, assistance; and—in what has become increasingly standard across the industry—the option to pre-board. While a nice gesture, pre-boarding can at times feel more like a two-second head start than a luxury. The good news is that you have options.

- **Board last.** Your first option is to pass on pre-boarding and instead wait until last to get on the plane. This works especially well for parents who aren't going to require a lot of overhead space, who find it stressful to be solely responsible for blocking other passengers from their seats, or who simply don't relish the idea of entertaining their infants in a confined seat on the plane for any longer than necessary.

- **Send ahead or go your separate ways.** This is what we like to think of as the (relatively) hands-free option. Whether you are traveling with another adult or need to seek the assistance of an airline employee working at the gate, consider sending someone ahead with your car seat, carry-on suitcase, stroller, or any other bulky items without which you can manage until closer to flight time. The extra few minutes this is likely to afford you and your baby in the gate area instead of being stuck in your seat(s) can make a bit of a difference—especially for an awake and demanding baby.

- **Stand up for pre-boarding.** If you definitely want to get on the plane and get settled in, don't be shy about taking the airlines up on their offer to pre-board. From what we've seen during our recent frequent travels, this still seems to be parents' preferred approach.

LIGHTEN YOUR LOAD: THE SHIP AHEAD OPTION

In this day and age of restricted overhead space and checked baggage fees, not to mention the long-standing challenge of juggling both kids and cargo during air travel, some parents nowadays opt to pack a box of travel supplies and ship it ahead. Compared to checking bags, this can actually prove to be cost saving, not to mention lighten your travel load. It just takes some advance planning to make sure your package is shipped in time to ensure it arrives on schedule at your desired location. Should you choose to ship ahead, just remember to carry on any must-have items (see Carry-on Contents section on page 255).

Please Remain Seated

You already know our strong bias toward having a purchased seat for your baby. If you have followed through and chosen to buy one, or just lucked out and taken over an unused seat, by all means make sure to use it during as much of the flight as possible. Often babies decide to voice their disapproval of having to sit in a car seat loudly enough that their parents feel obliged to remove them to stop the crying. Before you give in too easily, try to treat flying in an airplane as you would a trip in the car. Just as (we hope) you wouldn't dream of setting out for a drive without first securing your infant safely into his seat in the car, use the same approach on the airplane. Your baby will be safer and you'll increase the likelihood that, as he gets older, it won't occur to him to protest about being restrained on the plane.

Dressing for Success, Not a Flight of Fancy

Those of you who are frequent air travelers are undoubtedly well acquainted with the concept of dressing for the occasion. For one, there's the unpredictability of cabin temperature. We highly recommend dressing yourself and your baby in easy-on, easy-off layers so you are prepared for whatever in-flight conditions you may find. In making your selections, remember that easy access and comfort are key—even for you but definitely for your baby. If you consider this an opportunity to show your baby off in a frilly new dress or fancy new outfit, it will quickly become apparent that function was meant to overrule fashion when it comes to infant airplane attire (and, we would suggest, the rest of childhood). Simply put, elastic-waist pants, zip-up outfits, or easy-snap crotches are far easier than either tights or button-up-the-back onesies when it comes to diaper changing—especially when you are faced with doing it in cramped quarters.

TURBULENCE

According to the Federal Aviation Administration (FAA), turbulence is the most common cause of nonfatal injury in passengers and flight attendants; about 60 people per year are injured by turbulence while not wearing their seat belts. Turbulence can occur out of the blue, at any altitude, and in any season—even in clear blue skies. We therefore join the FAA in suggesting you pay just a bit closer attention than you might have in the past to the flight attendants as they do their safety briefing, including the part about what to do when you're traveling with a child. Use an approved child safety seat, and have the whole family stay buckled up at all times unless there's a good reason to unbuckle and/or get up.

Carry-on Contents

Believe us when we say it's well worth it to pack with your baby in mind. One of the major differences in traveling with kids is that you inevitably lose claim to a significant amount of space in your carry-on suitcase—at least until several years down the road. The basic goals underlying your suitcase-stuffing efforts should be that when you're done, you will be well prepared but, at the same time, weighted down by as few carry-on bags as possible. If everything you choose to bring along as carry-on items fits easily into your bag(s), it will significantly decrease the likelihood that you will leave a trail of belongings in your wake. That said, there are quite a few supplies you won't want to board without—the most important of which we have listed for you.

- **Diapering supplies.** When it comes to changing diapers on airplanes, expect the worst and don't assume the airline will have the supplies you need. If your baby usually poops twice a day, expect the pleasure of three or four poops. And if they're usually semi-formed, expect watery, leaky ones—just because good old Murphy (and his "it's bound to happen" laws) said so. We highly recommend giving priority in your carry-on or diaper bag to plenty of extra diapers, a hefty supply of wipes (both diaper and disinfecting), and some small plastic garbage bags (grocery-store plastic bags work quite well). If you don't end up needing them, that's great, but carrying them along with you is a small price to pay for not being caught empty-handed. Remember that flight attendants should not be expected to touch or discard diapers for sanitary reasons because they are the ones handling everyone's food. You can either dispose of the diapers—sealed in a plastic bag to minimize the odor—in the lavatory or pack them in your diaper bag to toss when you land. If you run out of plastic bags, the airsick bags work well as backup. Also, consider packing a travel-size antibacterial hand sanitizer in case you are unable to get to the bathroom sink to wash your hands.

- **Change of clothing.** Think about how many outfits your baby typically goes through in a day, double it, and make room for them in your carry-on. Then consider doing the same for yourself because you aren't likely to enjoy sitting in clothes that bear the fresh stains of parenthood any more than your baby would. Also, remember to leave space in your carry-on for any extra layers you and your baby may shed during the trip.

- **Additional supplies.** You will undoubtedly know your baby well enough to know whether leaving home without a pacifier is going to spell disaster. Making room for a favorite blanket, stuffed animal, or other attachment object is also a good idea if your baby is old enough to care about these. Be sure to also tuck in an adequate supply of tissues and paper towels, and then proceed to pack anything you might want for yourself in whatever space you have left.

IN-FLIGHT CHANGING CHALLENGE

The availability of pull-down changing tables in airplane lavatories is logistically invaluable for in-flight diaper changing. Unfortunately, however, they are fairly rare. If and when there is one, it tends to be on larger planes (for obvious reasons) and may only be located in one of the plane's several bathrooms, so be sure to ask a flight attendant.

Diaper-changing table or not, diapers will inevitably need to be changed in flight. The ability to change your baby's diaper on your lap will therefore be a handy skill to master in anticipation of any airplane flight. The underlying principles are essentially the same as those described in the diapering chapter (see The Art and Science of Diapering on page 133), but a few extra considerations will make in-flight diapering go more smoothly. First and foremost, for the sake of your fellow travelers, we strongly suggest you make every effort to limit your lap changes to significantly wet diapers and save the smelly ones for the lavatory. That being clearly stated from the outset, practice laying your baby on your lap with her head resting near your knees and her bottom toward your stomach. It is a particularly good idea to use the method of slipping a new diaper under your baby's bottom before taking the old diaper off when your lap is serving as the changing table. Now more than ever, you'll also want to keep "things" covered as much of the time as possible to avoid being caught in any cross fire. Have wipes and a bag readily available for quick cleanup and sanitary disposal, and for hygiene's sake, resist the urge to use an uncovered tray table as a diaper-changing table. As a sidenote, solo lap changing is entirely possible, but an extra pair of hands sure is nice for expediting the process and reducing the likelihood of a mess. Based on the rules of airplane etiquette, however, we suggest you refrain from seeking assistance from any of your in-flight neighbors unless, of course, they happen to be traveling with you.

In-flight Feeding

As hard as it already is to eat a meal comfortably on a tiny tray table if and when you're offered one, traveling with your baby likely adds to the meal-time challenge. The first challenge is managing to eat your own meal; the second is feeding your infant in cramped quarters with the likelihood of onlookers 6 inches away. You may find that this is all the more reason to get your baby his own seat, freeing up space for your own meal and a place to secure or hold him while he's eating. Be aware that tray tables rarely, if ever, can be put all the way down flat in front of a rear- and sometimes even a forward-facing car seat.

Breastfeeding in Restricted Airspace

Breastfeeding on airplanes presents its own unique set of obstacles. If your baby's car seat is in the window seat, you are in the middle, and a complete stranger is in the aisle seat and encroaching on your shared armrest (which isn't just a hypothetical scenario), breastfeeding comfortably may seem like an oxymoron. Here are a few suggestions that can help.

- **One-sided.** If the flight is short, nursing on the side farthest away from your seatmate(s) while saving the other for later, when you get off the plane, may prove to be a realistic option.

- **At an angle.** The close quarters greatly limit a breastfeeding mother's chance of privacy. Simply angling your body so that you're facing the window before trying to breastfeed can help minimize the degree of exposure.

- **Covering up.** For the sake of modesty or convenience, it is well worth your while to wear easy-access clothing, such as a breastfeeding shirt or a loose-fitting top layer over a button-down or untucked shirt.

- **Layering.** Use your outer layer, a blanket, or even the back part of your baby carrier as a practical way of obstructing the view.

- **Stalling.** Breastfeeding in the lavatory may seem like a reasonable last resort, but suffice it to say that it generally poses a huge inconvenience for fellow passengers and isn't exactly hygienic. In other words, we don't recommend it.

In-flight Formula Preparation

Short of taking along the more expensive but ready-to-feed formula (which can really slow you down in security), the best way to have plenty of easily prepared formula on hand is to put pre-measured amounts of dry powdered formula into several of your baby's bottles and seal them with nipples and lids. As an important forethought, be sure your bottles are completely dry before putting the formula into them, as a few drops of water left inside a bottle can make the powder stick to the sides in a manner reminiscent of cement and make future bottle cleaning a more challenging proposition. Once the pre-measured powder is sealed in dry bottles, tuck the bottles into your carry-on bag (or purse or diaper bag). Whenever it's time to feed your baby, simply add the appropriate amount of room-temperature water to each bottle.

Even though airlines may offer beverage service on just about all flights, you can't count on the timing. That's not to say that most flight attendants aren't accommodating, but there are inevitably going to be times (eg, during takeoff, landing, and periods of turbulence) when they are going to be unable to respond to your baby's urgent insistence. Instead, play it safe and bring along at least one extra bottle of water of your own. Simply purchase or fill one once you get through security. That way, you won't have to worry about refrigeration, heating, or timing of beverage service to be able to appease your suddenly famished child.

GOING WITH THE IN-FLIGHT FLOW

For anyone who has traveled by air in the past two decades, you're probably all too familiar with the requirement that all fluids packed as carry-ons must be in 3.4-ounce (100-mL) or smaller containers, all of which must collectively fit into a single quart-sized plastic bag. The good news for traveling parents is that the Transportation Security Administration (TSA) now allows for baby-related exceptions. What does this mean? It means that "medically required" liquids such as medications, baby formula and food, juice, and breast milk are allowed in reasonable quantities exceeding the usual 3.4-ounce limit, and they do not need to fit into the zip-top plastic bag. The TSA advises carrying on only enough for your baby's immediate comfort during the flight (which we recommend includes a little extra in case of delays). They also advise that in addition to x-ray screening, TSA "officers may ask you to open the container and/or have you transfer a small quantity of the liquid to a separate empty container or dispose of a small quantity, if feasible." For more details and current official guidelines, please visit TSA.gov.

In-flight Troubleshooting

As frequent fliers, we often received wary looks from fellow passengers as we boarded planes with a baby (or two or three) and took our seats. We're not sure which is more stressful: being the passengers who first realize they will be seated next to someone else's crying baby or being that baby's parent(s). Fortunately for all involved, many young babies actually travel well in flight; often it tends to be the crawlers and toddlers who get antsy and upset when confined, but that's a different book. For now, we want to focus our attention and yours on some of the more predictable in-flight infant challenges.

High-Altitude Crying

Babies of all ages cry for various reasons. When this natural occurrence takes place in the space constraints of an aircraft, try to be resourceful when trying to calm your crying child. As you do, take comfort in knowing that the drone of the engines usually limits how far a crying baby can be heard, as does the near-universal use of earbuds these days. Keeping your own cool can go a long way when you're trying to soothe your baby and have to remain seated. Check the usual suspects and respond accordingly: Is your baby hungry? Wet or dirty? Cold or warm? Bored? If it's bright outside, try closing the window shade; if your baby wants a view, show her the one outside the window or in the pages of the airline's magazine. If all else fails, try not to let a few dirty looks bother you, and be assured that most people sympathize with parents of crying infants. After all, everyone was a baby once, many have had to try to quiet one at some time in their traveling past, and you're unlikely to have to face the occasional less-than-understanding person ever again.

The Ears Have It

Before we discuss ear pain on airplanes, let us first offer you the reassurance that many babies never show the slightest signs of discomfort. Until you know that your own child (and you) will be spared, however, the thought of a baby screaming because of ear pain is easily and understandably one of the most dreaded aspects of air travel. And from firsthand experience, we can tell you it tends to be all the more disconcerting when that baby happens to be your own. Any of you who have flown before know that ears can be quite sensitive to changes in pressure. Switching to pediatrician mode for a moment, this is because the outer ear is separated from the middle ear by a thin membrane called the *tympanic membrane* or "eardrum." Experiencing a difference in pressure across this membrane causes a sensation that as many as 1 in 3 passengers (children more so than adults) experiences as temporary muffled hearing, discomfort, or even pain. Unfortunately, having a stuffy nose or a head cold can increase one's chances of ear problems. For an adult, chewing gum or yawning is often all that is needed for the middle-ear pressure to return to normal and make plugged-up ears "pop." Perhaps part of the reason that babies tend to be more vocal than adults about the changing pressure in their ears is because chewing gum is simply not an option, and we have yet to meet an infant who can yawn on command. If your baby has a cold or an ear infection, discuss with your pediatrician whether you should give an infant pain reliever. Unfortunately, decongestants have not been proven to help and, in fact, are not recommended for use in infants. For children with significant ear discomfort associated with a cold, an ear infection, or both, it may simply be best, if possible, to postpone flying. If your travel plans are not flexible enough to cancel because of a cold, just be aware of your increased odds of dealing with ear pain when you hop aboard.

Sucking Away One's Sorrows

Once on board, it's useful to know that there is a practical and realistic alternative to the traditional gum-chewing approach (which, for obvious reasons, is absolutely contraindicated at this age regardless of your level of desperation) that works very well for babies when it comes to relieving ear pressure. That alternative is sucking. Pediatricians, flight attendants, and seasoned parents alike commonly suggest offering a bottle, breast, or pacifier during the times when pressure changes in the cabin are likely to be greatest—takeoff and initial descent. You'll notice we said *initial* descent, not landing. That's because the pressure change is typically most noticeable as much as a half hour or more before landing, depending on a flight's cruising altitude. The higher up you are, the earlier in the flight the descent usually starts. If you generally don't tend to notice your own ears popping and the captain doesn't announce plans for the initial descent, you can always ask a flight attendant to let you know when it would be a good idea to try to get the sucking started. If sucking doesn't cut it and your baby seems to be bothered, stay calm and try rubbing his ears and singing a soothing song. Even if you find that nothing short of reaching solid ground (and normal air pressure) works to calm him down, remind yourself that you've done everything you can and that most babies who have difficulty with ear pain on airplanes tend to outgrow it.

OUT OF EARSHOT

Airplane cabin noise varies over the course of the flight. Levels can range anywhere from 60 decibels up to about 85 (at cruising altitudes) or even 100 decibels during takeoff and landing. Using cotton balls, noise-canceling headphones, or small earplugs may help to decrease the decibel level to which your baby is exposed and, as a result, make it easier for her to sleep or relax.

These Shoes Were Made for Wearing

As you make your way through airports and on and off airplanes, one thing's for sure: you'll be very grateful for comfortable shoes. And for those of you who were recently pregnant, just when you thought you'd seen the last of swollen feet, think again. Sitting for hours on a plane is a well-known cause of sluggish blood flow and swollen feet. Also misleadingly referred to as "economy class syndrome," poor circulation and blood clots (called *deep vein thrombosis, deep venous thrombosis,* or just DVT) resulting from air travel can affect people sitting anywhere in the airplane, not just in the coach (main) cabin. As you focus your attention on changing, feeding, soothing, and entertaining your baby, conventional wisdom suggests you keep your shoes on (lest you're unable to get them back on), be sure to stretch your feet and legs frequently throughout the flight, and even consider wearing designed-for-travel, knee-high compression socks, which are readily available at most drugstores or online.

24

choosing child care: insider tips for all parents who care

• • • • • •

As you sit down and enjoy the anticipation of bringing your newborn home, the last thing that may come to mind is the thought of turning around and putting your baby's care into someone else's hands. Yet the fact of the matter is that many of us are faced with doing just that, whether our parental leaves end at six weeks, six months, or even six years. That's why we decided it was important to include this chapter on choosing child care. In addition to both of us being pediatricians who have helped parents, including ourselves, navigate the world of child care, I (Laura) also happen to have some additional and relatively unique insights to share as the nine-year owner of a 200-student educational child care center providing care for children starting as young as six weeks of age.

Finding Child Care That's Right for You

The search for quality child care is hugely important—not only for reasons of health and safety but also because whoever cares for your baby ultimately stands to play such a key role in your baby's activities of daily learning (see Activities of Daily Learning on page 177). In this chapter, we help you better understand the various types of child care, know what to look out for, and, ultimately, how to recognize high-quality care when you see it. Of course, the challenge doesn't stop there because finding good child care isn't the same thing as being able to get your baby into it!

The Early Bird Gets the Crib

If you haven't already begun your search for child care, it's safe to say that now is the time—regardless of whether you've already welcomed your newborn into your family or you're newly pregnant. One of the most compelling reasons to focus your attention on your future child care needs now—regardless of what stage of pregnancy or parenthood you're in—is simply that finding the right child care can take time, and space is often limited. Let's face it: finding an infant spot in a high-quality child care setting or finding the ideal nanny can be downright competitive, not to mention pricey. At an amount of nearly $10,000 a year, child care costs are more than double that of in-state public college tuition. In some places around the country, babies' names are put onto waiting lists months before their anticipated arrival—sometimes before parents have agreed on a name (or, in some instances, even conceived!). Regardless of whether your child care plans involve employing the watchful eyes of friends or family, care in someone's home, or a child care center, we highly recommend starting your search and making preparations as far in advance as possible. While you may find this chapter seems to focus more on center-based care, most of the principles and standards of health and safety that we share with you can (and should) be applied to all child care providers and settings.

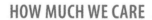

HOW MUCH WE CARE

The answer to just how many children in the United States today are in child care is simple: a majority. To elaborate, according to a US Department of Education survey released in 2016, this adds up to 60% (12.8 million) of all US children younger than six years attending some form of child care during any given week.

Who Cares?

There are several child care options from which you can choose. Here is a basic overview of each of the general types, along with some useful information about how each is structured, staffed, and regulated.

- **Child care centers.** Child care centers provide care for groups of children. They are typically defined as large or small, based on their maximum capacity. With only a few exceptions, child care centers, regardless of size, are required to be licensed by the state in which they're located. The minimum health, safety, and training requirements that must be met vary by state. While licensure alone doesn't guarantee quality, it can play an important role. Parents often turn to center-based care because there are multiple caregivers (which improves both safety and reliability) and regular inspections and because it affords additional space, equipment, and organized activities. Also of note, research has shown that children attending child care centers experience fewer injuries than those cared for at home. Prices for center-based care can vary significantly by center, location, and age of child (to give a few examples). If you are considering a church- or temple-based child care center or preschool, be aware that they may be exempt from your state licensing regulations, so be sure to carefully evaluate them as you would any other child care setting before enrolling.

- **Family child care.** In general, family child care providers offer child care services in their homes. This type of arrangement is also referred to as *non-relative home-based care.* As with child care centers, all states set minimum health and safety standards for family child care providers as well. Parents who opt for family child care are often those who find the homelike environment appealing and tend to favor the typically smaller numbers of children and single (or relatively few) caregivers characteristic of family child care. In addition, this type of care may prove to be a bit more flexible and less expensive than center-based care. Of note, children in this setting have been shown to have a higher incidence of injuries than in centers or in their own homes. While you may be tempted to choose a particular family care setting based on word-of-mouth recommendations from friends or colleagues, be aware that not all states require family child care providers to get criminal background checks or have ongoing training, so make sure you do your own checking. Also, be sure to check that any family child care provider you're considering is licensed and meets all health, safety, and care requirements.

- **In-home caregivers.** In general, this category of caregivers refers to nannies, au pairs, and housekeepers who provide care in the child's own home (although it's sometimes used to also describe what we've categorized separately as family child care in a provider's home). This type of child care isn't as well regulated and requires only minimal health and safety training. While it may seem quite pricey to enlist the services of an agency, nanny placement agencies (both local and online) typically provide extensive and very valuable services, including thorough background checks, reference checks, interviews, and more. Parents may find in-home care a more convenient arrangement than having to drop off their child elsewhere, and they are often willing to pay more for the convenience. However, the same issues of reliability and dependence on a single caregiver that arise with family-based care apply to in-home care as well. The fewer the number of caregivers, the more you'll want to have a good backup care plan in place. Also, keep in mind that in the government's eyes, hiring a caregiver means you have become a household employer, with all the many insurance, legal, tax, and payroll implications that come with it.

ACCOUNTING FOR IN-HOME CARE

Hiring someone to care for your child in your own home has some significant financial implications that are often overlooked by new, unsuspecting parents. That's because the Internal Revenue Service (IRS) requires household help—including nannies and babysitters—to pay taxes. You will need to not only take into account what sort of vacation pay or insurance coverage you're going to offer (and pay for) but factor in the government's expectations of you as well. According to the IRS, when you hire a household employee, there are a lot of things you must do, including (but not limited to) the following requirements:

- Find out if the person can legally work in the United States.

- Determine whether you need to pay state taxes.

- Withhold Social Security, Medicare, and federal income taxes.

- Get an employer ID number (often referred to simply as *EIN*).

- File and submit very specific tax forms.

To find out exactly what is involved in the process and to make sure you get it right, we strongly suggest you get informed guidance from a well-respected placement agency and/or obtain a current copy of the *Household Employer's Tax Guide* (IRS publication 926). You won't want to leave your baby at home in someone else's care without it!

- **Care by relatives, friends, or neighbors.** This type of care—often referred to as *family, friend, and neighbor care* or *kith and kin care*—is fairly self-explanatory. It's not characterized by any given location but rather by who is providing the care. Millions of families rely on this type of care. What may come as a surprise is that some states require friends and family members who are going to serve as caregivers to undergo a screening criminal history check, and several require minimal health and training safety similar to other forms of child care. Schedules, budgets, transportation, and a greater trust of friends or family members can all factor into deciding on this type of child care. While trust and familiarity can be a huge bonus with this type of care, be sure you still make it a point to sit down and discuss important aspects of your child's care to make sure you're all in agreement. While you'll certainly want to acknowledge what a great job your child's grandparents (presumably) did raising you or your partner, for example, also discuss how several important things have evolved since then—not the least of which include such important safety practices as back sleeping (see Safe to Sleep: Back Sleeping and Beyond on page 102), preventing exposure to secondhand and even thirdhand smoke, and using car seats (see Car Safety on page 219). Perhaps even share this book with them.

A LICENSE TO CARE

Of the roughly 12.8 million children younger than six years in child care, about 3 million are cared for in unlicensed and therefore unregulated settings. While not all forms of child care require a license, in general being licensed to care for children means meeting important requirements of and being monitored by a state licensing agency. While they can vary by state, according to Child Trends, licensing regulations generally include

- Health and safety measures to help protect your child from injury and illness

- Ratio and group sizes

- Background checks of adults who work in the child care facility

- Physical environment of the program

- Education and ongoing required training

- Program management

   With this information in mind, we recommend checking that the caregiver you choose for your child has a current license to provide child care services in your state.

Trust More Than Your Gut

Your gut instincts should definitely play a role in your search for someone you trust to be nurturing and provide your child with the best care whenever you aren't around. Word of mouth can also provide valuable insights. But don't stop there. Unless you take your child to a place where you are sure that all the background sleuthing has been done for you, always put in the extra time and effort necessary to ensure that your gut feeling rests firmly on additional and reassuring facts. In our book, these efforts should always include

- **Interviewing the caregiver.** Meeting potential caregivers face-to-face is critical. You get to ask your questions and gauge how comfortable you are, not only with the caregiver's answers but with the caregiver as a person.

- **Checking references.** You may feel as if you're just going through the motions, but you'd be amazed to learn what many parents (or employers) have discovered when they've called on references. Sometimes it's just the glowing feedback you'd expect. Sometimes you'll get an unexpected and eye-opening earful. Either way, at least two reference checks are a must. If you're considering a child care center, remember to ask other parents and staff about their experiences.

- **Going online.** For good or for bad, in this day and age we all have a digital footprint (see Preserving Your Child's Digital Footprint on page 374). When it comes to finding a trustworthy caregiver for your child, you'll want to make sure that he or she hasn't taken any concerning steps in the wrong direction. It takes almost no time at all to google someone or search out how one presents oneself on social media. While you certainly shouldn't rely on googling as your only screening measure, it's easy to do and can prove, at times, to be very telling.

- **Backing it up with a background check.** A nationwide background check doesn't come for free, but it can be invaluable. By working with a government or private agency, you can find out whether a prospective caregiver is listed in the child abuse or neglect registry or sex offender registry or whether that caregiver has any record of federal or state offenses. Remember, not all criminal background checks are created equal. Although all states conduct background checks as of 2012, requirements still vary considerably from one state to the next.

BACKGROUND CHECKS: WHAT YOU NEED TO KNOW

When it comes to placing your child into the care of others, it's of utmost importance that your chosen caregiver(s) check out okay. To help you have a clear understanding of how best to do this check, we share with you the following information, which is adapted from the Administration for Children & Families Office of Child Care, regarding exactly what you need to know about background checks.

Who should have a comprehensive background check?

- All adults living in a family child care home
- All child care center staff members, including directors, teachers, caregivers, bus drivers, janitors, kitchen staff, and administrative employees
- Every adult, including volunteers, who will have unsupervised access to your child
- Other adults who may come into the program and will have unsupervised access to your child, such as sports, art, or dance instructors

What are the federal background check requirements for child care providers?

Federal law requires all states to implement state and federal criminal background checks that include fingerprints of child care providers. The comprehensive background check must include a fingerprint check of the Federal Bureau of Investigation (FBI) database to ensure that providers do not have a history of convictions that could put children's health and safety at risk. In addition, potential child care providers must be checked to ensure that they are not listed as a sex offender and have not been found to have committed child neglect or abuse.

The following list has more details about the specific checks that are required. Ask your child care provider whether these criminal history checks are up-to-date for all adults who will have access to your children while they are in care.

1. An FBI fingerprint check.
2. A search of the National Crime Information Center National Sex Offender Registry.
3. A search of state registries, repositories, and databases in the state where the child care staff member lives, as well as each state where the staff member has lived in the past five years. These include the state criminal registry or repository (fingerprints are required in the state where the staff member currently lives and are optional in other states), the state sex offender registry or repository, and any state-based child abuse and neglect registries and databases.

(continues)

BACKGROUND CHECKS (*continued*)

How often must a background check be conducted?
Requests for a background check must be submitted before a provider is hired and at least once every five years.

How do I know whether the adults in my child care program have had comprehensive criminal background checks?
The federal law requires all child care providers to have a comprehensive background check. This requirement includes providers who are not required to be licensed but care for children receiving federal child care assistance. Any individual employed by a child care provider or who may have unsupervised access to children in care should have a comprehensive criminal background check. You can learn more about your state criminal background check requirements by contacting your state licensing agency.

If your child's caregiver does not have a license, ask for proof of a completed comprehensive background check. If the caregiver does not have this proof, ask him or her to complete a check, or conduct a background check yourself (contact your state police for information about how).

Qualifications and Considerations

Given all we now know about the importance of early brain development, early childhood education, and learning, we firmly believe that dedicated child care providers deserve to be treated (not to mention compensated) as professionals, and they should be well trained. The fact is that child care providers today are playing a hugely important role in shaping our children's first and very important experiences (see Activities of Daily Learning on page 177). The more education and training child care providers have, the more children have been shown to benefit.

- **A matter of degrees.** Ask whether caregivers have a degree in early childhood education or a related field, if they have done any sort of special training, and whether or not they routinely attend workshops or educational conferences. All these forms of professional development increase the likelihood that your child will be well cared for.

CDAs DEFINED

Some child care providers attain what is commonly referred to as a "Child Development Associate" (CDA) Credential. According to the CDA council, the CDA Credential is based on a core set of early childhood competency standards, and it is the most widely recognized credential in early childhood education. As of March 2016, this national credential includes several additional professional requirements.

- A minimum of a high school diploma or GED (or enrollment in a high school career and technical education program)

- A total of 120 hours of child care training in eight content areas that span everything from planning a safe and healthy learning environment and establishing productive relationships with families to emphasizing principles of early childhood learning, behavior, and development

- A total of 480 hours of experience

- Successful completion of a professional portfolio, verification visit, and CDA examination

    For more information, check out www.cdacouncil.org.

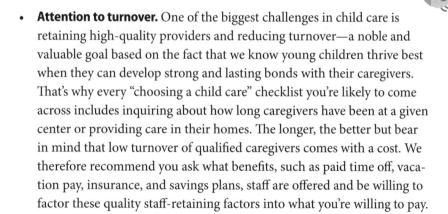

- **Attention to turnover.** One of the biggest challenges in child care is retaining high-quality providers and reducing turnover—a noble and valuable goal based on the fact that we know young children thrive best when they can develop strong and lasting bonds with their caregivers. That's why every "choosing a child care" checklist you're likely to come across includes inquiring about how long caregivers have been at a given center or providing care in their homes. The longer, the better but bear in mind that low turnover of qualified caregivers comes with a cost. We therefore recommend you ask what benefits, such as paid time off, vacation pay, insurance, and savings plans, staff are offered and be willing to factor these quality staff-retaining factors into what you're willing to pay.

- **Accreditation.** Child care accreditation generally indicates a greater commitment to health, safety, and the provision of high-quality care, as the voluntary standards required for accreditation typically exceed those required for licensure. The two largest organizations that provide child care accreditation are the National Association for the Education of Young Children (NAEYC) and the National Association for Family Child Care (NAFCC).

Child Care by Numbers

There are several important numbers you'll want to take into account in your quest for quality care.

- **Ratios.** If this is your first introduction to this all-important concept, *ratios* in child care simply refers to the number of children for which any particular caregiver is responsible. For example, one caregiver caring for one baby would give you the appealing ratio of 1:1. In general, the fewer children per adult, the better because young children thrive on lots of attention and require a lot of care. That said, unless you go the route of a personal in-home nanny or caregiver, your baby will most likely be sharing his caregiver's attention with at least two or three other infants. While a 1:3 ratio (one adult caring for three babies) is considered ideal, 1:4 is a more likely scenario, even in "high-end" centers. As you set out on your search, be sure to ask (and observe) how many babies are watched by a single adult.

- **Group size.** In the case of group size, bigger isn't better. Even if the overall ratio of adults to children is appropriate, younger children do better in smaller groups. In other words, an infant room that limits the group size to 8 babies (with 2 caregivers) is likely to be calmer and safer—and therefore considered better—than one that has the same 1:4 ratio but 3 teachers and 12 infants.

- **Cost.** No discussion of child care numbers is complete without a discussion of the cost of child care. While this is a broad subject that is affected by a whole host of other factors (including geography and type of care), in the context of ratios and group sizes, the reality is that fewer children and more dedicated staff members come at an expense. As you consider your options, it is important to keep in mind that all the numbers in the child care equation have to add up: if you want lower ratios, you'll undoubtedly pay more for them.

RECOGNIZING QUALITY WHEN YOU SEE IT

While a lot has been speculated, said, and written about how parents should go about determining which child care is best, research offers us a closer look at which characteristics, when put to the test, actually serve as the most reliable indicators of quality. Quite simply, if a child care provider or center consistently meets the well-defined guidelines listed in this box, children in their care are more likely to be safe and healthy.

- Appropriate supervision at all times and positive, consistent discipline

- Nurturing care

- Low staff to child ratio and group size

- Frequent handwashing and safe, hygienic diaper-changing techniques

- Qualified director and teachers who understand the needs of children and participate in ongoing staff training

- Well-established policies regarding safe storage and administration of medications, as well as immunization requirements

- Emergency plans that include regular fire drills and a reliable method of contacting parents in the event of an emergency

- Safety as a clear priority, as evidenced by such features as safe storage of any toxic substances and a safe outdoor playground

If you are interested in more detailed information, you can go to the Child Care Aware of America website at www.usa.childcareaware.org.

Health and Safety Considerations

Just about everything we've included in this book regarding your newborn's health and safety applies to not only you but *anyone* who will provide care for your baby. While the principles are generally the same, there are some health and safety topics specific to child care that we want you to be familiar with ahead of time.

In Sickness and in Health

Some of the concerns and fears we hear most often about child care pertain to germs and recurrent illnesses—the first signs of which can send child care–dependent parents into a panic. That's why we want to give you a healthy perspective on this topic. First, let us say that what you've heard is probably true: children who attend child care often get exposed to more germs and, as a result, get sick more often—by some estimate, on the order of 7 to 10 times a year, with more illnesses occurring during germ-sharing (cold and flu) season. It's worth noting, however, that this is a result not just of child care but of being around lots of other young children. Let's face it: young children (and even some adults) just can't be relied on to keep their germs to themselves. That said, there are definitely things that can be done to limit the spread of germs in child care, not the least of which is frequent handwashing (especially before eating and after wiping noses, playing outside, and taking trips to the bathroom or diaper-changing table), routine cleaning of toys, and well-defined exclusion criteria for when children (and their caregivers) are too sick to attend. Be sure these types of measures are in place and enforced. Also, take some comfort in knowing that children who've attended child care have also been shown to get sick less frequently when they get to elementary school.

Safe Sleep in Child Care

Safe sleep is something you'll definitely want to discuss before entrusting anyone to put your baby down to sleep. That's because all the infant safe sleep and sudden infant death syndrome (SIDS) prevention recommendations (see The Reality of SIDS: Creating a Safe Sleep Environment on page 103) pertain as much in the setting of child care as at home, if not more so; although nearly all (47) states have any sort of requirement that babies be put to sleep on their backs at child care centers, only 33 states require back sleeping in group child care homes. We feel obliged to emphasize this point because research suggests that infants in child care are disproportionately at risk for SIDS. Before you panic, rest assured that this is not an inherent risk of the child care setting itself but rather of inappropriate positioning of babies on their bellies who are accustomed to back sleeping at home. Our sound sleep advice: be certain that any and all of your child's caregivers are trained on and follow the exact same back sleeping and safe sleep recommendations (ie, those recommended by the American Academy of Pediatrics) that you do. This consistency really matters because if babies have parents who diligently put them to sleep exclusively on their backs only to have caregivers put them to sleep on their tummies for the first time, these previously unaccustomed belly sleeping babies have been found to be at significantly greater risk for SIDS.

Food for Future Thought

Having dedicated our time to writing an entire book called *Food Fights: Winning the Nutritional Challenges of Parenthood Armed With Insight, Humor, and a Bottle of Ketchup,* we are clearly committed to focusing attention on the expansive subject of childhood nutrition. For the time being, let us just say that in child care, what's on the menu matters. Even though solid foods may seem a long way off, just remember that it will be as important for your baby's other caregivers to pay careful attention to how much, how often, and what your child eats as it is for you. Nutritious meals and planned menus, along with attentive caregivers who routinely hold babies to feed them and staff members who sit to eat family style meals with older children, add up to a healthier feeding and overall more nurturing environment for your child.

Playing It Safe Outdoors

While the thought of your baby running, jumping, and sliding may admittedly seem a long, long way off, playground safety should nevertheless be on your radar screen as you set out to select a safe child care center. While playgrounds are vitally important in offering plenty of opportunity for physical activity and outdoor play, they are also one of the highest risk areas for injuries. For now, we'll simply say that sturdy playground structures, safe surfaces, good supervision, clean age-divided play areas surrounded by fences, and developmentally appropriate equipment are all worthwhile considerations.

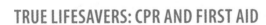

TRUE LIFESAVERS: CPR AND FIRST AID

Consider CPR (short for *cardiopulmonary resuscitation*) and first aid training to be an absolute must for anyone who cares for infants and children—yourself included. While states may require child care providers to have CPR certification and first aid training, be aware that in some states, only one trained caregiver is required to be present at any given time. We recommend you not only ask how many caregivers have completed CPR and first aid training but check to make sure that all certifications are current. Also, inquire about what sort of backup plan is in place if those who are certified are going to be absent.

SECTION

just for the health of it

· · · · · · ·

introduction

• • • • • • • •

No newborn parenting book worth its weight in diapers would be complete without an explanation of the most common medical aspects of newborn care, including a basic overview of the working parts, important signs of illness, and things you can do to keep your baby healthy. The fact that we are both parents and pediatricians puts us in the advantageous position of understanding what you likely want to know about ensuring the health and well-being of your precious new baby. For most new parents, this begins with the simple yet sometimes bewildering task of anticipating what you'll need and appropriately stocking your medicine cabinet with the necessary tools of the newborn parenting trade.

WHAT'S IN YOUR CABINET?

Stocking your medicine cabinet in anticipation of your baby's arrival will give you some extra peace of mind that you are well prepared to tend to whatever you may be faced with—from tiny toenails to first fevers and stuffy noses. While there are no hard-and-fast rules about what constitutes a well-stocked medicine cabinet, here's our streamlined list of suggested staples (with more detailed descriptions of their appropriate use included later in this section).

- **Baby nail clippers.** Adult-sized clippers are not advised. Emery boards are a worthwhile alternative or addition.

- **Cotton balls or swabs.** We can think of numerous uses.

- **Thermometer.** And yes, we mean the rectal kind.

- **Fever reducers.** Not to be given lightly, and it's definitely good to be prepared by having acetaminophen (eg, Tylenol) on hand for first fevers. Be aware that ibuprofen (the fever-fighting ingredient found in brands such as Advil or Motrin) is typically not recommended until six months of age.

- **Medication syringe.** Useful but not mandatory because infant medications come with measuring devices.

- **Nasal suction and saline drops.** It's best to avoid overuse of nasal suction devices, but when these are used appropriately, stuffy noses don't need to leave you feeling helpless.

- **Diaper cream.** Can wait but is certainly convenient to have on hand and likely to get used eventually.

- **Petroleum jelly.** Multipurpose, safe, and bound to be used on various occasions.

We also offer you the most pertinent medical information pediatricians want all newborns' parents to be familiar with before they head home—most notably, fever and jaundice. Having already included the obligatory disclaimer that we cannot and should not take the place of your own pediatrician, and having read far too many superficial checklists online and in parenting magazines on how to find your baby the "perfect" doctor, we decided to include this section of *Heading Home With Your Newborn* in order to offer you some more in-depth and practical insider advice. This includes how best to pick a health care provider you will be happy to call your very own and work in partnership with for at least the next 18 years!

CHAPTER

25

finding the right baby doctor: a view from the inside out

• • • • • •

As pediatricians and parents, we wholeheartedly agree with the current trend in which parents "interview" pediatricians to find the one who best suits them. After all, you can expect to pay a visit to your chosen health care provider at least 6 or 7 times during your baby's first year—and that expectation is taking into account only the standard number of well-baby visits (also known as *health supervision visits*)! It's worth starting out on your "mission" to find just the right one by keeping in mind that pediatrics, just like parenting, isn't always an exact science. When it comes to the art of pediatrics and parenting, you will undoubtedly come across a wide range of styles and opinions on what's best—whether you're discussing use of antibiotics, feeding, approaches to colic, or how to handle sleep problems. Beyond finding someone who is well trained in the science of pediatrics, it is to your advantage to make sure that the person (or group of professionals) you choose shares your personal parenting philosophy and style.

Your Quest for the Best

We have every intention of including the specifics of what you can and should look for in your search for the "perfect physician." Before we do, we thought we'd toss in a little reality check: there's no such thing. Perfect isn't possible because physicians are people too, and to date, we have yet to meet a person—ourselves included—without quirks and flaws (real and perceived). Just like everyone else, doctors have good days and bad. Some are superb communicators, and others are men and women of few words.

Some have families and children; some don't. Some have breastfed, while others don't have breasts (which, for clarification, is not a commentary on breast size but on the difference between the presence or absence of a Y chromosome). Some work part-time, while others put in unbelievably long hours and take calls 24/7. Yet none of these traits alone guarantee you that you've found a model of pediatric perfection. Instead, we recommend that you first take all of them into account and then factor in personality so that you end up finding someone you can really relate to. Remember, the doctor that seems perfect in the eyes of other parents may not be at all right for you. On a personal note, one of the hardest parts about beginning in private practice after finishing our pediatric training (aside from being bombarded with questions to which we were never taught the answers and trying to stick to some semblance of a schedule) was coming to grips with the fact that not everyone who came to see us was going to like us or our parenting approaches or our pediatric advice. Over time, we came to realize that it's just plain unnatural to see eye to eye with everyone—whether you're a parent or a pediatrician! The key is finding a good fit for everyone involved.

Let the Search Begin

The second or third trimester is an ideal time for you to start considering whom you want to serve as your baby's health care provider. Ask around to find out who in your area is well-liked, well trained, and conveniently located. You'll find that in addition to friends, neighbors, and family members, obstetricians are often a great source for recommendations. So are the nurses in labor and delivery and the newborn nurseries, many of whom interact with area pediatricians regularly and know which ones are the most skilled and which have the best bedside manners.

Choosing Among Health Care Providers

You will find that we tend to refer to babies' health care providers as *pediatricians* in this chapter and throughout the book as a matter of convenience. It's important to note, however, that several types of health care providers are qualified to care for babies and children.

- **MD and DO.** If doctors have an MD (short for *medical doctor*) after their names, it simply tells you that they attended a traditional medical school. Others have the initials DO (short for *doctor of osteopathic medicine*) after their names—a designation that tells you they are graduates of osteopathic medical schools. These medical schools train physicians, and both types of doctors can go on to do pediatric residency training, or specialization in the care of children. While there are some differences between these types of physicians, both are educated about normal human health and disease conditions.

BACKGROUND CHECK: THE AMERICAN ACADEMY OF PEDIATRICS

Now is as good a time as any to familiarize yourself with the American Academy of Pediatrics (AAP) because you're bound to come across this name (or these three letters) at just about every turn in your search for reliable information and all-around parenting enlightenment. The AAP is a professional organization of 67,000 primary care pediatricians, pediatric medical subspecialists, and pediatric surgical specialists throughout the United States, Canada, and Puerto Rico. If you happen to spot the letters *FAAP* after a doctor's name, they tell you that the doctor is a Fellow of the AAP—a title bestowed on pediatricians who pass the pediatric board examination (which we can tell you from personal experience is no cakewalk) and "made an ongoing commitment to lifelong learning and advocacy for children." As the authoritative source on health and safety issues for children, the AAP has the mission to attain optimal physical, mental, and social health and well-being for all infants, children, adolescents, and young adults. You can find out more about the AAP at www.aap.org, as well as find a wealth of pediatric and parenting information at the official AAP website for parents, HealthyChildren.org.

- **Board-certified pediatrician.** Board-certified pediatricians are physicians who have graduated college, completed 4 years of medical school, and have at least 3 years of on-the-job hospital- and office-based training (residency) in pediatrics. To become board-certified, pediatricians must also pass a rigorous examination given by the American Board of Pediatrics. To remain board-certified, pediatricians have to maintain ongoing education in pediatrics, demonstrate quality patient care, pass a general pediatrics board examination every 10 years, and hold a valid medical license. These certification requirements help ensure that certified pediatricians (including specialists) have sufficient knowledge and skills to provide quality care for children of all ages and adolescents.

- **Family physician.** Family practice doctors can be either MDs or DOs and, like pediatricians, also complete medical school and at least 3 years of on-the-job training in a family medicine residency. Like pediatricians, family physicians must also pass an examination and meet several criteria to become board-certified or renew their board certification. Unlike pediatricians, however, family physicians do not limit their practice to the care of patients from birth through adolescence. As their titles imply, they care for patients of all ages, including adults.

- **Nurse practitioner.** In some instances, you may find that your baby is scheduled to see a pediatric or family nurse practitioner. These health care providers are registered nurses with additional education. Those who specialize in pediatrics generally have specific advanced training in caring for children. Nurse practitioners may work in your doctor's office in conjunction with or under the supervision of physicians. While they are allowed to prescribe medications and to request medical services in all 50 states, the degree to which they can do so independently varies by state.

- **Physician assistant (PA for short).** Physician assistants complete 3 years of graduate-level training and hold a national certification and state license(s). They are able to make diagnoses and treat patients, but each individual physician assistant's scope of practice varies, as determined by state laws and the assistant's supervising physician.

Whomever you choose, make sure the professional has the training and experience to offer guidance on the health- and illness-related matters you may encounter—many of which are unique to childhood.

The Selection Process

Once you have found one (or a few) possible doctors, call the office(s) to see whether it is possible to schedule a prenatal or "meet the doctor" visit. You might want to also ask whether the visit is offered free of charge (because some doctors' offices charge a fee) or see whether it's covered by your insurance. While just about all parenting books, magazines, and posts we've read suggest bringing along a standard set of questions for the doctor, we have found that most parents are left not knowing exactly what to do with the answers. Furthermore, you may find that the specific answers you get are less important in your decision-making process than the physician's personal style and whether you felt like you clicked. Having said that, if you still feel the need to follow a checklist, we have included several points to consider under each commonly asked question that follows. Remember that you are not necessarily looking for the smartest doctor in your area, or the one with the most patients, but one who bases medical decisions on the best available information and, at the same time, is a good match for you, your family, and your parenting style. If at any point you feel this physician-patient relationship is not a good fit, even after you've already brought your baby home, we encourage you to discuss your concerns with your doctor and, if need be, to find another one.

The Issue of Insurance

Q **Does your office accept my insurance?** This question is worth asking even before you set up an interview because the reality of managed health care these days is that your insurance carrier may well dictate which physicians and practices you can take your child to and which ones you can't.

A Given the ever-increasing costs associated even with routine doctor visits, parents rarely decide it's worth going outside the system and paying out of pocket to see a particular doctor. With the uncertainties of what will happen with health care reform at the time we are writing this book, we strongly suspect that knowing what your costs and coverage will be up front will continue to be useful to you. Some parents also find it more convenient, more cost-effective, or both to explore concierge, subscription, and cash-only practices.

WE'VE GOT YOU COVERED

As you plan for the arrival of your newborn, don't forget to check with your insurance company to find out what you need to do or submit to have your baby added to your insurance policy. Then just be very sure to have any and all necessary forms submitted within the required number of days after your baby is born (usually 30 days, but first double-check and then follow up)—a crucial task you will not want lost in the shuffle of new parenthood.

How Privileged Is Your Professional?

Q Do you have hospital privileges at the place where we plan to deliver?

A While this information is worth knowing, we've found that it rarely factors into a parent's decision about your baby's health care provider unless the parent feels very strongly about seeing that particular person in the hospital. If you decide to take your baby to a health care provider who does not have hospital privileges where you plan to deliver, your baby will still be seen and evaluated by a qualified physician at the hospital. At discharge from the hospital, you can proceed to arrange all your well-baby visits with your chosen professional.

Q Where do you admit infants and children in the event that they require hospitalization?

A The answer to this question is important only if you or your insurance company has a strong preference for one hospital over another because your pediatrician will naturally admit your child to the hospital at which that physician has privileges. Some physicians have privileges at multiple hospitals, which may give you some flexibility. Others refer to hospital-based physicians (commonly referred to as *hospitalists*) whenever one of their patients needs to be admitted.

Asking About Availability

Q What are your office hours and location(s)?

A While you're probably like most parents in that you'd be willing to drive to the ends of the earth for your newborn, chances are good that when given the choice, you'd rather not have to drive across town, much less all over creation, every time your baby needs to see the doctor. As with nearly everything from real estate to diaper pails, location will most likely play some role in your decision. You'll also want to find out whether the practice you're considering has office hours that actually suit your needs. If your schedule is flexible, extended hours may not be such an important factor. For those of you who can barely make it to the bank during banker's hours, much less set up camp in your doctor's waiting room on a workday, you may want to look around for a practice that offers weekend hours or stays open late on weekdays. Also, find out about the parking situation, whether it's paid or free, so that you're not stuck driving around or searching for a spot if there isn't a dedicated lot.

Q **How does your office handle scheduling appointments, answering patient phone calls, and after-hours emergencies? How difficult is it to get an appointment for a sick visit? For a routine checkup?**

A We don't feel it's necessary to cross doctors off your list simply because they are not always available to answer your questions personally and timely in the middle of a busy workday. You'll just want to make sure that qualified members of their staff are ready, willing, and able to help you during regular business hours. The office should have a well-defined mechanism to contact the doctor and clear instructions as to where to go in the event of an after-hours question or emergency. Again, this is some good basic information to have about your chosen or considered practice, but it's not likely that you'll be told something that makes you decide to look elsewhere. In reality, you're more likely to find out after you've started going to a particular practice whether your wait time is repeatedly and unacceptably long, whether you're able to get advice by phone or schedule appointments relatively easily, and whether you're happy with the overall workings of the office.

Q **Is timeliness next to godliness?**

A Here's what we can tell you from personal experience: being a punctual pediatrician is much easier said than done. That's because pediatricians never know how long any one visit is going to take until they are in the room. This uncertainty makes scheduling a best-guess attempt. Having said that, factoring a doctor visit into what is likely to be your own less-than-predictable and very demanding schedule is not any easier. So you and your doctor should each do your best to show up on time yet be willing to cut each other some slack every now and then in acknowledgment of the strenuous jobs you both have. That said, if your doctor routinely runs late—not just 15 to 30 minutes every now and then but regularly more than an hour—it's worth considering whether something is wrong with the way appointments are scheduled.

Tricks of the Scheduling Trade

To give you your best shot at avoiding the pediatric practice rush hours, traffic delays, and peak travel days, we suggest the following tips:

- **Be the first out of the gate.** Ask for the first appointment of the day, or pick a time right after lunch whenever possible. These are the times when things are less likely to have backed up. We have no insider knowledge to share with you about how to avoid days when your doctor arrives unexpectedly late from making rounds at the hospital in the morning or runs late despite working through lunch; in those situations, all bets are off.

- **Schedule midweek.** Mondays and Fridays are notoriously busy in the doctor's office because parents come on a Friday in anticipation of a weekend without convenient access or as soon as they can on a Monday after going it alone with a sick child over the weekend.

- **Avoid holidays, vacations, and predictable events.** Rush-hour traffic on the road may slow down considerably on national holidays and during vacation times, but this slowdown is often a time when parents can opt to bring their kids into the doctor without having to take a day off from work. It's not that you shouldn't set out to visit your pediatrician on, say, Presidents' Day; you are just not likely to be alone. On holidays when your doctor's office is open, hours may be reduced and they may be short-staffed—both factors that increase your likelihood of a longer wait. For future reference, there also tends to be a bit of a mad rush at the end of the summer, when kids all but flood in for mandatory school physical examinations and immunizations.

- **Anticipate extended visits.** If you anticipate needing extra time with your baby's doctor, ask whether you can be scheduled additional time for the visit. Consider taking the last appointment of the day when your doctor won't feel the pressure of lots of other patients stacking up behind you.

Training and Experience

 What is your training background and level of experience?

 Our first response to you on this question is to figure out how much you really care. As practicing physicians, we all have diplomas hanging on our walls and have had to go through the careful scrutiny of the state licensure board before hanging a shingle. And to be board-certified in pediatrics, everyone has to pass the same test and meet the same requirements regardless of where they trained. Some new parents conclude that the older and more experienced a pediatrician, the better. Plenty of others, however, find themselves interested in taking their babies to someone younger who they feel shares more of their contemporary attitudes or perhaps has children of a similar age.

Going Solo?

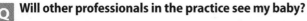 **Will other professionals in the practice see my baby?**

This is a legitimate question, and it shouldn't surprise you if the answer is yes. While still a fair number of solo practitioners are out there, there has been a definite trend toward group practice. If you are considering a group practice, you may be better off by asking how many days a week the professional you're interested in seeing works and whether you'll be able to request visits with that person whenever that person is in the office. Given that pediatricians are just like everyone else and occasionally take days off, get sick, or go on vacation, you'll also want to make sure you are comfortable with the other professionals in the group who will take over when yours is not available.

Seeing Eye to Eye

What is your philosophy about particular medical treatments or parenting strategies such as circumcision, use of antibiotics, spanking, or potty training? What is your approach to breastfeeding? Sleep problems? Colic?

If you don't have strong feelings about child-rearing or definite opinions regarding your child's medical care, you'll be able to focus your attention on other factors, such as those just listed, when you are selecting a pediatrician who will be the best fit for you. More often than not, however, parents and pediatricians alike have strong feelings about certain approaches to raising children. If you are dead set against using formula or pacifiers, for example, you will definitely want to find out which professionals in your area are the most supportive of and experienced in the practicalities of breastfeeding. For certain topics for which the research and science are well established, such as the importance of immunizations, be aware that some pediatricians may find it difficult to support or even accept into their practices families who choose to go against well-established guidelines.

Personal Characteristics

Your search for a pediatrician need not be entirely scientifically based or logical. It is perfectly reasonable to also take into account personal qualities in your quest. Depending on your own comfort level or the gender of your child, you may prefer a male pediatrician instead of a female (or vice versa). It may be a priority for you to have your child treated by someone who has firsthand experience as a parent, shares your cultural or religious background, or has an authoritative style instead of a more laid-back, collaborative one (or again, vice versa).

A Room of One's Own

It's worth discussing the feature of separate waiting rooms (separating patients who are sick and those who are well) if for no other reason than because it seems to have become standard for parenting books and magazines to recommend finding a practice that has them. We wholeheartedly agree that in an ideal world (or at least in an ideal doctor's office), it would be very nice to keep those who happen to be coming to the doctor because of an illness away from those who have yet to catch one—especially when those who are well include you and your baby. We want to point out that it's not exactly realistic to think you can successfully dodge all illnesses—in or out of the doctor's office. After all, people tend to be most contagious *before* they develop symptoms, and we all live in a world full of bacteria and viruses. To be honest, we've never actually known a parent to choose a practice because it had one waiting room instead of two. In our experience, parents are usually more concerned with how long they have to wait to be seen than where.

Our thoughts on the matter: ask whether it's possible for you and your newborn to wait in an empty examination room if the waiting room arrangement doesn't allow for separation of sick children from well children. Other than that, we suggest using common sense just as you would when you are taking your baby out anywhere in public: limit the amount that others are allowed to come in direct contact with him, shield him from the direct line of fire if someone nearby is coughing or sneezing, and use criteria other than architectural design to determine whether a particular pediatrician or practice is right for you.

WAITING ROOM WISDOM

The last thing you want to come away with after a doctor visit is a parting gift of germs you didn't come with. That's the rationale behind guidelines from the American Academy of Pediatrics (AAP) that are focused on minimizing the spread of an illness in pediatricians' offices. In addition to the usual hand hygiene and cough or sneeze etiquette that should be used in any public setting, the most recent AAP recommendations suggest

- Keep 3 feet of separation between patients who are sick and those who aren't (6 feet for those with underlying conditions that make them more at risk, such as cystic fibrosis).

- Minimize the sharing of objects such as toys, especially those that are difficult to clean.

Our advice is to simply bring your own forms of entertainment to keep yourself and your kids occupied during doctor visits, which can be predictably unpredictable in length.

In the End

When it comes to the bottom line and making a decision, we hope we've persuaded you that there's more than one "right" answer to each question and that you are well equipped to figure out your own right answers. When all is said and done and you've weighed all your choices, remind yourself that while you're not exactly searching for a new best friend, you certainly want to find a doctor whose style best suits your needs and is going to be a supportive partner in your exciting and educational journey through parenthood.

26

head to toe and in between

· · · · · ·

Ever wish that parenthood came with a tour guide and your newborn came with an instruction manual? Given that we are determined to serve as helpful tour guides and this book is, in many ways, meant to play the role of an instruction manual, we certainly don't want to neglect any of the nuts and bolts of baby care. This chapter is an up close and personal look at all the involved parts—a handful of which are unique to the newborn period, such as the shriveled up umbilical cord and the soft spot on top of every newborn's head. Others we discuss not because they would otherwise be unfamiliar to you but because the context has changed. Chances are good that you've never paid so much attention to or been solely responsible for someone else's fingernails, tear ducts, or nose before. In the spirit of arming you with useful baby body basics, let's get started with the head-to-toe tour.

From the Beginning: How Far Things Have Come

A Quick Glance Back

You may find that part of the wonder of your beautiful new child is trying to comprehend just how he or she could possibly have come to be—not just the birds and the bees stuff but the fact that a single fertilized egg can grow and develop into a newborn in a matter of a few short months. When you think about it, becoming a parent is nothing less than miraculous. Yes, we know that referring to the many long weeks of pregnancy as "short" may lead you to question whether we've actually experienced the joys of pregnancy before, but we assure you we have. It's just that in the grand scheme of things, the reality of what was once a microscopic blur now taking the form of a newborn represents the fastest rate of growth that we as humans ever experience over the course of our entire lifetimes.

As you prepare yourself for what lies ahead, here's a quick look at how far you and your baby have come or, for those of you reading this in anticipation, how far you stand to go.

- At 4 weeks: Your baby probably measured no more than a large grain of sand.
- At 9 weeks: Your baby is about the size of an olive.
- At 14 weeks: About the size of a fist.
- At 24 weeks: Around 1 pound.
- At 32 weeks: Half his or her ultimate birth weight.
- At birth: Your baby is an average weight of 7½ pounds and roughly 20 inches long.

Sizing Up the Situation

Many parents are greatly relieved to find out that it is perfectly normal for just about all newborns to lose some amount of weight—typically 5% of birth weight for those who are formula-fed and 7% for breastfed. This characteristic weight loss tends to be more pronounced in newborns who are breastfed (see Breastfeeding on page 5) than for those who are bottle-fed—sometimes reaching as high as 10% of birth weight before they start gaining it back. In either case, all newborns are expected to turn the corner, stop losing weight, and start gaining back ounces all within the first week or so, a turning point that should result in newborns ultimately regaining or exceeding their birth weight by two weeks of age. Monitoring day-to-day weight changes (and even comparing before- and after-feeding weights) serves as a relatively good indicator of whether newborns are getting enough to eat. You'll therefore find that your baby's pediatrician pays close attention to your baby's day-by-day numbers in the hospital and in the days after discharge. This will be especially true while you are waiting for your milk to "come in" and if your newborn gets off to a sleepy start, is uninterested in eating, or is simply a poky eater.

"Parts Is Parts"

Taking It From the Top

As you've undoubtedly noticed, newborns have little to no head control, at best mustering up their resolve to briefly pick up or turn their heads. In part, this is because it requires a fair bit of strength, and the muscles involved simply need time to develop. Babies also have another factor working against them when it comes to holding their heads up high, and that is their heads' sheer size. While your baby's head may not seem all that big to you, take a moment and compare it to the size of the rest of his body. Now make the same comparison between your own head and body. Your baby's head is proportionately much bigger, making him unquestionably top-heavy. On a practical note, we thought we'd point out a point of parental interest: newborns' big heads don't require extra attention just by new parents. Clothing manufacturers have also taken note and figured out how to accommodate them as well, designing infant clothing with expandable and stretchy wide collars or adding snaps, zippers, or buttons to narrow necklines.

WEIGHT LISTS AND HEIGHT PREDICTIONS

In the first few days, most newborns lose several ounces but usually no more than 10% of their birth weight. That means a baby who weighs 7 pounds at birth may well drop the scales instead of top them, reaching a weight as low as 6 pounds 4 ounces or so before turning things around.

In the first few weeks, babies gain up to an ounce per day or as much as a pound per week.

Subsequently, a baby is likely to double her birth weight by 4 months of age and triple it by the time her first birthday rolls around.

For the sake of looking ahead, it is possible to roughly estimate a boy's adult height by simply doubling his height at 2 years of age. For a girl, double her height at 18 months. You can also calculate your child's *mid-parental height* by taking the average of the parents' height and adding 3 inches for boys or subtracting 3 inches for girls. This calculation is far from precise, however, and may be off by 4 inches in either direction!

Room to Grow

The fact that the bony plates that make up your newborn's skull won't join together for many months is quite fortunate. By remaining open and expandable, they allow your baby's brain to grow. You will find that your pediatrician routinely monitors this growth by measuring the distance around the largest part of your baby's head and recording it on a head circumference growth curve alongside her weight and height. On average, your newborn's head should

- Increase in circumference by as much as 2 inches over the next two months.

- Reach about 90% of adult head size by the time your child turns three years old.

HEAD HANDLING WITH CARE

On a more serious note, head size, along with a distinct lack of head control, leaves babies very susceptible to injury. This is why it is so important to never shake a baby. Doing so has potential to cause much more serious harm than it would in older children or adults. As for the soft spot, it's not as vulnerable as one might think, but it still warrants being handled with care (see The Soft Spot later on this page).

The Shape of Things to Come

The topic of a cone-shaped head is particularly directed toward those of you who have been mistakenly led to believe that all newborns are born picture-perfect, with pretty little round heads. Let us just say that for anyone who has gone through or will experience vaginal delivery, it is nothing short of a blessing that a newborn's skull is made up of soft bony plates that are capable of compressing and overlapping to fit through the narrow birth canal—a process referred to as *molding*. For some babies—such as those who "drop" well in advance of being born (in other words, settle themselves headfirst deep into their mother's pelvis long before delivery) or those who must endure long labors and narrow birth canals—the result is often a newborn head shape that more closely resembles a cone than a nice round ball. If you run your fingers over your newborn's skull, you may even find early on that you can feel ridges along the areas where the bony plates of the skull have overlapped. In short, slightly misshapen heads are quite common right after birth. Fortunately, over the next several weeks, the bones of your baby's skull will almost assuredly round out and the ridges will disappear, assuming, that is, that your baby doesn't spend too much time on his back with his head in any one position—a common but easily avoidable cause for development of a flat back or side of the head, known as *plagiocephaly* (see Safe to Sleep: Back Sleeping and Beyond on page 102).

The Soft Spot

You will notice one to two areas on your baby's head that seem to be lacking bony protection. These soft spots, referred to as *fontanelles* (*anterior* for the larger one in the front, *posterior* for the smaller and typically less noticeable one in the back), are normal gaps in a newborn's skull that will allow your baby's brain to grow rapidly throughout the next year (**Figure 26-1**). Many parents are afraid to touch these soft spots, but you can rest assured that,

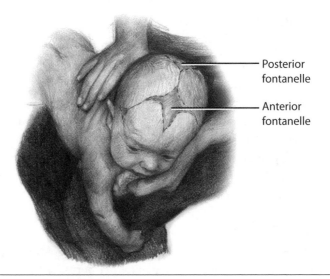

Posterior
fontanelle

Anterior
fontanelle

Figure 26-1. Soft spots, or *fontanelles*

despite their lack of a bony layer, they are well protected from typical day-to-day baby handling by a tough, fibrous membrane. Here is a list of other practical things to know about the soft spot(s).

- In young infants, a sunken soft spot combined with poor feeding and dry diapers can suggest dehydration. Our advice to you: don't read too much into this because it can be a subtle finding or can sometimes be present in healthy babies. Instead, make sure you have a good grasp on how to recognize dehydration (see What Goes In Must Come Out on page 71) and check with your baby's doctor if you have any concerns—with or without a sunken soft spot.
- In some instances, the soft spot on top of your baby's head may seem to be pulsating. There is no need to worry; this movement is normal and reflects the visible pulsing of blood that corresponds to your baby's heartbeat.

A BIG HEAD USUALLY MEANS…A BIG HAT

While there are certainly some instances when a big head can signify an underlying medical problem, it's reassuring to keep in mind that the most common cause of a big head is genetics; in other words, the tendency toward "big headedness" simply runs in the family.

Cover Up

Ever wonder who was in charge of determining what's the latest style in newborn headwear in the newborn nursery? Well, before you spend too much time laying blame, we figured we'd point out that those typically uninspired polyester knit newborn caps aren't given out just for looks.

Newborns not only have proportionately bigger heads but don't regulate their body temperatures as well as adults or even older infants do and therefore stand to lose a significant amount of heat from their heads if left uncovered. This is the real reason that it's generally recommended that you put a hat on your baby's head during the first few weeks—especially in cool weather or drafty rooms.

Bumps and Bruises

In addition to molding, a bit of swelling or bruising of the scalp immediately following delivery is not uncommon for newborns. The swelling is usually most noticeable at the top back part of the head and is medically referred to as a *caput* (short for *caput succedaneum*). When bruising of the head occurs during delivery, the result can be a boggy-feeling area, called a *cephalohematoma*. Bruising and swelling are usually harmless and go away on their own over the first days and weeks, but they can be a contributing factor for jaundice (see Seeing Yellow: Jaundice on page 335).

Gone Today but Hair Tomorrow

Sure, babies are sometimes born with full heads of hair, but it's far more likely for them to be born with little to none. And those with hair today are likely to find it gone tomorrow. That's because any hair your baby is born with is likely to thin out significantly over the next few months before ultimately being replaced with "real" hair. It is also entirely possible that whatever hair your newborn does have may change color by as much as several shades and several times over his lifetime.

Cradle Cap

Although *seborrheic dermatitis* is the technically correct term for cradle cap, parents faced with scaly newborn scalps tend to agree that it should more appropriately be called "cradle crap." Cradle cap is one of the earliest and most common forms of seborrheic dermatitis. It tends to show up anywhere from 2 weeks to 12 months and, in addition to the scalp, involves the forehead and face, behind the ears, and the diaper area, the armpits, and other skin folds. Cradle cap resembles the baby equivalent of dandruff and, despite being harmless, nevertheless tends to drive some parents nuts. This is most often because cradle cap can be a nuisance to get rid of—especially for babies who have a lot of it. While you can certainly try the commonly recommended approach of massaging affected areas with a little baby oil, mineral oil, or baby shampoo followed by gently removing the flakes with a soft brush (some use soft-bristled toothbrushes), we strongly suggest you don't lose any sleep over it. Your pediatrician can give you additional advice regarding the use of an over-the-counter cradle cap hair wash or medicated dandruff shampoo if you're determined to conquer your baby's cradle cap. Otherwise, we've found it's best to simply let cradle cap run its course, as it usually goes away over the course of the first year.

The Eyes Have It

Do You See What I See?

When it comes to baby vision, the eyes don't really have it all until three to five years down the road—about the time when 20/20 color vision is thought to set in. That does not mean, however, that your newborn can't see anything. Here's a glimpse of what your newborn can see.

- **From a distance.** Because of their limited range of vision—estimated to be around 20/400—newborns tend to pay closest attention to objects near their faces. At birth, your newborn should be able to blink in response to light and see a good 12 inches in front of him fairly clearly—the perfect distance from which to gaze at your smiling face while you hold him. By the time he reaches three months, he should be able to not only see but also follow light, faces, and objects as they move in front of him.

- **In contrast.** Early on, babies are rumored to prefer items with contrasting colors. While this serves as a good explanation for the popularity and marketing of red-white-black infant toys, the truth is that babies aren't thought to have full color vision until around five to seven months of age, and you really don't need to go out of your way to offer your newborn a healthy daily dose of visual stimulation. Your everyday interactions and commonplace baby objects (such as books, pictures, or rattles) will more than suffice (see Activities of Daily Learning on page 177).

- **Gaining control.** While it is common for babies younger than four months or so to appear cross-eyed on occasion, they should develop better eye-muscle control relatively quickly. Normal eye alignment and the ability to focus are key factors in developing normal eyesight, so be sure to mention any unusual eye movements you notice, especially if they continue beyond the first few months, to your baby's pediatrician.

NO MORE TEARS…YET?

Anecdotally, babies don't typically shed tears in the first month or two after birth. That said, even babies born prematurely reportedly produce enough tears to coat and lubricate their eyes. Best explanation we could find? Simply that making tears is different from shedding them. The amount of tears newborns typically make apparently isn't enough to send them rolling down cheeks until they are at least one month old.

Duct Work

Your newborn has tiny tear ducts located in the inner corner of each eye that drain into the nose and, when functioning properly, play an important role in draining tears (**Figure 26-2**). We liken this drainage system to a sewer system: if and when babies become stuffy, those who happen to have been born with narrower than usual or blocked tear ducts—a condition that applies to as approximately 6% of newborns—may experience a noticeable backup in the "sewer system." In fact, this sort of blockage (also referred to as *congenital nasolacrimal duct obstruction* or *dacryostenosis*) is the most common cause of persistent tearing and eye discharge in infants and young children. Unable to adequately keep up with the normal ebb and flow, tears back up, resulting in a watery and/or goopy eye). If you and your pediatrician determine that your baby has a blocked tear duct or two, you can clean off any goop that accumulates around your baby's eyes by gently wiping the lids with a warm, damp, clean towel or tissue. We should point out that eye goop often seems to bother parents much more than it does newborns. When the going gets goopy, we recommend you resist the temptation and limit your wiping to when things get really nasty.

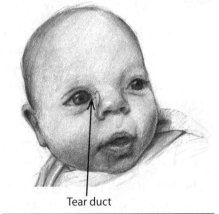

Tear duct

Figure 26-2. Location of tear duct

Although its usefulness has, in the past, been debated, the current first line of treatment is massage. By using a clean finger, tissue, or towel to lightly press and gently massage the area between the corner of the eye and the nose downward 2 or 3 times a day, you can presumably help relieve any obstruction in the duct and get things moving. Most blocked ducts get better by the first birthday. Those that don't clear up on their own generally necessitate a trip to a pediatric ophthalmologist, who may deem the careful use of a small probe necessary to open up the uncooperative ducts.

PINKEYE

While blocked tear ducts end up being solely to blame for a good many goopy eyes, it is nevertheless going to be important for you to be aware of and on the lookout for pinkeye. Although *pinkeye* (often used interchangeably with *conjunctivitis*) technically refers to any eye that appears pink (or red) regardless of cause, the term is most often used to describe eye infections. Although it's easy enough for us to tell you that true infections—especially those caused by bacteria—often have a thicker yellow or greenish discharge and are more likely to be accompanied by some degree of swelling and/or redness, distinguishing between the two is easier said than done. Because it is particularly important for eye infections in newborns to be diagnosed and treated without delay, any suspicions you may have should be promptly followed up with a phone call to your pediatrician. Even if your baby has already been diagnosed as having a blocked tear duct, you'll want to watch carefully for signs of infection because infants who have blocked tear ducts are more prone to developing them.

What's Going to Make Those Brown Eyes Blue?

What you see when you gaze into your newborn's eyes is not always what you'll ultimately get when it comes to eye color. Not only are the genetics of eye color quite complex, but predicting a baby's future eye color before birth is relatively unreliable. We can tell you, however, that a baby's eye color depends on how much of a particular pigment is in the colored part of the eye, or the *iris*. The more of this pigment—called *melanin*—there is, the darker brown a baby's eyes will appear. Conversely, babies with blue eyes have very little melanin. Anywhere in between results in varying shades of brown, hazel, or green. With that in mind, it makes more sense that if your baby is born with brown eyes, nothing short of colored contact lenses is likely to change her eye color to blue. However, babies who are blue-eyed at birth have the potential to produce more melanin over time and end up with eyes of a different color (usually by six months of age or so) than they were born with. Interestingly, some older kids and adults also continue to see changes in their eye color as they age (even without the help of fashionable contact lenses).

Seeing Red

Ever end up with red eyes in photographs? If so, you're already familiar with exactly the same reflex your pediatrician routinely looks for when he or she shines the light from an ophthalmoscope into your newborn's eyes—the red reflex. What may be a nuisance to photographers happens to be a very reassuring sign for pediatricians when it occurs in newborns. The red reflex not only reflects the presence of normal retinas at the back of your baby's eyes (appearing red because of the many blood vessels located there) but also tells us that light can make its way all the way in and back out again unobstructed. An absent or white reflex, in contrast, may mean there is a problem with the eye.

We're All Ears

Setting the Sound Stage

Did the latest playlist of classical music for yet-to-be-born babies catch your attention? Perhaps you came across parents-to-be who religiously read books to the soon-to-become newborn in their arms. Well, as tempting as it may be to get a head start on a baby's education, we suggest that expectant parents sit back and relax during their pregnancies because there will be plenty of time for teaching later. With that said, if your idea of relaxing happens to include listening to calming music or taking a few practice runs through *Goodnight Moon* before bed, your efforts are not likely to be in vain—at least not after your sixth or seventh month. That's because although the earliest signs of hearing begin around 18 weeks, by 28 weeks fetuses have been shown to respond consistently to sound in utero.

SOUND ADVICE FOR ALL NEWBORNS

Whereas an adult can typically hear sounds at around 13.5 decibels (the level of a soft whisper), a fetus at 27 to 29 weeks is able to detect sounds at a level closer to 40 decibels—the average sound of a running refrigerator or the flow of light traffic. By the time a baby reaches full term, his ability to hear will have matured to such an extent that he can hear sounds similar to those heard by adults. However, anywhere from 1 to 6 babies out of every 1,000 will have childhood hearing loss. Given these numbers and the fact that hearing plays such an important role in a baby's language and cognitive development, universal newborn hearing screening is recommended for *all* newborns. According to HealthyChildren.org, "[t]he goal is for all babies to have a newborn screening by one month of age, ideally before they go home from the hospital; identified by 3 months of age and enrolled in early intervention or treatment, if identified as deaf or hard of hearing, by the age of 6 months."

Accessorizing

It may (or may not) surprise you that one of the most frequent ear-related questions we get is "How soon can I get my baby daughter's ears pierced?" Unfortunately, actual research on the subject is relatively sparse. That said, our response seems to be quite aligned with many of our pediatric colleagues: if you can wait until your child is less susceptible to infection, is less likely to swallow the tiny (and not generally size-appropriate for children younger than three years) parts inherent to wearing earrings, and is better able to care for her own ear piercings and even until she is old enough to decide for herself, we highly recommend doing so, even if it means waiting until she is in elementary school or later. If, however, you feel compelled to have your infant's ears pierced during infancy, you'd be well-advised to wait until at least after she gets her six-month shots so that she'll be better protected against tetanus and infection. Then try to find an experienced professional piercer who uses sterile equipment and, if possible, has experience piercing baby earlobes. As with many things, you'd be wise to check with your pediatrician first. Some actually provide this service themselves, while others may be able to steer you in the direction of someone they feel is careful and trustworthy.

Your Baby's Nose Knows

Despite the fact that mouth breathing seems as though it should be a perfectly reasonable alternative, babies, for the most part, preferentially breathe through their narrow little noses from birth until about three to six months. Knowing that, it should make sense why many newborns develop noisy breathing with the slightest amount of stuffiness or dryness. Add a snotty-nose cold and congestion to the picture, and the effects become more noticeable and challenging—especially at feeding or sleeping time. Given what a challenge this can pose, we have included some of the basic techniques recommended for ridding your baby of unwanted snot and congestion in hopes of keeping everyone breathing easy.

THE AIR MOVES IN, THE AIR MOVES OUT

Every now and then, a baby's nasal passageway doesn't develop and open up the way it's supposed to. A quick and easy way to determine whether air is able to make its way into and out of your newborn's nose as expected is to take a tissue or thin piece of cotton (stretch out the tip of a cotton swab or part of a cotton ball) and hold it just in front of one nostril while lightly pressing the other nostril closed. You should see the tissue or cotton move gently each time your baby breathes out.

- **Nose drops.** Often referred to as *saline nose drops,* nose drops work by simply moistening and loosening up mucus. They are inexpensive, sold over the counter, and readily available just about anywhere that sells basic baby supplies. They can be used alone to moisten or loosen up dried mucus or followed by a bulb suction. If you are so inclined, you can even make your own by mixing ¼ teaspoon of salt in 1 cup of warm water. Use just 1 to 2 drops (or 1 to 2 sprays) of the saltwater solution in each of your baby's nostrils.

- **Bulb suction.** We've included this option not because we think it always works but because some new parents are quick to reach for their bulb suctions when in search of fast relief. While we readily admit that they can and do serve a purpose for babies younger than around six months of age (and their parents) in their snottier times of need, we suggest you take a moment to consider what it feels like to have a piece of rubber or plastic inserted, however gently, up your nose. After factoring in this not-so-comfortable thought, we recommend you limit your use of a bulb suction to times not only when your baby seems to be truly congested and has a big blob of mucus in clear view but when the snot actually seems to be interfering with her ability to eat, sleep, or breathe. If and when you reach for the bulb suction, squeeze the bulb first. Then insert the tip gently into the nostril, and slowly let go of the bulb. As you do, the small amount of suction should help remove (suction up) the obstructing mucus. If, however, the mucus is just hanging out, minding its own business, and not really bothering anyone (save for its appearance), consider giving your bulb suction a rest and grab a tissue instead.

SUCCESSFUL SUCTIONING

If and when you need to use a bulb suction to remove mucus, it's generally a good idea to limit your attempts to about 3 times a day, as more frequent use can irritate your baby's nasal lining and make him even more congested. For best results, press down lightly on one nostril to hold it closed while you gently suction the other side, keeping in mind that the middle part of each nostril tends to be the most sensitive to probing.

- **Vaporizers and cool-mist humidifiers.** Running a cool-mist humidifier is almost a knee-jerk reaction of parents everywhere when faced with a baby who has a stuffy-nose cold. While you may not always see a hugely noticeable response, there are definitely times, such as when your baby won't sleep or eat because she's congested and irritable, when you'll probably agree that every little bit helps. Adding moisture in the form of cool mist to the air is certainly one small step in the right direction. To get the most benefit, be sure to place it as close to your baby as you can—while still remaining safely out of reach. Also, be sure to clean it carefully to keep mold and bacteria from contaminating your efforts. As a note of caution, hot-water vaporizers are not recommended (because of the risk of hot-water burns). Instead, you may find that running a hot shower with the door closed and then sitting in the steamy bathroom with your baby, a safe distance away from the actual spray, can also help improve the drainage.

Sneezing

Newborns typically sneeze a lot. You can save yourself a lot of unnecessary worry if you remember to chalk the sneezes up to sensitive reflexes rather than overinterpret them as a sign of illness. Most babies outgrow this tendency to sneeze in response to the slightest tickle within a few months—at about the same time as they begin to gain control over their other reflexes (see Reflexes on page 324).

A Word of Mouths

Most new parents have few, if any, concerns about their newborns' mouths—that is, unless they see something they think doesn't belong there. If you find anything in your baby's mouth that surprises you or that you're just not sure about, be sure to bring it to the attention of your pediatrician. Typical in-mouth sightings can include

- **White or clear bumps.** Whitish bumps are sometimes found or appear on the gums, lips, or roof of the mouth. Generally harmless, they often serve to fool parents into thinking a tooth is erupting months before one pokes its way through the gum.

- **Newborn (or natal) teeth.** On rare occasion, teeth decide to erupt ahead of schedule—sometimes even showing up at birth. If your baby's doctor doesn't notice them first, you'll want to point them out because they may, in some instances, need to be removed.

- **Sucking blisters.** Babies can develop blisters just from sucking—something they obviously do a lot of in their first weeks and months. They appear most often on the lips but sometimes on fingers or even toes as well, if and when newborns manage to reach and get them to their mouths. Sucking blisters generally require no treatment and end up going away on their own.

- **White coating.** If you start to see white on the inside of your newborn's mouth, you'll want to consider two major causes—(1) lingering breast milk or formula or (2) thrush. The white spots of thrush (a yeast infection found in the mouth) tend to appear most often on the tongue and hidden in the nooks and crannies of the mouth, commonly tucked between the cheeks and gums. Thrush is often overlooked or written off as residual formula or breast milk until it persists and spreads. As a rough rule of thumb, any white spots or patches in a newborn's mouth that don't easily wipe off with a damp washcloth or cotton swab should be evaluated for thrush and treated accordingly.

Thrush Attack

Thrush is caused by a type of yeast (*Candida albicans*) that commonly lives in the intestinal tract and is also responsible for some diaper rashes. Unlike the red spots and patches it is known to cause on a baby's rear end, *C albicans* forms spots or patches of white in the mouth that don't easily wipe away and slowly spread. While many parents consider thrush to be a pain in the butt, in most instances, it is fortunately not a pain in the mouth; it is simply a nuisance. Your baby's pediatrician can help make the diagnosis and set you up to remedy the situation. Good ways of treating thrush include

- **Liquid yeast medication.** This comes as a prescription solution called *nystatin* that is suitable for putting into your baby's mouth. While you'll want to follow your doctor's recommendations—typically putting one dropperful inside each cheek 4 times a day—the underlying approach to treatment is even more straightforward: look for white spots, and try to get your medicated solution on them (we prefer to use a clean cotton swab). Once you do, try to wait at least 30 minutes after applying before feeding your baby so that the medication has time to do its work.

- **Thinking outside the mouth.** You aren't likely to rid your baby of thrush unless you address the problem outside her mouth, as well as in it. It can take a good boiling (or sterilization) to kill the yeast that hang out on pacifiers and baby-bottle nipples. And for those of you who breastfeed, be forewarned that *C albicans* doesn't limit itself to "artificial nipples." If your baby has thrush or you experience a burning, irritated feeling on your nipples, check with your baby's doctor about treatment of yourself as well so that you don't pass the infection back and forth (see What's Behind Burning Nipples on page 22). This typically involves the use of an over-the-counter anti-yeast cream, such as *clotrimazole* (eg, Lotrimin), applied several times a day to the nipples. It's recommended that the cream should just be washed off before nursing.

- **Persistence.** Thrush isn't always easy to get rid of. It not only hides out in hard-to-reach places but has an annoying habit of popping back up again just when you think you, your bottle of yeast medication, and your boiled pacifiers have conquered it. Even when the coast seems clear, keep your guard up and watch for any new white spots to appear. Sometimes, getting rid of thrush requires a stronger antifungal medication (such as *fluconazole*) for treatment.

Tongue-Tied

We're all born with a little tissue called a *frenulum* that connects the bottom of our tongues with the floor of our mouths. Babies are occasionally born with a frenulum that extends as far out as the tip of the tongue, an extension seeming to "tie" a newborn's tongue, limit its ability to stick out past the lips, and potentially interfere with sucking and feeding. This condition, known as *ankyloglossia* or "tongue-tie," has generally been considered harmless by pediatricians. That said, a significant number of lactation consultants who were surveyed expressed concern that it can cause breastfeeding problems. While some studies have shown that tongue-tied babies who were having difficulty latching on to breastfeed benefited from having the frenulum cut (typically a simple office procedure called a *frenotomy* or *frenulotomy*), there's still a lack of a definitive answer as to whether this procedure is a necessary or beneficial treatment. As we write this, new recommendations from the American Academy of Pediatrics are due to be released in the near future—reinforcing that your best approach to tongue-tie involves discussing any breastfeeding challenges and up-to-date treatment options with your pediatrician.

Smiling

No one knows exactly why newborns first begin to smile when they are sleeping and wait a few weeks before they carry these smiles over to the daytime. Nor is it easy to say exactly when during the first month your baby's new smiles will become more intentional. If you ask us, does it really matter? We don't find it worthwhile to spend much time debating the meaning of a smile because we think any newborn smile should be enough to melt a parent's heart. And by three months of age, your baby should have developed an undeniably social smile that he will happily share with those around him.

Chest

A Breath of Fresh...Fluid?

Take a moment and consider the fact that babies actually practice breathing well before they're born. It is not exactly intuitive, given that their lungs are filled with amniotic fluid right up until the day when they decide to leave their cozy uterine surroundings, enter the outside world, and take their first big breath of fresh air. This fluid, found in the lungs of all babies through-out pregnancy, is essential for healthy lung development. So is time. For the first month and a half of pregnancy, fetal lungs take on their basic shape and structure. If you think of the lungs as a tree, this is the period when the trunk and major branches are formed. Up until the 25th week, smaller branches form and the smallest "leaves"—known as *alveoli*—start to develop and take on the structure ultimately necessary to breathe in oxygen. By the time a baby reaches full term, he is estimated to have anywhere from 50 to 150 million alveoli. This number continues to increase over the first several years, an increase burgeoning to a total of about 300 million alveoli in adulthood.

Baby Breaths

For anyone not already familiar with some of the notable differences between the way adults breathe and the way newborns breathe, some of the character-istic newborn breathing habits may make you more than a little nervous. In the interest of sparing you unnecessary angst, we want to familiarize you with two of the more common (and normal) tendencies.

- **Picking up the pace.** Perhaps one of the most common questions we get about the newborn breathing style is if it's "normal" for them to breathe so fast. The answer is yes, it can be. Even at rest, otherwise healthy newborns breathe considerably faster than adults in addition to having faster resting heart rates.

- **Taking a break.** The tendency of newborns to take several breaths in rapid succession followed by a few seconds of rest—referred to as *peri-odic breathing*—is common and often disconcerting to parents caught previously unaware. As long as newborns remember to limit their pauses to no more than a few seconds and experience no accompanying color changes—especially anything resembling a shade of blue—periodic breathing is considered a normal, harmless habit.

Breasts

We're willing to bet that many of you out there were hoping there were going to be at least a few body parts you could put off thinking about until puberty. We want to be sure to mention, though, that baby girls and baby boys alike are, on occasion, born with enlarged breasts. That's right, the swelling of one or both breasts can vary from subtle to fairly pronounced and is thought to be the result of babies' exposure to their mothers' hormones during pregnancy. Some newborns even have some milky white breast discharge to go along with the swelling, something you may have heard referred to as *witches' milk*. The good news: you don't need to do anything about the swelling or discharge. Swollen newborn breasts generally disappear on their own within a few weeks to months.

"IT'S A NUBBIN"

Nubbins, extra nipples, supernumerary nipples, accessory nipples—whatever you want to call them—these so-called third nipples are extra breast tissue found on the chest below the level of a baby's two nipples (and as low down as on the abdomen). Brought into the national spotlight on a memorable episode of the classic hit show *Friends* (Chandler had one), they're hardly ever of any medical significance, rarely change during puberty, and in most cases are small enough and flat enough to either go unnoticed or look like birthmarks. Some babies, however, are born with a third nipple that more closely resembles a normal nipple. If an extra, out-of-line nipple becomes a source of embarrassment for your child later in life, take comfort in knowing it can be removed.

The Care and Keeping of the Cord

The umbilical cord is one of the new baby body parts that seems to get the most attention. After serving for so many months as a vital connection between mom and baby, it quickly becomes unnecessary once your baby is born and starts breathing and eating on her own. You can expect your newborn's umbilical-cord stump to dry up and fall off within a few weeks (typically anywhere from one to three, to be more precise). In the meantime, you may be relieved to know that the blood vessels that once ran through it are now closed off, and your baby's umbilical cord and belly button are no longer a direct connection to anywhere.

Letting Go

Many new parents are very tentative when it comes to caring for their newborn's umbilical cord. For the most part, dealing with the umbilical cord means keeping it clean and waiting for it to fall off. In days past, a type of infection-preventing purple dye or rubbing alcohol was frequently used. Since 1998, however, the World Health Organization (WHO) has advocated for doing nothing except keeping the cord clean and leaving it exposed to air (or loosely covered). Of course, if it does become soiled, the recommendation is to simply clean it with soap and sterile water as needed. The reason for this shift to a "dry umbilical-cord care" approach is because when left alone, most umbilical cords will just fall off by themselves. We've found that intermittently and gently pushing down the skin surrounding the umbilical cord so that the base of the stump gets some exposure to air can help speed up the drying process a bit. In case you're worried about hurting your baby, you'll be relieved to know that no nerve endings are on the cord itself, and babies don't feel any pain or discomfort with careful handling of the cord. Every now and then, you might see a little blood at the base of the cord—an admittedly disconcerting sight that is usually the result of a cord stump becoming detached a bit too soon (like a scab pulled off before the underlying skin is entirely healed). The most useful approach to cord care is for you to let the cord fall off all on its own, and until it does, avoid undue moisture to the cord (see Prelude to a Bath on page 154). Be sure to call your baby's doctor in the unlikely event that you see any signs of infection, including yellow drainage or any redness or tenderness of the skin around the cord.

UNCOOPERATIVE CORDS

Some of you may benefit from a little forewarning: not all cords cooperate according to plan. Some of the more common inconveniences we come across include

- **Hanging on.** Some cords are persistent, clinging on for dear life despite daily encouragement to fall off. While the normal range is as long as five weeks, it's worth discussing an obstinate cord with your pediatrician to see whether something can be done about it or if it warrants further evaluation.

- **Oozing.** After the umbilical-cord stump falls off, the belly button tissue may take its own sweet time to heal. If it continues to ooze or develop a little pink, moist bump that doesn't dry up, your pediatrician may apply a touch of a chemical called *silver nitrate* to quicken the healing process. Rarely, pus may ooze from the belly button or surrounding skin may become red and swollen. If either happens, show your baby's doctor without any delay because any and all potential infections warrant immediate attention at this age. True infections of a newborn's umbilical site generally require medical management, antibiotics, and close observation.

- **Bleeding.** When your newborn's cord comes off, don't be surprised if there is a little bleeding to go along with it. The best way we've found to explain the bleeding: it's like when a scab comes off and pulls a bit at the normal skin as well. There's bound to be a little short-lived bleeding.

Innies Versus Outies

Ever look at your own belly button and wonder why it was that your doctor didn't do a better job of giving you a cute little "innie" when you were born? Well, you'll soon discover, if you haven't figured it out already, that the innie versus "outie" status of your newborn's belly button is completely out of anyone's control. Ultimately, how much or little your newborn's belly button will stick out depends on how the umbilical-cord scar heals or, in the case of an umbilical hernia, how the gap between the two abdominal muscles closes up (something that usually happens on its own by five years of age).

BANKING ON CORD BLOOD

Cord blood—blood that courses through the umbilical cord right up until a baby is born—has been found to contain cells that can successfully cure a wide range of genetic, blood-related, and immune system disorders, as well as some types of cancer. This makes cord blood of great interest in the medical world, offering hope for treatment of such potentially devastating diagnoses. Fortunately, collection of cord blood is relatively quick, easy, and pain-free, and it is typically done just before or just after delivery of the placenta.

Several types of cord-blood banks, including both public and private, exist worldwide and allow for the long-term storage of these lifesaving cells. With the existence of cord-blood banking, expectant parents are now faced with an important decision: whether to invest what can be a significant amount of money into storing their babies' cord blood in a private, for-profit cord-blood bank. While the idea of reserving your baby's cord blood exclusively for potential personal or family use in the future is understandably tempting, the actual likelihood of needing to do so is medically unlikely. Unless you already have a child or another family member with a known medical condition that could directly benefit from a cord-blood transplant, private storage is not currently recommended. That said, allowing your baby's cord blood to be collected and stored in a public blood bank and made available in a national registry is recommended, should the option be available to you.

Back to Basics

Sacral Dimple

It's adorable to see babies with dimples on their cheeks, but on occasion, they show up on a baby's backside in the area just above the buttock crease, called the *sacral area* (**Figure 26-3**). Most sacral dimples, when present, are very shallow and simply look like a little indentation in the skin. While they may also seem cute, it is well worth making sure they're carefully evaluated by a health care provider because every now and then, they serve as a sign that what lies underneath didn't develop quite according to plan. Most notably, this can include the potential for sacral dimples to extend deeper below the surface and possibly affect the spine or surrounding structures or potentially become infected.

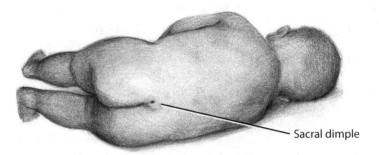

Sacral dimple

Figure 26-3. Sacral dimple

Genitals

Now to address those parts of your newborn's body that new parents tend to have questions about but often hesitate to ask. When it comes to learning about your newborn's genitals, we strongly believe that "down there" just won't suffice (nor should it), and there may well be some information or details that are new to you, regardless of whether you have a baby of the same or opposite sex as you.

BOY OR GIRL

Along with pregnancy comes the inevitable question "Are you going to find out?"—a question that refers to the modern-day luxury of being able to find out months ahead of time by ultrasound, or even more definitively by chromosome testing, whether you're destined to have a boy or girl. Even though you may not be finding out, the early period of genital development is referred to as the "indifferent stage" for good reason. That's because there is no difference in appearance of the external genitals between boy fetuses and girl fetuses until around the 14th week. So if you (like us) are among those who couldn't wait to get a sneak peek, rest assured that your obstetrician was not just trying to teach you a lesson in patience by making you wait until somewhere between your 16th and 20th week to get an ultrasound.

Baby Girls

Girl Parts

Before we talk about some of the anatomical details unique to baby girls, we figured it would be useful to review a bit of basic terminology. The *vulva* consists of the external, visible parts of the female genitals. These parts include the *labia majora* (sometimes described as the outer "lips" or "flaps" of skin), the *labia minora* (also known as the smaller, inner "lips," just inside the labia majora), the *mons pubis* (the mound-like area just above the labia majora), the *clitoris* (the small, sensitive part that sits at the top of the labia), and the *vestibule* (the area between the labia, where the urethra and vaginal opening are found).

Keeping Clean

Unless poop is involved, there is no need to scrub thoroughly in all the nooks and crannies that make up your newborn girl's vulva (**Figure 26-4**). In fact, when cleaning your baby girl, soap is not always considered necessary. You can use plain water, a baby wipe, or a damp washcloth or cotton ball to wipe from your baby's front to her backside. Too vigorous cleaning can irritate the labia and actually cause the flaps of skin to stick together.

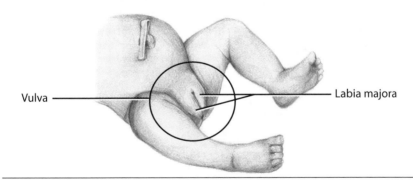

Vulva ———————————————————————— Labia majora

Figure 26-4. Vulva

LABIAL ADHESIONS

Infants and young girls sometimes develop what are called *labial adhesions*. This is a condition where the folds of the labia minora fuse or stick together, either partially or completely. In most instances, a large enough opening remains to allow pee to come out normally. Labial adhesions are caused by irritation of the labia, with subsequent fusion of the tissues during the healing process. This condition usually goes away on its own once a girl reaches puberty because the higher estrogen level helps lubricate the tissues. For newborns, your pediatrician may advise you to apply petroleum jelly (eg, Vaseline) or a prescription estrogen cream to help separate fused labia.

Vaginal Discharge

Newborn girls often have clear or white discharge from the vagina. This discharge helps protect the vaginal area from sticky poop and the like. During diaper changes, you can gently wipe away excess discharge, but you don't need to dig deep or scrub hard to get rid of it all. Call your pediatrician if the discharge becomes yellow or green or develops an odor, because such changes may suggest the need for further evaluation or treatment.

Vaginal Bleeding

Some newborn girls seem to have mini menstrual periods with bloody discharge from the vagina. Although you may find it disconcerting, this is a normal effect of exposure to mom's hormones before birth that usually goes away within a few weeks.

Baby Boys

Boy Parts

Newborn boy anatomy is a bit simpler to visualize, as both the *penis* and the *scrotum* are clearly visible and easy to identify. Additional parts include the *foreskin,* which is the layer of skin that covers the end of the uncircumcised penis, and the *testes,* which are the small oval-shaped objects that should be located inside each side of the scrotum. Although in everyday terms the words *testes* and *testicles* are often used interchangeably, technically, *testicles* is defined as the *testes,* the *vas deferens* (the "stalk" that connects to each testes), and the *epididymis* (a small coiled structure that sits on the back of each testes), collectively.

Penis Care

Whether or not you decide to circumcise your baby boy, the routine newborn care is the same: gently clean the penis (**Figure 26-5**) during baths, pulling the foreskin back only as far as it will go. For uncircumcised boys, you will only be able to see the opening at the tip of the foreskin. It will be a few years before the foreskin will loosen enough to pull behind the head (or glans) of the penis for cleaning. For circumcised boys, your goal is to keep the head of penis clean and prevent any foreskin from causing adhesions by sticking to the glans.

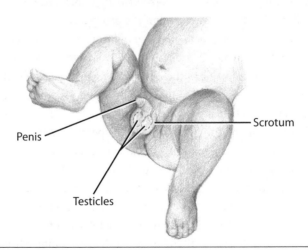

Penis

Scrotum

Testicles

Figure 26-5. Penis, scrotum, and testicles

HYPOSPADIAS

In the condition known as *hypospadias,* the foreskin won't look quite right, and the opening of the urethra where the pee comes out (also called the *meatus*) may not be right at the tip of the penis, where it's supposed to be. Recognizing hypospadias at birth is especially important for parents who plan to have their newborn sons circumcised because circumcision should be delayed and performed by a urologist at the same time as correction of the hypospadias.

To Circumcise or Not to Circumcise

While some recognized health benefits outweigh the risks to removing the foreskin of the penis—such as decreasing the already low risk of cancer of the penis, the likelihood of urinary tract infections in men, and the spread of sexually transmitted infections—the American Academy of Pediatrics has deemed them not significant enough to recommend routine circumcision for all newborn boys. The decision to circumcise is felt to be solely up to the parent and should be based on your personal, religious, and cultural beliefs.

Except for babies born small, prematurely, or with hypospadias, circumcisions are generally done within a week or two of birth. This procedure may be done in the hospital or your pediatrician's office and is typically performed by either your baby's doctor or your obstetrician. Babies feel pain, so be sure to ask about options for limiting pain of the procedure, as sugar water, acetaminophen (eg, Tylenol), or a local injection of lidocaine is routinely given. Also, be sure to ask whether your insurance company covers the cost of the procedure because not all do. Outside of the newborn period, a urologist may perform medically necessary circumcisions (usually around six months of age) when risk of adverse events from the surgery and general anesthesia is lower.

Following a circumcision, the head of the penis may appear purple-red or swollen for up to a week. You can also expect a moist or even goopy-looking scab to form and remain on the head of the penis while it heals. A little Vaseline, antibiotic ointment in the form of Bacitracin, or lubricant such as K-Y Jelly often helps keep the scab from sticking to the diaper and is therefore most useful while the circumcised area is still raw. In general, parents should avoid giving their newborns full baths until the penis has healed completely (see Prelude to a Bath on page 154). Contact your pediatrician if you think you see pus or notice any bleeding that leaves a spot of blood bigger than a quarter on your baby's diaper.

When to Call a Foul Ball

There are a few commonly mentioned conditions involving a baby boy's scrotum and testicles with which you may want to familiarize yourself. If your baby's testicular area doesn't look quite right, he may have

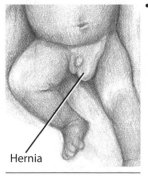

Hernia

Figure 26-6. Hernia

- **A hernia.** Hernias (**Figure 26-6**) tend to be more common in babies born prematurely and are 10 times more likely to occur in boys than in girls. This is a condition where a small opening in the belly wall allows part of the intestine to creep down into the scrotum, or testicular sac. This can actually occur in the groin area of girls as well. When a baby boy has a hernia, his scrotum or groin area may appear full and larger than normal. The bulge of a hernia tends to appear or enlarge when babies cry because crying puts more pressure on the belly. If you suspect that your baby has a hernia, contact your pediatrician. Surgery will usually be required to make sure the intestine doesn't become stuck, twisted, or swollen.

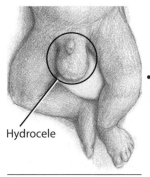

Hydrocele

Figure 26-7. Hydrocele

- **A hydrocele.** Excess fluid surrounds the testicle(s) and makes the scrotum look large (**Figure 26-7**). This fluid *transilluminates,* meaning if you hold a flashlight against the scrotum, it "glows" and appears fairly translucent. Hydroceles usually disappear by 1 year of age without any intervention. They occur in about 10% of baby boys.

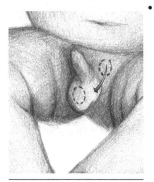

Figure 26-8. Undescended testicles

- **Undescended testicles.** Over the course of fetal development, a baby boy's testicles move down from the abdomen and ultimately settle themselves in the scrotum (**Figure 26-8**). Sometimes the testicles (one or both) are slow to descend, taking their own sweet time to move down into the scrotum during the first few months. Other times the testicle does not descend and therefore does not develop as it should and won't function properly if left to fend for itself in the abdomen. If and when surgery is indicated, it is recommended as early as 6 months of age but no later than 18 to 24 months.

On the Surface: Your Newborn's Skin

Visualize what happens to skin that has been soaked for a long time in a tub full of warm water. It gets shriveled and soft and has a tendency to become a bit dried out afterward. Now if you consider that your newborn has been soaking in an amniotic fluid bath for nine months, you'll better understand why her skin looks like it does—most likely dry, cracked, or peeling. If you think about it, it's amazing that a newborn's skin doesn't look worse than it does after delivery. While we find that almost all new parents come to us in search of a way to remedy the dry skin situation, there's not much to be done except exercise patience. Moisturizers only serve to temporarily slick down the dead, flaky skin that is destined to be sloughed off anyway, and given that some young babies have sensitive skin to begin with, we suggest avoiding unnecessary use of lotions in the first month unless otherwise directed by your baby's doctor.

Rashes

Newborns frequently develop rashes on the skin, most of which are common and harmless. In an effort to familiarize you with what you may be faced with (because many newborn rashes tend to show up on the face), we have put together the following list. Whether caused by maternal hormones or tiny pores that are easily clogged, these common newborn rashes rarely require anything more on your part than patience and a hands-off approach, with the exception of an occasional wipe with a wet washcloth.

- **Baby acne.** Although baby acne doesn't tend to show up until a month or so of age, we're listing this first because it tends to be the most concerning for parents. Just as in puberty, these pimples appear because of the effect of hormones on the oil glands, only this time, it's mom's hormones from pregnancy that are the culprit. Baby acne tends to come and go for a few months before going away and may worsen before finally getting better. Do your best to refrain from poking or popping, as this only stands to make things worse. Try to take advantage of good-skin days to get some pictures of your blemish-free little one.

- **White bumps (*milia*).** These tiny bumps are usually found on newborn noses and usually disappear within a few weeks without requiring anything on your part.

- **Erythema toxicum.** This red, splotchy, bumpy rash with little blister-like lesions in the center can make newborns look as if they've been attacked by fleas. "E tox," as it is often called (short for *erythema toxicum*), often appears shortly after birth—within hours or days—and can be expected to go away within about a week. Individual spots can come and go within hours (similar to hives) and should not be poked, prodded, or popped. Because any blister-like rash needs a doctor's evaluation, be sure to get confirmation that it's E tox you're dealing with.

- **Heat rash.** Warm clothes or sweat can cause fine pink pimples on your baby's skin—most commonly on the face and in and around skin folds. Try to keep him cool and dry to avoid heat rash or to get rid of it once it appears.

- **Eczema.** While eczema tends to show up before five years of age, it's uncommon for babies to develop their first symptoms for at least the first couple of months. When it does, eczema usually appears as rough, dry, red areas of skin in the folds of the elbows, backs of the knees, cheeks, or scalp. And while the cause is not always clear, eczema-like rashes can be triggered by certain soaps, detergents, or foods in a breastfeeding mom's or older infant's solid food diet.

Birthmarks by Color

- **Pink or red.** Splotchy, flat red or pink spots on the eyelids, forehead, or back of the neck and scalp are called "angel kisses," "salmon patches," or "stork bites" (the technical term is *nevus simplex*). These often fade over the first few years, and they tend to get brighter when your baby cries. Darker red areas on the skin are called *port-wine stains* or *nevus flammeus*. Hemangiomas are bumpy strawberry-like collections of blood vessels that may be found anywhere on the body and can be of any size. They may not appear until after birth, and they typically grow in size during the first year before gradually shrinking over the next several years. Most disappear on their own, while a few may require laser or steroid treatment or even surgery.

- **Blue.** Mongolian spots are bluish green, flat birthmarks often seen in babies with darker skin. They are frequently located on the lower back or buttocks but can be found on other body parts as well. They tend to fade with time, but until they do, it's a good idea to make sure their presence is documented in your baby's medical record to decrease the likelihood that they will be mistaken for unexplained bruising.

- **Brown.** Flat, light-brown birthmarks are called *café au lait spots*. These usually require no intervention but, on occasion (usually when someone has six or more of them), can be associated with other symptoms or, rarely, neurological conditions. Spots called *moles* or *nevi* may also be brown but tend to be darker and, in some cases, raised.

Blue or Mottled

Because babies don't have great circulation, you may well see your fair share of mottled or even bluish skin, especially of your newborn's hands and feet. If you notice this, simply make sure your baby is warm enough by covering up cool extremities and repositioning her to get the blood flowing. On the other hand, should your newborn's lips, gums, or skin around the mouth appear blue, contact your pediatrician without delay because this more centrally located blueness may mean your baby is not getting enough oxygen.

Fingers and Toes

Not a whole lot to say about fingers and toes: it's usually a matter of counting ten of each and you're done. Well, almost. Every now and then, a baby is born with an extra digit or with a toe that curls a bit more than normal—neither of which is likely to be a big deal in the grand scheme of things and both of which tend to run in families. If either situation applies to you, discuss it with your pediatrician. We've found that the real story from a practical standpoint is not your newborn's fingers and toes but what lies in store for you on the tips of them. What throws some parents for a loop is the recurrent challenge of nail management.

Nails, Nails Everywhere

Did you know that fingernails grow an estimated 0.1 millimeter each day and grow faster in young people, in males, and in the summertime? Well, neither did we until we looked it up, but that is apparently the case, and it certainly doesn't surprise us. While that may not seem like much on the surface, let us assure you that it will keep you busy. Keeping up with your newborn's nails as they continually grow can be a very demanding task. As far as we're concerned, the real purpose baby nails serve is to break you into parenthood. They will likely require trimming or filing at least once a week because long nails on the hands of newborns with little to no control of them predictably result in stray scratches. If you happen to fall behind on your nail clipping, your baby will inevitably remind you (and make you feel guilty) by scratching his face when his nails get too long (or if you leave sharp corners or points when clipping).

Hand Exploration

Many parents cover their newborn's hands with baby mittens or socks to prevent wayward nails from scratching their faces. As your baby develops over the next several weeks (and you become more skilled at nail clipping), it's a good idea to allow your baby plenty of time during which he can freely explore with his hands. If scratches continue to be a problem, we suggest limiting covered time to when your baby is sleeping.

Curved Legs and Feet

It's not surprising to find that after being curled up in her mother's body for nine months, a newborn's legs and feet come out a bit footloose and fancy-free—appearing to be curved. These positional effects gradually improve over the first months and years. A few babies will have more significant problems with the bones of their feet, which may require casting or surgery. Make sure your pediatrician checks your baby's feet, especially if they seem rigid or curved and can't be straightened out on physical exam.

THE BABY MANI-PEDI

A handful of parents are intimidated by the prospect of having to cut their baby's nails and would probably opt for a professional manicure-pedicure if only it was generally available. No such luck. If you're lucky, your hospital nurse will be able to help demonstrate the correct technique, but some hospitals discourage their personnel from doing so (we can only presume because any unintentional injury may be a liability problem). And while we aren't exactly recommending it (or admitting to doing it ourselves), we're well aware that some parents opt to bite or peel off their newborn's nails rather than fiddle with clippers or scissors. Be aware, however, that doing so can potentially lead to infection. Because clippers and scissors can trim nails in a more controlled fashion, you'll be much better off using one or the other (or both) or simply using a nail file to keep things under control. For best results,

- Trim or file your baby's nails when she's asleep and her hands are less of a moving target.

- Push down on the fingertip skin so you can get the clipper or scissors around both sides of the nail and avoid cutting your baby's finger (or toe).

- Then, just as a professional manicurist would, finish off any sharp or rough edges with an emery board and…voilà! Not so bad after all, once you get the hang of it.

Reflexes

Reflexes are actions that happen automatically. Newborns are born with several of them, many of which they grow out of as their nervous systems develop and take control over the next several months. We've listed some common (and entirely normal) reflexes that you'll probably come across.

- **Grasp.** We consider the newborn grasp reflex to be one of the most endearing. It causes your baby to grasp tightly to your finger if you place one into the palm of his hand. Pressing on the bottom of his feet will also cause his toes to curl up.

- **Sucking.** The sucking reflex is present even before birth, as witnessed during many prenatal ultrasounds. You'll find the reflex is so strong that your baby may want to suck even if he's not hungry. Rather than overfeed him, consider offering a pacifier or clean finger to satisfy his urge (see Sucking Sense and Sensibility on page 67).

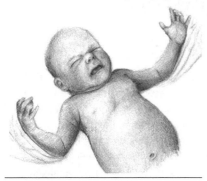

Figure 26-9. *Moro* or "startle" reflex

- ***Moro* or "startle" reflex.** When newborns are startled by loud noises or sudden changes in position, they may well throw their arms and legs out and even start to cry (**Figure 26-9**). You can chalk up this entire sequence to what is known as a *Moro* or "startle" reflex.

- **Fencing pose.** We included this reflex only as a point of general interest. Watch your newborn as he lies on his back. Whichever side his head is turned to is likely to be the side he reflexively extends his arm, while the opposite arm will bend at his side, resembling the pose of a fencer (**Figure 26-10**).

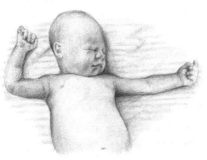

Figure 26-10. Fencing pose

27

fever: trial by fire

· · · · · ·

As you're probably well aware, fever is a hot topic that applies to everyone—young and old. We all get plenty of firsthand experience with it long before we reach parenthood, yet there's nothing quite like a baby's first fever to make even the most well-prepared parents feel a bit hot and bothered themselves. Whether it happens at one and a half weeks, months, or years of age, fever can admittedly be quite unnerving. As pediatricians, we are committed to making sure you develop a healthy respect for fever—especially in the first few months after your baby is born. As parents, we're also convinced that having a good understanding of what causes fever, its implications, and what may (or may not) need to be done about it will help prepare you to manage your baby's first and future fevers safely and confidently.

Fending Off Fever

Before you read up on what to do in the event that your newborn gets a fever, here are some simple strategies for putting off your first run-in with fever for as long as possible.

- **Limiting exposure.** You may find you have many well-wishers waiting in the wings even before you get home from the hospital. While you should be sure to express your gratitude for their support, be selective about whom you allow to share their best wishes in person. By coming over to see or hold your baby, they may share their viruses as well. Be aware that until newborns are old enough to be fully protected by vaccines (see Getting to the Points: Vaccines, Your Baby, and You on page 343), exposure to anyone who is unvaccinated can pose an additional risk that, for many parents, is a risk not worth taking.

- **Handwashing.** Now is not the time to be shy about requiring that anyone and everyone who wants to lay hands on your susceptible bundle of joy has to wash their hands first. All rules of in-law etiquette aside, don't hesitate to postpone all hugs and cheek pinching for as long as possible but at least long enough to ask for a show of clean hands first.

- **Don't go looking for trouble.** There's nothing inherently risky about taking an appropriately dressed newborn out of the house, but it's wise to be a bit choosy about where you go. Crowded areas and small closed-in spaces are perfect places to come into contact with unwanted germs. If you can't avoid them altogether, try to stay at least 3 to 6 feet away from anyone obviously coughing or sneezing. Alternatively, taking a walk outdoors or sticking to wide-open spaces will decrease the likelihood that your baby will be coughed on, sneezed at, or touched by people who are sick.

- **Help is only a wipe away.** Despite all your best fever-fighting efforts, you may find at some point in the not too distant future that someone, somehow, has managed to break through all lines of defense and touch your baby with the same hand recently used to hold a snot-filled tissue or cover a cough. Given that this situation can and has happened to the best of us, we suggest keeping a handy supply of baby wipes nearby to wash off the "contaminated" area at your earliest convenience. Even though we don't have hardcore evidence proving that this works, the basic principles of infection control strongly support such a simple effort, and we therefore consider it well worth a try.

Fever in Newborns

Instead of venturing into great detail about what causes fever and whether it truly warrants your fear and respect, we first want to point out what we consider to be our most important take-home message: discussing what needs to be done about a newborn with a fever is *very* different from fever considerations for older infants and children. The reason is straightforward: the younger the baby, the less prepared her immune system is to fight infection. Therefore, the best way to sum up a new parent's healthy approach to fever is that it's *always* better to be safe than sorry. You should never wonder about whether to "bother" your newborn's doctor about a fever; just make the call. Sure, most fevers during the first few months are likely to be caused by the same common cold viruses that plague the rest of us, but a newborn's risk of more serious problems from an infection, while relatively small, is nevertheless real. It is for this reason that *any baby with a fever during the first few months should be brought to the immediate attention of a doctor.* What happens from there depends on the age of the baby and the circumstances. In some cases, babies with fevers simply need close observation. In others (especially in the first month), you should be prepared for your baby's doctor to check blood, urine, and even spinal fluid for signs of infection. In general, the younger a baby is and the sicker she seems, the more likely she is to require hospitalization and treatment with antibiotics in addition to the tests just mentioned.

IN THE ABSENCE OF FEVER

While new parents are routinely warned to take fevers very seriously, some infections have the potential to cause little or no fever in newborns. In fact, it has been estimated that only half of newborns with an infection get a fever. In the absence of fever, babies who seem to be more irritable or less responsive than normal—anywhere from a bit listless to downright lethargic—or are having problems eating need to be taken just as seriously as those with fevers and evaluated to determine the cause. If you ever find yourself concerned about your baby's health, don't waste any time sitting around waiting for a fever to show up before consulting with your baby's doctor.

Overcoming the Fever Fear Factor

Now that we've done our duty in delivering the "take all fevers seriously in your newborn" warning, we also feel obliged to give you a bigger picture perspective and point out that there's a fine line between taking fevers seriously and living in constant fear of a rise in your baby's temperature. We hope that the information that follows helps eliminate the fever fear factor and better prepare you to rise to the occasion.

The Body's Built-in Thermostat

You've probably heard it on the news or read it in print: fever serves a purpose. While we won't belabor this point and make you suffer through all we learned on the subject in our own medical training, it's worth reminding yourself every now and then. Fever not only acts as a warning sign for infections but also is thought to help the body in its effort to fight germs. A part of the brain called the *hypothalamus* is responsible for regulating body temperature—similar to the way a thermostat controls the temperature in your house. In general, infants and young children have more sensitive "thermostats" than adults. When viruses, bacteria, or other fever-causing agents trigger the hypothalamus to raise the body's set point, body temperatures rise. You can therefore think of fever as the body's equivalent of having its thermostat setting turned up.

Fever Defined

The natural question that begins most discussions involving fever is "Exactly what temperature is considered a fever?" You'd think you could get a straight answer to such a seemingly straightforward and commonly asked question. But chances are good that if you asked around, you'd get a wide range of answers starting anywhere from 99°F on up to 100.4°F or more. That's because several factors go into defining fever.

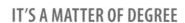

IT'S A MATTER OF DEGREE

"Normal" body temperature is generally defined as 98.6°F. A rectal temperature of 100.4°F or higher is typically used to define a fever in newborns and always warrants a call to the doctor. How the numbers that fall in between are interpreted tends to vary considerably. In part, that's because body temperature fluctuates normally over the course of any given day, generally rising a bit in the afternoon and evening. The degree of variation is thought to increase with age; while a child's or adult's temperature can vary as much as 2°F over the course of the day, you should expect your newborn's normal temperature range to be much smaller.

Using Thermometers for Good Measure

Back in the day, pretty much everyone used a glass mercury-containing thermometer. While we'll spare you a long-winded discussion of the potential dangers of broken glass and the risks associated with exposure to spilled mercury, suffice it to say, these thermometers are not just out of style, but they are not recommended. From a practical standpoint, this change is also a good thing, as we have yet to talk with anyone who found mercury thermometers to be easy to read. In contrast, the readily available digital thermometers currently in vogue are (almost) foolproof. Put them in (or on) the right spot and the numbers just appear.

Hot Spots: Fever by Location

The easiest way to categorize thermometers is according to the part of the body where the temperature is taken (*axillary* for underarm, *tympanic* for ear, *oral* or *pacifier* for mouth, *temporal artery* for forehead and temple, *temperature strips* for forehead, and *rectal* for…well, it's self-explanatory). Temperature strips, albeit temptingly easy, are generally frowned on as being notoriously inaccurate. Even using some of the more accepted temperature-taking routes, such as placing a thermometer in a child's mouth or armpit, can result in temperatures that vary quite a bit. That's why the definition of fever usually includes some reference to the location in which the temperature was taken.

FEVER ON LOCATION

The following temperatures represent the ones typically used to define fever:

- 99°F axillary
- 100°F oral
- 100.4°F rectal

When reporting a temperature to your pediatrician, there's no need for you to add, subtract, or otherwise mathematically manipulate the results according to where you took the temperature. Instead, just be sure to mention how and where you measured it.

You should be aware that many doctors recommend using rectal thermometers only for babies up until the age of about three months (with some recommending continued use until up to three years) because the resulting readings have long been considered the most accurate measure of a newborn's core body temperature.

Bottoms Up: Taking a Rectal Temperature

While you're certain to find plenty written about the ins and outs of using each type of thermometer, we decided that your time and ours would be best spent focusing on the rectal approach. There's no way around it: rectal temperatures are considered the gold standard of temperature taking, especially for babies younger than about three months. When it comes to figuring out whether your newborn has a fever, you should settle for nothing less. If you are now squirming at the thought (which we're pretty sure some of you are), take a minute to get used to the idea and then we'll walk you through the process. Despite the dread many new parents seem to experience, you just have to believe us that taking a baby's rectal temperature is not all that difficult or uncomfortable—for the baby or the parent. In fact, many parents sweat their way through taking their first temperature only to be pleasantly surprised when their babies don't seem to mind. Some even sleep right through the whole "ordeal"!

INNOVATIVE THERMOMETERS

Ear and temporal artery thermometers are marketed to parents as quick and easy alternatives to rectal thermometers and have both been shown to be relatively accurate methods of measuring temperature—just not yet standardly recommended for newborns. The temporal artery thermometer simply involves sliding the thermometer across the forehead, while ear thermometers require a good fit and angle in the ear. If you already happen to have one of these types of thermometers, you don't need to get rid of it; just be aware that it's a good idea to reach for the rectal thermometer until more definitive recommendations come out or your baby reaches at least three months of age for temporal artery thermometers and six months for ear ones.

The easiest way to get set up is to lay your baby on a comfortable but firm, flat surface. Place him across your lap if you like, or consider using a changing table or sofa or the floor—whatever you find easiest and most convenient. You can either put him onto his belly or lay him on his back. If you opt for the back, hold up your baby's legs as you would if you were changing his diaper (**Figure 27-1**). Or place him face down with his hips and knees slightly bent. Be forewarned that regardless of how you approach it, taking a rectal temperature has the potential to trigger pooping—especially in young infants—so you might want to place a towel or changing pad underneath your baby in advance. Disposable probe covers are optional but can make cleanup much easier. You may also want to dab a little lubricating jelly (such as Vaseline or K-Y Jelly) onto the short, rounded metal tip of the thermometer first. Then carefully insert the tip into the rectal (anal) opening just until the metal tip

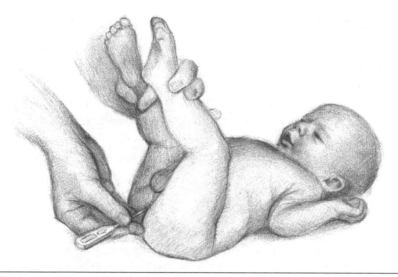

Figure 27-1. Taking a rectal temperature

is no longer showing (usually between one-half and 1 inch). Then all you need to do is keep the thermometer in place by gently squeezing your baby's butt cheeks closed around it until a reading has been made. Once you're done using the thermometer, remember to give it a good wash with some hot, soapy water, especially if you didn't use a probe cover. Be sure to put it away somewhere handy along with a written or mental note that this is now designated "for rectal use only"—not that it couldn't technically be used for any other type of temperature taking, but the thought of mistakenly doing so tends to cause people to cringe.

Over-bundled = Overheated?

It is a commonly held belief that over-bundled infants can end up with an elevation in their temperature. On the one hand, there is a certain degree of truth to this belief because babies' skin temperatures have been shown to rise noticeably with bundling and cool down again once they are unbundled and their temperature rechecked. Rectal temperature, on the other hand, is thought to be relatively unaffected by bundling, especially if you get a reading of 100.4°F or higher. Bottom line: never write off an elevated rectal tempera-ture as simply the result of too many layers of clothing or blankets—especially if the temperature doesn't come down on their removal.

Getting a Feel for Fever

Forgoing a thermometer in favor of feeling your baby's forehead is never considered an acceptable measure of fever in a newborn. Even for older children, for whom this thermometer-less method of temperature taking has been shown to be a decent way to tell whether they are hot, you still cannot rely on your hand alone to determine just how hot. In other words, parents may well be accurate in saying that their older children have fevers simply because they feel hot, but estimating just how hot—101°F versus 103.5°F, for example—is always best left to a thermometer.

CLIMATE CONTROL

Interestingly enough, there doesn't seem to be a definitive answer to the question of what temperature to set your thermostat at for the sake of your newborn's health and well-being. In general, however, consensus among parenting experts seems to be that a comfortable room temperature for babies is anywhere from 68°F to 72°F. When it comes to what is appropriate indoor attire for the youngest members of the household, some feel that babies are adequately dressed when wearing the same number of layers as everyone else. Others recommend an additional layer of clothing. We really don't think it makes that much of a difference either way and simply suggest that if your baby seems to be uncomfortably warm or cool, just be sure to adjust her clothing, your thermostat, or both accordingly.

Understanding Febrile Seizures

Febrile seizures are seizures caused by fever. While somewhere between a reassuring 95% and 98% of all children *never* have a febrile seizure, we've nevertheless found that the very idea causes most parents a certain degree of anxiety—much of it unnecessary—now and throughout parenthood. And that's why we thought we'd give you a bit of perspective on the subject to carry with you in the months and years to come. For purposes of easing your current state of mind, we want to start by pointing out that the statistics are quite comforting: newborns are unlikely to experience this type of seizure because febrile seizures typically occur between 6 months and 5 years of age. Long thought to be triggered more by a rapid rise in temperature than by the ultimate height of the fever, this long-standing theory regarding the underlying cause of febrile seizures is not clearly supported by evidence. What does seem to hold true is that if a child is destined to have a febrile seizure, it will most likely occur early on in the course of the fever, usually in the first 24 hours, rather than days into an illness. And finally, to set the record straight, febrile seizures by themselves don't cause permanent damage and are rarely predictive of a long-lasting seizure disorder. That said, seizures in babies always need to be fully evaluated to determine whether there are any underlying causes before concluding that it was a febrile seizure.

TOO MUCH OF A GOOD THING

Having done our best to inform you about the gravity of fever, let us now do our best to spare you and your newborn a lot of unnecessary probing. Given that most babies actually make it all the way through the first several months without ever needing to have their temperature taken, there is definitely such a thing as taking a baby's temperature too often. Quite a few new parents pay heed to all the abundant cautionary advice about fever in the newborn period and are consequently under the impression that they need to take and record their babies' temperatures daily (or even more frequently). We can think of very few, if any, reasons that would warrant such routine measurements in the absence of any suspicious symptoms. Big picture perspective: some of you may benefit by giving your new thermometer a break (figuratively speaking, anyway), whipping it out only for good reason (ie, make sure you didn't skip Overcoming the Fever Fear Factor on page 327).

Treating a Fever

It is short and easy to tell you how to treat a newborn's fever: if you suspect your newborn has a fever, your immediate course of action is to seek medical advice and/or attention. Everything you may know or have heard about fever medications, lukewarm baths, or the potential benefits of fever takes a back seat during the newborn period. End of discussion.

Okay, so we aren't really going to leave it at that, but we definitely mean it when we say that you don't have to bother yourself with the information in Fever Medications (the following section in this chapter) right now if you don't want to. In fact, we seriously considered not including it because we didn't want to give any of you the impression that there is any room for interpretation of fever in newborns without involving your pediatrician. Then we gave it a second thought and decided that when it comes to parenthood and fevers, there are a lot of inquiring minds out there who undoubtedly want to know more—if only for future reference.

Fever Medications

We don't intend to tell you when and how much fever medication you should use for your newborn because

1. This book is not about our practicing medicine.
2. We've already told you the golden rule—that you should first and foremost be talking with your baby's doctor.
3. Your baby's doctor, in turn, will tell you which medication to use and how much, if any (both of which will depend on your baby's age and weight).

Instead, we've listed some of the basics of fever medications that we think every parent should know.

*   Just about all medications commonly used to treat fevers in newborns and throughout childhood contain either acetaminophen (eg, Tylenol, Tempra, FeverAll) or ibuprofen (eg, Advil, Motrin).
*   Fever medication meant for use in infants comes in liquid form (concentrated drops or suspensions) or as rectal suppositories.
*   Fever medications are always dosed according to a baby's weight.
*   Different sizes of droppers are used to measure liquid fever medication. As a result, one dropperful can mean different amounts, depending on which type and brand of infant drops you're using, so always pay very close attention to the markings, and use only the dropper that came with the bottle.
*   Infant drops may be much more concentrated than the children's suspension form. Always make yourself double-check that the dose you are using is correct for the type of medication you're using.
*   Be sure to read the fine print on the label about how often the medication can be given and take it very seriously! Acetaminophen is not to be given more often than every four to six hours. Ibuprofen (not generally recommended for infants younger than six months) should be repeated only every six to eight hours. Diligent record keeping—whether you use pen and paper or opt for an app (see At-Home Record Keeping on page xxix)— is always important, especially if multiple caregivers will be giving the medication.

28

seeing yellow: jaundice

* * * * * *

In our humble but medical opinion, all new parents should add the color yellow to their list of newborn traits to be familiar with, watch for, and be poised and ready to bring to medical attention if and when it shows up. That's because most newborns during their first weeks stand a good chance of turning at least a light shade of yellow—in other words, developing some degree of jaundice. While jaundice by itself is not, in fact, a disease, it is a visible indication that extra bilirubin is in a baby's bloodstream. And while not nearly as common, it's worth being aware that in large amounts, bilirubin can cause problems. In most cases, however, jaundice is harmless. In some cases, it requires treatment. In any case, you'll want to be prepared to recognize jaundice and discuss its appearance with your pediatrician without delay.

Behind the Scenes

We thought it would be useful to provide you with a basic understanding of what lies just below the surface of yellow-tinged skin. To do that, it helps if you understand what bilirubin is. From birth and throughout our lives, our bodies are responsible for continually breaking down and getting rid of old red blood cells, all the while replacing them with new ones. Bilirubin is simply a normal breakdown product of red blood cells. Our livers are given the ongoing task of processing bilirubin, which is ultimately disposed of by the intestines in the form of poop. Jaundice results when, for whatever reason, too much bilirubin accumulates in the body.

Who Gets Jaundice?

While bilirubin is an antioxidant and having small amounts can be a good thing, having too much can cause health problems. A baby's genetics can also influence the amount of jaundice that is present. There are several straight-forward reasons why healthy, full-term newborns develop higher than normal levels of bilirubin and end up looking yellow. Not only do newborns have a proportionately larger number of red blood cells than adults—inevitably requiring more in the way of breakdown and processing—but it can take a baby's liver several days or even weeks after birth before it is able to rise to the occasion and function at full speed. Ultimately, the two main factors involved in bilirubin removal include

1. How much of it there is
2. How efficiently it's being cleared out

Here are examples for each.

It's in the Blood

- **More blood.** As we mentioned, babies are born with a higher concentra-tion of red blood cells than adults and older children have. This places a greater demand on a newborn's liver.

- **Bruising.** Many newborns experience some degree of bruising or even develop what is called a *hematoma* (an egg-like swelling of blood, most commonly in the scalp), which typically results from the pressure of child-birth (see Bumps and Bruises on page 298) or from the use of forceps or a vacuum during the delivery. As these additional collections of blood cells are broken down in the body, there is a resulting increase in bilirubin level that the newborn's body must then clear.

- **Blood type differences.** Jaundice is sometimes caused when mom and baby have different blood types. For the most part, a mother's blood remains separate from her baby's throughout pregnancy. During delivery, however, some of it manages to pass through the placenta and umbilical cord and make its way into the baby's bloodstream. Recognizing these stray red blood cells as foreign, the baby's body swiftly reacts against them by breaking them down, posing the potential for a more rapid accumula-tion of bilirubin.

Getting the All Clear

- **Catching on.** Babies tend to have slow liver function at first and may have some evidence of jaundice as they wait for their livers to mature and catch up.

- **Slow to go.** Newborns who are slow to figure out how to eat or are not getting much fluid in the early days of breastfeeding may in turn be slow to poop. There may be other medical reasons for why a newborn has problems with pooping. Either way, the end result is that bilirubin stays in the body instead of being pooped out.

- **Problems with processing.** Far less commonly, a baby may have a more serious problem with the liver. Certain disorders can cause the liver not to function properly, resulting not only in a buildup of bilirubin but the appearance of pale-colored (almost white) poop.

From the Top Down

Whenever bilirubin builds up in the bloodstream, regardless of cause, more of it inevitably makes its way into the skin and causes it to appear yellow. Interestingly, the yellow tends to show up in a fairly predictable head-to-toe fashion—first showing up on the face and then gradually spreading down toward the toes. How far down on a newborn's body the yellow goes is thought to be roughly indicative of how high the bilirubin level is in the blood. In other words, the lower down on the body the yellow extends, the higher the bilirubin level is likely to be. As a sidenote, the shade and intensity of the yellow can be deceiving and can't be relied on to offer any sort of definitive clue as to just how high the bilirubin level actually is.

Time Course

Most babies who are born at full term reach their peak levels of jaundice within 3 to 5 days before improving completely; bilirubin levels in babies born prematurely, however, often peak a few days later. In either case, after the bilirubin level peaks, an otherwise healthy baby's jaundice should resolve within a few weeks. Newborns who appear to develop jaundice earlier or whose jaundice persists much longer than is typically expected may have an underlying medical problem that should be evaluated by a pediatrician.

- **Early jaundice.** Any jaundice that appears within the first 24 hours after birth needs medical evaluation. Sometimes it can indicate a problem with the liver or a baby's blood cells that needs to be addressed, but in all instances, it suggests that the bilirubin level needs to be watched closely and treated appropriately.

- **Typical jaundice.** Regular newborn jaundice (also called *physiologic jaundice* or *non-pathological jaundice*) appears gradually after the first couple days. The bilirubin level generally peaks by about 5 days after birth for full-term babies and about 1 week for those born premature.

- **Late jaundice.** Newborns with what is referred to as *breast milk jaundice* may not reach their most yellow until 2 weeks of age, and their level may take anywhere from 3 to 12 weeks to return to normal. Fortunately, breast milk jaundice in an otherwise healthy baby who is breastfeeding and gaining weight well does not require that mom stops breastfeeding, but you'll certainly want to talk with your pediatrician before coming to any conclusions about whether you think your baby might have this type of jaundice.

- **Persistent jaundice.** Regardless of when jaundice sets in, babies whose livers can't keep up, for whatever reason, get progressively more yellow. In some babies who have liver conditions, a baby's poop can also lose its color and become pale. This is one of the many reasons why pediatricians routinely express sincere interest in the color of baby poop (see The Many Colors of Poop on page 77). Another sign to be on the lookout for in conjunction with jaundice is poor growth because just about any underlying medical problem can cause newborns to gain weight more slowly than expected. On occasion, red blood cell abnormalities are also known to cause the type of jaundice that lasts for longer than a few weeks. Before you assume the worst, read on because good old-fashioned, run-of-the-mill jaundice can certainly take a while to fade away.

EASY COME, SLOW TO GO

Jaundice appears fairly predictably from head to toe as bilirubin levels rise. However, the yellow color does not always disappear in reverse as bilirubin levels subsequently fall, and it can take weeks for jaundice to fade away completely. In general, the whites of the eyes are usually the last things to return to normal.

Spot-checking for Jaundice

Just as with fever in the newborn period, trust us when we say that your baby's doctor will want to know if you're seeing yellow in your baby's eyes or on her skin. While some babies become unmistakably yellow, a development easily alerting parents and pediatricians alike that they need to be evaluated, we have found that others pose more of a challenge. That's because the color changes of some newborns' skin can be more subtle—whether due to varying underlying skin tones, ruddy complexions, dim room lights, yellow clothing, sleep deprivation, or yellow-painted walls or simply because jaundice has a way of gradually creeping up on new parents unnoticed. To be more effectively on the lookout for jaundice, we suggest you

- Move to a well-lit area, preferably one that offers you natural light.
- Gently press on your baby's skin and then remove your finger.
- Before blood flow returns and makes the skin appear pink again, take a look to see whether the underlying area appears yellow. If you're not sure, compare it to a spot much farther down on the body using the same technique.
- If the first area you check appears to be yellow, make your way down your baby's body—the upper chest first, the nipple line next, and then the belly; continue to spot-check until you find a level at which the jaundice stops. Report (or show) your findings to your baby's pediatrician.
- Keep a watchful eye to see if the jaundice increases—an admittedly unreliable visual sign that tends to go along with other important signs of concern such as increased sleepiness or lethargy, and poor feeding.

Measuring Bilirubin Levels

Skin color changes can offer parents and pediatricians the first hint that bilirubin levels are on the rise. Subsequently, the rate at which the yellow color spreads from head to toe can give us a vague idea of how fast the bilirubin level is increasing. Whenever the degree of jaundice is in question, a simple blood test is currently considered the most accurate way of determining where things stand. If your baby becomes jaundiced, don't be surprised if he is subjected to one or more heel pokes or blood draws to collect the necessary sample(s) to determine how much bilirubin is in his bloodstream. How many bilirubin levels your baby's doctor decides to check will depend on not only what's causing your baby's jaundice and how many days old your baby is when it appears but also how high the first level is, how fast it seems to be rising, and how likely it is to be effectively cleared. Also available is a technology called *transcutaneous bilirubin monitoring* (TcB) that determines bilirubin levels by using a special form of light applied to the skin's surface. Although some studies have shown TcB monitoring to be equally accurate, and it is generally more readily accepted because it is noninvasive (ie, no bloodletting is involved), when in doubt, pediatricians still consider the blood test to be the gold standard. Your pediatrician may refer to resources such as http://bilitool. org to determine what type of intervention, if any, is recommended.

Taking Care of Business: Treating Jaundice

Getting Pooped Out

Because we know bilirubin is primarily cleared out of the body in poop—something that some newborns produce in much more abundant supply than others—it only stands to reason that newborns who get off to a slower start with pooping may in turn become a bit more yellow than those who fill their diapers early and often. When it comes to jaundice, the more you can do to encourage feeding (and therefore pooping), the better. You may have been advised to feed your baby at least every three to four hours, or, in the case of breastfed babies, at least 10 times per day. But if your baby is interested in eating even sooner, go ahead and feed her more frequently, as this can help clear out the bilirubin. If possible, feed your baby slightly more milk at each sitting (such as by adding a few more minutes per side if breastfeeding or by offering an extra ounce or so if bottle-feeding) to help increase the poop output.

LET THE SUNSHINE IN ON JAUNDICE

Rumor has it that in the 1950s, an observant nurse noticed that babies placed near the window in the newborn nursery were less likely to become jaundiced than their (relatively) in-the-dark colleagues on the other side of the room. Whether this story is actually true, we're not sure because we didn't devote any time to checking it out. What we do know is that while sunlight can change bilirubin into a form the body can dispose of more easily, exposure to direct sunlight is not recommended because of the associated risks (namely, sunburn, hyperthermia, dehydration, and potential long-term skin damage). Just be aware that although commercially tinted film to selectively filter harmful rays may be recommended as an alternative to direct sunlight, you'll want to make sure the room temperature is such that your baby won't get too cold while undressed.

Let the Lights Begin

After further study of the "let the sunshine in" principle of treating jaundice, a particular wavelength of blue light has been shown to speed up the bilirubin breakdown and elimination process without causing sunburn. As a result, light therapy (also referred to as *phototherapy*) is the most common medical treatment of newborn jaundice. Phototherapy simply makes use of this blue wavelength in the form of a "bili blanket" or special lights to treat babies with high bilirubin levels easily and effectively. This lighting may be done in the hospital, especially if the level of bilirubin is very high or becomes elevated quickly. More often than not, however, jaundice appears after babies have been discharged. For otherwise healthy babies whose jaundice shows up when they are at home or ready for discharge, it's often possible to have the phototherapy equipment set up at home for the few days they need it. Of course, for significantly high levels, it's safest to be treated in the hospital.

A Positive Perspective on Rising Bilirubin Levels

While we have done our best to prepare you for the possibility of jaundice, we are well aware that facing a yellow newborn with rising bilirubin levels requiring repeated trips to the pediatrician's office (or blood work in the hospital) all in the first week or so of parenthood can be quite challenging. In fact, some new parents find jaundice to be so concerning—even when it's well under control—that it makes them feel that their new babies are unhealthy and that they themselves are ill-equipped for the demands of parenthood. We therefore want to make sure to give you a more positive big picture perspective. Remember, not only is jaundice not a disease, but bilirubin is actually thought to be protective so long as it doesn't reach too high a level. While it is true that extremely high levels of bilirubin, when left untreated, can have serious effects on babies such as hearing loss or brain damage, severe jaundice is rare and generally tends to occur in babies born prematurely or who are critically ill. We are fortunate that modern-day medicine allows us to recognize and treat rising bilirubin levels long before they reach dangerous levels. In addition, any poking, prodding, repeated doctor visits, phototherapy, or hospitalization necessitated by bilirubin levels on the rise is usually done to keep bilirubin levels from ever getting to the point where they could pose a more serious risk.

29

getting to the points: vaccines, your baby, and you

● ● ● ● ● ●

We'd like to think this chapter won't be your first exposure to the topic of vaccines. If nothing else, we hope by the time you finish reading it, you're convinced it shouldn't be your last. That's because vaccines are recognized as one of the most lifesaving public health achievements of the past century and have become a mainstay of modern medicine, pediatrics, and parenthood. The fact is that your child will receive plenty of vaccines over the next several years (and on into adolescence and adulthood, for that matter), all of which help prevent the serious and life-threatening diseases of decades past. Whether you have recent memories of getting a flu vaccine, or older recollections of your own childhood immunizations, a lot has changed with today's vaccines. Here's an overview you won't want to skip, starting with a look at vaccines and ending with a quick but sobering reminder about the devastating diseases themselves—diseases we now have the power to prevent.

What Exactly Are Vaccines?

To answer the fundamental question "What exactly are vaccines?" let's start with a brief background on the immune system and how it works. We are all born with an immune system made up of cells, glands, organs, and fluids. These components work together throughout the body to fight bacteria and viruses and other threats to our health. The immune system's job is to be on the lookout for any germs that enter the body, recognize them as foreign invaders (commonly referred to as *antigens*), and make weapons specifically to fight against them (*antibodies*). One of the most important features of the immune system is its memory. Your immune system not only is capable of making antibodies against a whole host of antigens but learns from its experiences. This learning allows our immune systems to better defend us in the future against antigens we've been exposed to in months, years, and even decades past. Simply put, this is how we develop *immunity.*

PUTTING VACCINES INTO PERSPECTIVE: HOW FAR WE'VE COME

1796	Edward Jenner notices that milkmaids exposed to cowpox seem to be protected from getting smallpox—an extremely deadly disease that at the time accounted for up to 10% of all deaths worldwide. His observation leads to the development of the first successful vaccine.
1955	Jonas Salk, MD, develops the first polio vaccine.
1963	The first measles vaccine is licensed, followed in 1967 by the MMR (measles-mumps-rubella) vaccine.
1964	A committee is established by the Centers for Disease Control and Prevention (CDC) to provide expert advice on the use of vaccines. The Advisory Committee on Immunization Practices continues to do so ever since.
1979	The world sees its last case of smallpox. Its eradication is heralded as one of the greatest achievements of modern medicine.
1988	The World Health Assembly launches a global attack on polio at a time when the virus was still found in 125 countries on 5 continents and paralyzed more than 1,000 children each and every day.
1990	VAERS (Vaccine Adverse Event Reporting System) is created as a national system to monitor vaccine safety. It still exists today.
1991	Hepatitis B vaccine is recommended for all newborns and infants.
1999 to 2001	Thimerosal is phased out of use as a preservative in the routine childhood immunization series as a precautionary measure. It is later found not to cause any harmful effects. Even so, only a few of today's childhood vaccines use thimerosal in the manufacturing process (which is then removed), while most contain no thimerosal at all.
2006	Fewer than 2,000 cases of polio a year are reported worldwide. The fact that this number is so close to 0 is attributed to the monumental polio eradication effort that began in 1988 and resulted in the immunization of more than 2 billion children.
2014	Federally supported vaccination of children born from 1994 to 2013 has or will prevent nearly 750,000 deaths.

Vaccines—also commonly referred to as *immunizations*—help prevent dangerous germs from causing diseases by preparing the immune system to recognize them. In fact, vaccines are composed of the very same antigens (or parts of them) that cause diseases. Unlike germs themselves, however, vaccines are made of either killed antigens or significantly weakened live antigens. The trick to making vaccines is making sure they're strong enough to teach the immune system to create antibodies, memory cells, and, therefore, immunity but not strong enough to cause diseases. While most vaccines are given as shots, certain vaccines can be given by mouth (orally, such as the rotavirus vaccine) or in the nose (nasally, such as one of the current flu vaccines). And for those of you who are needle averse, be aware that emerging vaccine technology may soon yield innovative new ways to give vaccines that are just as effective but do not require a shot. As for us, we're still holding out hope for the long-rumored vaccine-producing banana plant and other forms of edible vaccines that stand to present more palatable possibilities for disease prevention.

Getting Right to the Point

Let's get to the point that many new parents seem to worry about most: the one that is used to give shots. Yes, it's a needle. And no, we don't personally find the actual process of getting a shot to be pleasant. Given that shots' reputation almost invariably precedes them, it only makes sense that many pediatricians we know spell the word s-h-o-t, tiptoe around the concept of it, and/or do their very best not to say the word *shot* any more than necessary. But to put things into perspective for you and all parents with whom we've discussed vaccination over the past two decades, we like to point out that a quick needle poke is actually preferable to many well-tolerated discomforts we can think of, including paper cuts. Unlike a paper cut, however, the poke of a needle serves a very clear and potentially lifesaving purpose.

A BOOST BEFORE BIRTH

Did you know that mothers can take credit for giving their babies' immune systems their very first antibody boost? Although a newborn's immune system can take a good six months after birth to get up to full speed, antibodies can cross over from the mother to the baby through the placenta months before birth. While antibodies shared between mom and baby during pregnancy provide newborns with valuable protection against many infections, they unfortunately don't protect against some serious and vaccine-preventable illnesses, such as whooping cough (*pertussis*). In addition, their ability to protect wears off within one month to one year. These limitations are both good reasons why vaccines are given as early as possible in childhood and why it's so important for moms and other caregivers who are in close contact with babies to get themselves vaccinated against influenza and to get the Tdap vaccine. They are also the reason why breast milk (which contains antibodies) helps keep breastfed babies healthier during the first year (see A Breast a Day Keeps the Doctor Away on page 12).

With that in mind, let's focus our attention, as well as yours, on some simple yet effective ways you can support and soothe your baby as she gets her shots.

- **A show of support.** We have observed over the years that how babies react to getting shots often reflects how their parents react. If you tremble and quake, your baby will definitely be able to sense your stress. Our suggestion? Take a deep breath, remind yourself that shots are over and done with quickly, and offer your baby a strong show of support by staying calm, close by, and ready to hold and console her. This approach will serve you well for the many shot-related visits that lie ahead. You should also apply the same principle of calm when your baby turns into a toddler and spends her days toddling, tripping, and bumping into things. When she feels any pain, she will undoubtedly look to you for a reaction. If you can remain relatively cool and supportively collected, you'll help ensure that each and every head bump or up-and-over attempt at walking (of which there will be many) doesn't turn into an unnecessarily melodramatic experience.

- **Hold tight…not only figuratively but literally.** Realize that your physical contact, whether it's holding your baby in your lap, hugging her, holding her hands, or stroking her head, can go a long way toward making the actual shot much more bearable. By helping make sure your baby doesn't move during the process, you can help ensure that the shots are over and done with more efficiently *and* safely.

- **Be soothing.** While getting a shot is no walk in the park, the procedure itself is over very quickly and typically leaves babies surprised and a bit indignant more than anything else. After your baby receives a shot, we recommend you hold, talk to, sing to, or otherwise soothe her right away and then move on to something else, such as breastfeeding or giving a bottle, or going for a brief walk outside the examination room.

Taking the Edge Off

One dose? Two doses? Three doses? Four! One of the most immediate questions parents typically pose after all the shots are said and done is whether they can, should, or need to give their newly vaccinated infants any acetaminophen (most commonly in the form of Tylenol). In our experience, any pain from injections is usually short-lived, although some babies have soreness at the site of the shot for a day or two. After receiving any vaccine, there's also a chance babies may develop a low-grade fever (up to 100°F or 101°F), and some may be a little fussier or sleepier than usual for the rest of the day. While these symptoms can be disconcerting to new parents, they can also mean the vaccine is having the desired effect. While we both tend to fall into the wait-and-see-if-it's-really-warranted camp, you should discuss with your baby's doctor if and when to give any pain reliever or fever reducer after shots have been given, as parents and pediatricians alike vary in their philosophies. Methods of medicating range from all or nothing to somewhere in between.

- **Wait and see.** This approach means you choose not to give any acetaminophen in anticipation of unwanted symptoms before or after immunizations are given but rather sit tight and wait to see whether any signs or symptoms truly warrant it.

- **A dose for good measure.** This middle-of-the-road approach involves giving a single dose of acetaminophen after your baby gets shots "just in case" and then waiting to see whether any additional doses are needed. While some parents and pediatricians used to opt to preemptively premedicate *before* the shots, concerns have been raised about whether doing so actually decreases the body's desired immune response. For this reason, giving acetaminophen *before* shots or symptoms has gone out of favor.

- **Covering your bases.** As far as we know, not too many parents these days opt to give their babies acetaminophen every 4 to 6 hours for the 24 or so hours after shots. And if you ask us, that is probably a good thing. Although acetaminophen has been shown to decrease the degree to which babies get fevers after shots, a recent study also raised the question of whether acetaminophen has the potential to lessen the effectiveness of shots. Given that most babies really seem to do well without the benefit of any medication, we recommend minimizing how much you give unless your baby is fussy, feverish, or uncomfortable, in which case you should discuss the symptoms with your baby's doctor.

Regardless of the approach you choose, we want you to always be sure to consult with your pediatrician and your vaccine information statements (see VIS = Very Important Sheets on page 352) about adverse effects your baby may experience. Ask whether giving acetaminophen is warranted, and if it is, make sure to find out the proper dosage for your baby, based on her current weight (see Fever Medications on page 334).

YOUR FIRST SHOT AT PREVENTION: HEPATITIS B

According to the American Academy of Pediatrics (AAP), all newborns should be given their first shot at vaccines even before leaving the hospital. According to the updated 2017 AAP policy statement, the first dose of hepatitis B vaccine (also referred to as "Hep B vaccine," or HBV for short) is recommended to be given within the first 24 hours after delivery because doing so maximizes the effectiveness of the vaccine in preventing newborn infection. Although a baby's risk of infection with hepatitis B virus is relatively low, it is a risk well worth protecting against. The hepatitis B virus is known to cause serious liver disease that can lead to liver failure or cancer later in life. Fortunately, the vaccine is considered to be one of the most effective vaccines available and has been shown to be both safe and effective when given as a first, or "birth," dose to all medically stable newborns weighing 4 pounds 6 ounces or more. If you want to put the hepatitis B vaccine's protective powers into perspective, consider this statistic: since routine vaccination began in 1991, infection rates among children and adolescents have dropped by more than 95%.

The Childhood Immunization Schedule

Each year, leading pediatric and infectious disease experts put together the standard childhood immunization schedule. This schedule is admittedly a busy one, involving a master multiyear rollout plan for your baby's many vaccines. While this would be the time when we'd ideally proceed to lay out a nice, simple timeline for you to follow, the reality is that this timeline changes a bit each year based on the latest scientific information available, and the schedule is created with a certain degree of flexibility. What we can tell you is that you can pretty much expect at least one immunization—and probably more—at each of your baby's routine well-child visits (also known as *health supervision visits*), typically scheduled at 1, 2, 4, 6, 9, 12, 15, and 18 months of age. Here are some additional factors that play a role in scheduling vaccines.

- Vaccines are given early in childhood, based on the principle that the sooner we protect babies, the better. That's because many of the infections that immunizations are so effective in preventing are deadliest during infancy.
- Figuring out when to give each vaccine depends on scientific research that tells us when children's immune systems will be able to rise effectively to the challenge.
- Vaccines given in combination, such as the MMR (measles-mumps-rubella) vaccine, have been shown to be at least as effective, if not more so, than when each component vaccine is given separately.
- Most childhood vaccines require more than one dose to ensure that your child develops immunity. There is always a required wait time between one dose and the next.

While there are occasional exceptions, the official childhood immuniza-tion schedule is a good starting point for most children because most "alter-native" vaccine schedules have not been studied for safety and effectiveness, and many pediatric practices only accept patients who have been vaccinated according to the schedule recommended by the Centers for Disease Control and Prevention (CDC). In large part, this is because having unvaccinated children in a pediatric office can put infants and other children with weak immune systems at risk. If you are determined to follow a different schedule that involves postponing or foregoing certain vaccines, you may be asked to sign a document stating that you understand the risks and consequences of not vaccinating your child. Should you have any questions or concerns about vaccines, discuss them with your baby's doctor.

For the (Immunization) Record

What we can share with you from experience, as pediatricians and as parents, is the advice to keep good records about every vaccine your baby gets, starting from day 1. Sure, this may seem like stating the obvious, and yes, your baby's doctor is required to document all of them as well. But given that you will be asked to provide this information many, many times over the upcoming years—for your child's entry into everything from child care to elementary school, a new doctor's office, a foreign country, college, and beyond—we can't stress enough how glad you'll be to have handy a neatly documented, up-to-date list of the names and dates of all your child's vaccines in one easy-to-track-down-later place. Whether this information is in a baby book or updated online, stored for safekeeping in your computer files or on a state registry, having a backup of your child's meticulously maintained immunization record will prove to be exceptionally useful, if not downright mandatory.

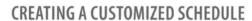

CREATING A CUSTOMIZED SCHEDULE

If you like to stay on top of things and want to create your very own customized immunization schedule, look no further than the Centers for Disease Control and Prevention (CDC) website. The only part of the process that requires your patience will be entering the Web address needed to take you directly to its very cool Childhood Vaccine Assessment Tool (www2a.cdc.gov/vaccines/childquiz). Once there, all you have to do is enter your baby's birth date (which, for the record, is not shared or stored) and…voilà! You have a printable schedule of all currently recommended vaccines and the calculated date on which your baby will be due to get each of them. There is even a column for you to record the actual date your baby receives each vaccine.

Reliable Resources

It's only natural that parents want to know as much as possible about the safety and effectiveness of vaccines. The best trick to staying informed about all your child's future vaccines is knowing where to get the most current and accurate information. We suggest you start by making it a habit to discuss vaccinations with your baby's doctor and taking time to read the Vaccine Information Statements (VISs) you will receive every time your child gets a vaccine.

If you'd like additional information, here are some of the reliable organizations and websites we share with our own patients, friends, and family members.

- **HealthyChildren.org, the official American Academy of Pediatrics (AAP) website for parents**
  - www.healthychildren.org/immunizations
  - The AAP and its 67,000 members play an integral role in assessing, revising, and delivering information about vaccines and have created a parent-friendly website to give you direct access to this useful information.

- **The CDC**
  - www.cdc.gov/vaccines
  - Here you'll find a wealth of information you can trust about everything from safety and schedules to details about the diseases themselves.

- **The Immunization Action Coalition**
  - www.vaccineinformation.org
  - This national nonprofit organization is dedicated to the prevention of disease through immunization by way of creation and distribution of educational materials for the public (as well as for health care providers).

- **The Vaccine Education Center at the Children's Hospital of Philadelphia**
  - www.chop.edu/service/vaccine-education-center
  - Here you'll find Parents PACK (which stands for Possessing, Accessing and Communicating Knowledge), a program designed to give parents access to up-to-date information and a place to go to ask questions and have an informed dialogue about vaccines. The easiest way to find it is to simply use the search option on the website and type in "PACK."

VIS = VERY IMPORTANT SHEETS

Okay, so technically, *VIS* stands for **V**accine **I**nformation **S**tatement. However, these sheets are not only informative but unquestionably important—so important, in fact, that federal law requires that VISs be handed out before most vaccinations are given. Carefully written by the Centers for Disease Control and Prevention (CDC) and available in nearly 50 languages, they conveniently contain the most current information about the benefits and risks of each vaccine, as well as a description of any potential adverse effects condensed into a relatively easy-to-read single sheet of paper. While you will certainly have plenty of VISs provided to you over the next several years, you can access them for yourself at www.immunize.org/vis.

Out of Sight but Never Out of Mind

While we hope you will now be better prepared to oversee your child's immunizations, we want to close out our overview with a quick reminder of why it is that vaccines are so important. That most new parents (and younger pediatricians) in the United States today have never seen, much less experienced, a case of polio, mumps, or rubella, for example, is both good and bad: good because this lack of exposure means we've been incredibly successful in combating devastating diseases of the past but bad because it has made it all too easy to get swept up in the day-to-day details of new parenthood and forget about diseases that are now largely out-of-sight. But with the exception of smallpox, they are not gone. To keep them from being out of mind, we're leaving you with a brief but important look at some of the diseases we're all working together to prevent.

- **Polio.** This is a contagious viral illness that affected up to 20,000 Americans a year before widespread vaccine use. Some people infected with this virus (including former President Franklin Roosevelt) were left with paralyzed arms, paralyzed legs, or both. In others, however, the virus paralyzed the muscles necessary to breathe and resulted in death.

- **Measles.** Measles not only can cause rash, cough, runny nose, eye irritation, and high fever but can also lead to ear infections, pneumonia, and—most concerning—seizures, brain damage, or death. Before a vaccine was available, nearly everyone in the United States could be expected to get measles, and 450 died each year of the disease. While there has been a truly dramatic decrease in measles cases in the United States—from millions down to hundreds of cases per year—rates of infection run the real risk of surging every time vaccination rates go down. If the vaccine was no longer available, there's every reason to believe that the highly contagious virus causing measles (*paramyxovirus*) would return to infecting US children by the millions and cause an estimated 2.7 million annual deaths worldwide.

- **Mumps.** In addition to the more common symptoms of fever, headache, and swollen glands, the mumps virus is known to cause deafness, meningitis, painful swelling of the testicles or ovaries, and (more rarely) infertility or death.

A CONCERNING BUMP IN MEASLES AND MUMPS!

To say that measles and mumps are "out-of-sight" is untrue, *and* allowing them to become "out of mind" is proving itself to be a very risky proposition. Before a vaccine was introduced in 1968, a total of 3 to 4 million people were infected by the measles-causing virus (*paramyxovirus*) every year, resulting in about 500 deaths. After being declared eliminated in the United States in 2000, measles resurfaced; there have increasingly been pockets of outbreaks mostly caused by international travel and communities with groups of unvaccinated individuals. After a record number of measles infections in 2014 (644 reported cases in 27 states), 2015 saw an outbreak of measles thought to have started at Disneyland that in the first two months of the year had already infected 173 people in 17 states. In the year 2019, we saw the greatest number of measles cases since 1992, with 1,250 cases reported in the first nine months. Although measles was reported in 31 states, more than 75% of cases were in New York state, and most were in people who had not been vaccinated.

Similarly, intermittent mumps outbreaks have occurred in the United States as recently as 2014, as well as two large outbreaks in 2009 to 2010, involving more than 3,000 people, and a 2006 multistate outbreak that sickened more than double that many.

Outbreaks such as these serve as harsh reminders of the need to protect our children against vaccine-preventable diseases and, more specifically, that the benefit of the MMR (measles-mumps-rubella) vaccine is as important as ever.

- **Rubella.** While the rash, mild fever, and arthritis characteristic of rubella may not seem too serious, the rubella virus poses a great risk to unborn babies. If a pregnant woman gets infected, a miscarriage or serious birth defects can result.

- **Diphtheria.** Diphtheria is caused by bacteria that have the ability to create a thick covering over the back of the throat and cause breathing problems, paralysis, heart failure, and death—particularly in infancy.

- **Tetanus.** This potentially fatal infection results when bacteria get into the body through open cuts or wounds. It doesn't take more than stepping on a rusty nail or cutting yourself with a dirty knife to become infected. Tetanus is commonly referred to as "lockjaw" because it causes painful tightening of the muscles, including the jaw, that can make opening one's mouth or swallowing impossible. Of those infected, 2 out of every 10 die of tetanus.

- ***Haemophilus influenzae* type b.** You are probably familiar with this bacterium only by its abbreviated name, *Hib*. It can cause pneumonia, severe swelling in the throat, and infections of the blood, joints, bones, and heart, and it used to be the leading cause of bacterial meningitis in the United States in children younger than five years. Before Hib vaccine became available in 1985, this bacterium was responsible for more than 20,000 severe infections and 1,000 deaths a year.

While there are many more diseases science can claim to have conquered, we'll stop here and let you learn more about them, as well as the vaccines that prevent them, by using the resource list we've provided.

SECTION

thanks for the memories

• • • • • • •

introduction

· · · · · · ·

Time Flies, So Catch It!

Time certainly may not seem to fly by when you're anxiously awaiting the birth of your baby or knee-deep in diapers and facing your umpteenth night of interrupted sleep. But one of the almost universal insights parents gain with time is just how fast the days, weeks, months, and years go by. A cliché? Yes, but one definitely worth taking note of at the start of your parenting career and then making sure to capture in the form of meaningful moments preserved for posterity along the way.

Reality Check

Before we jump right in to our advice about how best to approach creatively capturing and archiving your parenting memories, we feel the need to share a bit of historical perspective. When we set out to write the first edition of *Heading Home With Your Newborn* more than 15 years ago, we felt the need to disclose that neither of us came close to qualifying as Martha Stewart disciples when it came to craftiness (although Laura on occasion had to curb her urges). Nevertheless, we found that our own relatively simple creations and suggestions we'd collected over the years about how best to preserve childhood memories ranked high on the list of our most popular advice. Fast-forward to today, and not even Martha Stewart can compete with the vast array of Pinterest-worthy creations now readily available and at your fingertips 24/7. In light of this virtual plethora of crafty ideas—from books to bloggers and beyond—we have come to the revised conclusion that the most important insight we now stand to offer you, rather than a mere handful of suggestions, is foresight. Once you've given just a little advance thought to what piques your interest and appeals to your tastes, at the very least, we hope to help you think up or find enough ideas to keep you from joining the ranks of the parents before you who have found themselves regretfully saying, "What a great idea! If only I'd thought to do it myself…sooner…with my first child…when I had time!"

CHAPTER

30

birth memories

• • • • • •

Whether the birth of your baby has yet to become a reality or is an event so recently ingrained in your memory that the possibility of forgetting any detail seems unlikely, we want to forewarn you that even birth memories tend to fade and blur over time. That's fine for those of you content with simply remembering the date and time of the big event along with a few random details interjected into the picture. If you aim to remember more—for your own sake and to share with your child someday—you will want to continue reading this chapter. The suggestions and reminders we've included are admittedly simple and straightforward, yet while you're swimming in all the novelties of parenthood, you might not otherwise think of them.

Keys to Photographic Success in the Delivery Room

The birth of your baby will undoubtedly be a momentous occasion—one worthy of capturing for posterity (if you are so inclined). However, it's one thing to envision the perfect photo (or video) of your baby's grand entrance in the delivery room and another to actually get it. Also worthy of consideration is figuring out exactly how much of "the moment" you want to capture, how you're going to go about doing it, and how much of it you intend to share with others.

- **Plan ahead.** If and when you fall into delivery preparedness mode and pack your suitcase in anticipation of your trip to labor and delivery, don't forget to charge whichever photographic device you hope to use (and bring along any chargers, batteries, memory cards, or other accessories they may require, if you opt for anything more than the camera on your phone). Even beyond showing up with your phone or other camera equipment of choice, we suggest you take a few minutes between breathing exercises and obstetrician appointments to discuss a simple photographic game plan. First and foremost, be sure to find out if your hospital has photographic restrictions. If there are any, you'll want to factor them in as you think about your photographic goals. If you've got your heart set on capturing a particular shot, the odds of getting it will be better if you make your wishes known ahead of time to whomever you plan on having in the delivery room with you. Don't forget to figure out a place to keep your camera of choice that's out of the way but easily accessible. While all this advance planning may seem a little extreme to some of you (especially those of you less "into" photography than we are), trust us when we say the resulting photos will speak for themselves.

- **Delegate.** If you don't consider yourself much of a photographer, have no desire to rise to the occasion and focus your efforts on capturing the moment, or just anticipate having too many other things on your mind when you deliver, we (and the realities of childbirth) suggest you delegate. If you plan on having family or friends in the delivery room, pick one you consider to be the best photographer and who's least likely to be overcome with emotion when it's time to push the button, click the shutter, or start the video rolling. Then clarify which shots you hope to have captured when all is said and done. Also make sure your designated photographer is comfortable using whichever camera equipment you plan to have on hand, as well as prepared to charge it, swap out memory cards, or replace batteries. In short, the delivery room isn't a great place to sit down for the first time and attempt to figure out someone else's phone or the latest in digital photography and technology.

- **Use discretion.** You don't have to have gone through labor and delivery or witnessed a baby being born before to realize there's not a whole lot of privacy involved in the process. That does not, however, mean you can't control the degree of exposure evident in the commemorative photographs. I'm sure you all know what we're talking about because you inevitably have to give at least some thought to how to take pictures of a baby being born *without* getting what seems crude to say, but has nonetheless been best described as, the infamous "crotch shot." Fathers-to-be (or other family members or friends) who might otherwise find themselves caught up in the moment often do well in their role as photographer if you've not only delegated the job ahead of time but made it very clear what you do and do not want to see revealed in the family photo album or posted online for all of eternity. The fact that digital photographs can quickly and easily be edited or cropped helps, but you'll still want to make sure ahead of time that nothing gets shared socially without your approval first.

- **Consider composition.** Now you may be thinking to yourself, "Who has the time to consider composition? I'm just focused on maintaining some degree of composure." But that's why it's worth mentioning the concept to you now and not in the delivery room. After all, many new parents have regretted not discussing photographic discretion in advance of the big event, much less having the designated photographer give some quick thought to such photographic challenges as the fact that open curtains on a bright sunny day can ruin even the best new baby pictures. How much forethought you choose to devote to this subject will depend purely on how important the photographic end result is to you.

THE PERFECT POSE

Before you deliver, you may want to set your sights on what continues to be our favorite delivery room picture. While not all deliveries are conducive to being captured on film, the cutting of the cord is a pose well worth a shot. Now, before you laugh this photographic feat off as an impossibility, let us assure you that it can be done—if not by you, at least by someone else in the delivery room. Long before I (Laura) went into labor, someone suggested I try to take a photo of my baby on the delivery room scale so I could use it as my birth announcement photo (see Tipping the Scales on page 364). Having made that a personal goal, I instructed my husband to keep track of our camera and to give it to me as soon as I delivered. Little did I expect to find myself with camera in hand well before my son made his way to the scale—in time to snap photos of my squawking baby in the obstetrician's arms as his father did the honors on the cord. Thrilled with what I considered to be the ultimate once-in-a-lifetime photo, I decided to try again with my next child. Two years later, I ended up with an even better photo of my husband cutting the cord—this time complete with a clock in the immediate background bearing witness to the momentous event.

- **Digital distribution.** There's no question that as a society, we're now fully embedded in the digital age. When it comes to sharing the joyous news (and photos and videos and texts and tweets) of your baby's birth, this means the opportunity to do so almost instantaneously. That said, we recommend you figure out your game plan ahead of time. Some parents prefer the good old-fashioned method of compiling an email list ahead of time and sending out an email announcing the arrival. Others find it easier and faster to post photos and updates on Facebook, upload photos to photo-sharing websites, or make use of Twitter, Instagram, or any of the rapidly multiplying, ready-made venues for sharing news with accompanying photographic documentation. For those who are digitally adept and so inclined, you can even create your baby's first digital footprint in the form of a dedicated web page or blog—ideally spending some time setting it up *before* you get preoccupied with new parenthood.

LOOK WHO IS SPREADING THE NEWS

If you want to increase your chances of being the first to break the news about your new arrival, consider taking some precautionary social media measures. In this day and age of instant sharing, we've heard of many instances in which congratulatory messages are posted online before new parents can even find the time to post an announcement themselves (let alone notify their family first). On Facebook, for example, you can keep this from happening by simply changing your settings so that you get to review all posts before they appear on your timeline. If you'd prefer, you can even opt to prevent people from posting to your wall altogether until you have the chance to spread the word. Once you're done fine-tuning your Facebook settings, remember to find out options for doing the same for any other virtual channels that may interfere with your first-to-report plans. And, of course, make your wishes known to those who might otherwise beat you to the post.

Video

It used to be that a new video recorder topped just about every expectant parent's wish list. Nowadays, with almost every smartphone equipped with impressive video capabilities, the most important decision is whether you want to record the events of the delivery room or ban all live coverage of the event. This is purely a matter of personal preference. Just remember that the considerations we discussed for photographs in the delivery room apply to video as well—only more so. Unless you plan on doing a whole lot of editing, whoever is in charge of filming should be well versed in discretionary limits, not to mention the use of common sense when deciding when to put the camera down and get out of the way. If nothing else, we will close by once again suggesting you put a ban on instant uploading because it is our firm belief that those being filmed as the events of delivery unfold should have the ultimate say (as well as absolute veto power) when it comes to sharing the associated sights and sounds.

31

commemorative
birthday creations

· · · · · · ·

Having started out this section of the book by acknowledging that we are
not prepared to go head-to-head with what's readily available online when it
comes to offering a comprehensive list of commemorative creation options
for the day your baby is born; we nevertheless feel it would be both fun and
worthwhile to share a few of our own popular, tried-and-true suggestions,
as well as recommended resources for finding others.

Saving Time in a Bottle (or Box or Book)

Timeless Bouquets

Even if you've never dried and preserved flowers before, here's your chance
to create a great keepsake that is inexpensive to make and priceless. If you
happen to receive roses or other flowers in recognition of your baby's birth,
remember to take them home with you and hang them upside down (or put
someone else in charge of doing so) until they are *completely* dry. Especially
if you have no prior experience with flower drying, please pay particular
attention to our emphasis on the word *completely*. Trust us when we tell you
from experience that anything short of fully dried flowers has a high likelihood of turning into a progressively moldy bunch of old flowers sealed in a
jar. Fortunately, most flowers can be left drying for as long it takes you to spare
a few extra minutes (a process that, from personal experience, can admittedly
take a couple of months). Then simply get a glass jar that has a tight-sealing
lid, cut the stems off the flowers, and carefully place them into the jar along
with any additional small mementos you might have saved or purchased (such
as pink or blue confetti or ribbon). Next seal the jar so that it's airtight. A bow
around the outside of the jar (pink, blue, or another of your choosing) makes

for a nice finishing touch. While it is quick and easy to make, this keepsake is likely to become far more valuable than the minimal time and effort you put into it. We hope you'll be thanking us for years to come.

Tipping the Scales

We have yet to meet any parents who haven't appreciated the thus-far timeless suggestion of taking a picture of their newborn on the delivery room scale as the perfect way to capture both their baby and his official birth weight in one shot. This relatively easy-to-get and likely-to-be-treasured picture makes a great stand-alone keepsake. Better yet, it makes the perfect choice if you're considering a photo birth announcement. Just be sure to consider whether you (and your child, when he looks back) really want one with all baby parts exposed. Our recommendation: use one that factors in a degree of modesty (such as in **Figure 31-1**).

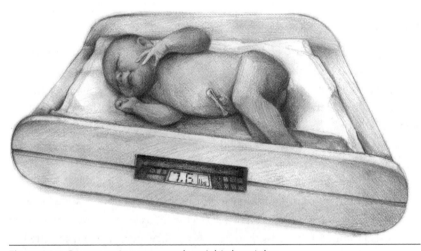

Figure 31-1. Documenting your newborn's birth weight

Once Upon a Time on the Day You Were Born

It may seem hard to imagine as you settle into a routine of caring for a newborn that one day, in the not too distant future, this same child will ask you as many questions as she can come up with about more subjects than you can presently imagine, including the day she was born. As we mentioned at the beginning of this chapter, your memories of childbirth and the events surrounding it may seem so vivid immediately following the grand event that you'll figure you can afford to wait a while before taking the time to record them. Well, we suggest you learn from our mistakes and spend a few minutes writing down, recording, or otherwise documenting for your child what will certainly become a cherished gift—your account of the day she was born. Whether you choose to use video for a more eloquent storytelling component or simply jot down a list, include as many details as you can, no matter how trivial they may seem now. You'll be surprised to find out which details your future four- or five-year-old (not to mention your future self!) considers to be the most entertaining, whether the detail is the pre-labor dinner that didn't sit so well during delivery or that she peed on her daddy the first time he held her. We suggest, however, that you censor out the details that might be deemed too much information by future viewers and simply stick to what was surprising, amusing, wonderful, endearing, and/or memorable about the day.

Box Things Up and Put the Day on Display

The beauty of creating a good old-fashioned shadow box frame that displays all the paraphernalia you collect from the day your baby is born is that just about anyone can do it quite easily with only a little forethought, at very little expense, and in a relatively sleep-deprived state. It also gives you something to do with all the hospital and delivery-related odds and ends you otherwise don't know what to do with but can't quite bring yourself to throw away.

- **Collecting memorabilia.** This is where the forethought comes in because you'll want to remember to gather up as many small items as you can think of that relate to the day your baby was born. While you can certainly look online for additional examples, some suggested items to get you started include

  - Baby hat from the hospital

  - Hospital clothing or outfit your baby wears home from the hospital

  - Cord clamp

  - Hospital name card (usually attached to baby's crib throughout hospital stay)

  - ID bracelets

  - Birth announcement

  - Dried flowers

  - Recent ultrasound picture

  - Headlines and date cut out from the local newspaper (if you happen to be one of the increasingly few people who actually still get one!)

  - Any souvenirs of the day, such as movie ticket stubs or a take-out menu from a restaurant

- **Purchasing supplies.** You can either wait and purchase the necessary supplies after your baby is born or plan ahead and purchase them when your hands aren't yet so full. We've found that the planning ahead option increases the likelihood that you'll have your project ready before your baby's first birthday. Either way, as long as you manage to gather the memorabilia, it's not as important *when* you get inspired and find the time to sit down and work on putting together your shadow box display. When you do, useful supplies to have on hand include

  - *A shadow box.* While there's no reason you can't get this whole project done professionally, it's quite easy (and less expensive) to buy a shadow box from a craft store or frame shop. Choose your frame size according to how many mementos you intend to include.

  - *Decorative paint or paper.* Many craft store shadow boxes come with only an inset made of white cardboard. If you're content with a plain white background, you can skip ahead. Otherwise, look for some nonfading craft paper—pink- or blue-checkered paper seems to be quite popular—grab some paint, gather some fabric, or get some new baby wrapping paper to line the inside of the shadow box.

- *Supplies.* Simply grab some scissors, tape, glue, or staples. Just be sure to check with your local craft store or read up online regarding which types of tape and glue are best suited for this type of project.

- *Additional decorations.* Using additional items in your shadow box such as ribbon, tiny decorative flowers (pink or blue if you so choose), or new baby confetti (which most commonly comes in the shape of tiny rattles and baby bottles) can add interest and spruce things up.

The rest is really quite easy. After you figure out what you want to use as a backdrop—whether it's plain white cardboard, the day's newspaper headlines, your baby's birth announcement, or decorative paint or paper—and prepare the inside of your shadow box accordingly, play with the layout of your trinkets until they look good to you. You may want to consider using photocopies of newspaper headlines or ultrasound photos because the originals will likely start to yellow over time. Regular tape may do the same thing, so consider asking an associate at any scrapbooking store what your longer-lasting options are for securing your assorted items for posterity. Then simply secure your memorabilia, along with some decorative ribbon, confetti, or flowers, and... voilà! Or, alternatively, simply engage someone at your local frame shop and get the project done professionally. Either way, without it requiring much in the way of artistic skills, you'll have a commemorative creation worth displaying in your home for years to come.

First Steps Toward Creating Digital Footprints

In the highly connected digital world we now live in, it's important to take a moment to consider how the digital footprints babies are all but born with stand to virtually follow them for the rest of their lives. This footprint can be a great thing, when it is comprised of memories captured, shaped, and shared. In some instances, however, it can be less than desirable. While it's only natural to get caught up in the moment of having a new baby and want to snap photos and share the news, we want to provide a few considerations to help ensure you capture memories without undesirable aspects.

- **Know your audience.** Consider with whom you really want to share photos, details, and otherwise private cherished moments. If you have a large following of not-so-close Facebook or Instagram friends, for example, you may want to limit how much you share. If only your immediate family and friends follow you on social media, post away.

- **Look to the future.** Remember that what you post now stands to be part of the virtual world for decades to come. Decide whether birth details that seem innocuous now, for example, may prove to be decidedly embarrassing for you or your child in the future. Thinking ahead can also mean reserving email addresses, URLs, and other social media accounts in your child's name for future use (or even for sharing news or tales or blogging in your child's voice until he is old enough to continue the tradition himself!).

- **Protect identifying information.** We suggest you err on the side of caution when sharing any identifying information or unnecessary details. For example, many parents opt not to show their children's faces and make it a point to refer to their children only by their initials in the shared virtual world rather than disclose their full names. Similarly, remember that it's not considered such a great idea (ie, it's a bad idea!) to share children's birth dates in public forums.

- **Live in the moment.** As a final thought that will apply to your baby's birth date and every day thereafter, we like to remind parents that just being present and cherishing the time you spend with your baby is and will always be invaluable. While capturing these moments (whether digitally or otherwise) can be fun, don't let your desire to click, record, document, commemorate, or share them interfere with actually experiencing and appreciating them in the moment.

MEANINGFUL THANK-YOUS

Once you've had a baby, you'll find that the gifts just keep on coming with the passing of each holiday and birthday. While your baby can't exactly be counted on to deliver the proper thank-you, as his parent you can help provide his gift givers more meaningful thanks by photographing or filming him lying on, wearing, reading, or using each gift and sending the photo or video clip to whichever friend or relative was kind enough to give it. As your child gets older and can play a more active role in expressing his appreciation, continue in the tradition of capturing special moments, events, trips, or gifts from others and remembering to send the photos or videos as a more meaningful way of saying, "Thank you."

Additional Pinterest-Worthy Picks

Having shared a few of our own personal favorites, we would be remiss if we didn't also steer you toward Pinterest for many more ideas on how to create customized baby-related crafts. Unless you've lived under a craft-free rock since Pinterest first launched in 2010, you're probably well aware that this online bulletin board offers a virtual smorgasbord through which its millions of contributors can tack up favorite pictures of food, clothing, crafts, home decor, travel sites, and more. For those of you who aren't already active on the site or who have yet to venture into its baby-specific boards, here are just a few of the many potential newborn categories we want to "pin" for you to get you started. Should you choose to undertake any of these or any of the other zillions of creative parenting crafts you come across, consider taking a picture and sharing it with others.

- **Birth ornaments.** Consider getting a plain, transparent ornament at any craft store and tucking small items such as your newborn's hospital wristband, bassinet ID card, and hat inside for safe and decorative keeping. You can also order these and a plethora of other personalized mementos (such as a picture of constellations in the night sky on the day your baby was born) on websites such as Etsy and Amazon.

- **Handprint and footprint art.** On paper or pottery or put into a shadow box, there are endless possibilities to what you can do to be reminded of just how tiny your newborn once was. As a friendly reminder, we suggest using washable ink or nontoxic paint or inkless printing kits (also see Big Before You Know It on page 372).

- **Newborn photo opportunities.** From posing with teddy bears to sitting in a basket to resting on a favorite blanket, get plenty of ideas ahead of time on cute accessories, custom outfits, or creative composition you can use to snap some adorable newborn photos, then save them all to print in a photo book from a drugstore photo service, Shutterfly, or any number of other services.

- **Shared holiday sentiments.** If your baby is born on or near a holiday (as all three of Laura's were!), look for creative ways to commemorate both occasions, whether in a seasonal costume or by turning upside-down footprints into ghosts for Halloween or right-side up footprints into reindeer for a customized winter holiday greeting card.

CHAPTER

32

capturing moments along the way

• • • • • •

Before going any further, we feel obliged to tell those of you who may have skipped the previous chapters and aren't already aware, there are entire craft books, blogs, and websites—not the least of which include Pinterest—dedicated to the subject of preserving childhood memories and many people who profess to be experts in this field. While experts we are not, we have more than enough years of experience in dealing with the regrets and missed opportunities of other parents (and, at times, our own) that we decided to offer you an additional sampling of suggested ways you can continue to preserve in time some of your child's proudest (or most amusing) moments.

A Word About Baby Books

Perhaps one of the easiest ways to start out is with a baby book—whether you reach for the traditional paper kind or choose the more contemporary option and go digital. Our advice to you is this: get off to a good start by documenting some of the early details of your child's life for posterity, and simply continue the habit later in life. Those of you who are still more comfortable putting pen to paper and didn't get a baby book as a shower gift should have no difficulty finding one that suits your tastes—anything from a calendar-style book (in which you can fill in the blanks for everything from the birth weight and head circumference to the first visitor, first smile, first tooth, and first birthday) to a book with blank pages that you can fill in as you please. Those of you who are more technologically inclined can just as easily keep an online baby journal, with plenty of options for turning your digital document into a printable book later on. Fortunately, the virtual explosion of digital options has continued since we first wrote about it in previous editions. Now available to new and seasoned parents alike are virtually unlimited templates, creative ideas for digital baby books, photographic baby book options, and more. Explore your many options (ideally, ahead of time), and go with what best suits you.

Big Before You Know It

The reason we thought to so prominently include the suggestion of preserving your child's footprints and handprints is because we can't tell you the number of times parents have thought that the idea of doing so was great and marveled at another parent's footprint creation but never got around to creating one themselves. After all, who hasn't looked at a little pair of shoes, a birth certificate with imprints from a newborn's tiny feet, or a toddler's handprints on a piece of construction paper and wistfully remembered the days when their own child was that small? It's quick, it's easy, and there are more than a few retail products out there that eliminate any need for creative talent. Some suggestions include

- Simply frame a piece of paper with your baby's handprints or footprints on it. Adding your baby's name and birth information or putting the prints onto decorative paper is an easy way to embellish your work of art. We suggest making the extra investment in nonfading paper.
- Place your baby's first pair of shoes into a shadow box alongside a footprint made when the shoes were worn.
- Make an imprint or 3-D plaster mold of your baby's hand or foot. Mold kits, some of which allow you to adorn, paint, or otherwise enhance your creation, are readily available at most craft shops or stores that sell baby products.
- Go to a pottery painting store and use baby-safe paint to preserve your baby's handprint or footprint on a dish, a serving plate, a tile, or any of the large number of other pottery pieces that are generally available.
- Create a handprint (or footprint) photo frame.
- Consider repeating your print craft(s) of choice more than once, as they can serve as fun comparisons of how your child has grown over the years.

HELPFUL HANDPRINT HINTS

It's easiest to get a good handprint if you wait until your baby is asleep before attempting it. You may also find the activity to be less challenging if you wait a few weeks or months before choosing hand over foot because newborns are notorious for keeping their hands in tight fists—both when they are awake and asleep—much to the dismay of their handprint-seeking parents.

Journaling

While many of you may not have ever contemplated the idea of keeping a journal, and most of you probably don't consider yourself to be storytellers, this section is still worth reading. Perhaps one of the cutest things we've seen when it comes to capturing the memories created during new parenthood came from my (Laura's) newborn nephew. Okay, to be honest, the weekly updates sent via his very own email address were technically penned by his mother. But each update had offered up, in first-person narrative, all sorts of details about his preceding week of acclaimed accomplishments, memorable milestones, and amusing mishaps. Family and friends (especially those who live too far away to share in the day-to-day experiences) generally enjoy reading and receiving regular updates (especially early on, as well as for new grandparents), and down the road, these updates are sure to become an invaluable and highly entertaining compilation of preserved memories. If you've never been much of an enthusiast of journaling before, maybe this contemporary, digitally derived approach will be as compelling a reason as any to start! If digitally sharing your musings isn't exactly your style, it's still perfectly acceptable to reach for a baby book or fancy hardbound journal. Even a notebook or a simple Word document will do. After all, it's going to be the thoughts you capture that count.

PRESERVING YOUR CHILD'S DIGITAL FOOTPRINT

In this day and age of high-tech everything, it is often said that our children start creating a digital footprint from the day they are born. With that thought in mind, we want to share with you a practical, tech-savvy new-parent tip, courtesy of Laura's very tech-savvy twin sister. Once your baby's name has been set in stone—by mutual agreement, birth certificate, or both—check to see whether your chosen name is available as an email account, social media account, domain name (or any combination of those) and register it. By doing so you will be staking your baby's first claim to a dedicated space in the digital world. (See also First Steps Toward Creating Digital Footprints on page 367.)

parting insights

• • • • • •

You have now reached the end of this book, but you are only just starting your lifelong adventure. We thought long and hard about what parting
insights we wanted to leave with you because in the end—all diapers and
joking aside—we love being parents and want you to enjoy this noblest of
professions as much as we do. When we tried to think of how to finish things
off in a meaningful way, everything that came to mind seemed to have been
said before—mostly in the form of clichés. The one we feel is nevertheless
worth repeating is that you will soon become the person who knows your
baby best—what she wants, needs, likes, and dislikes. This expertise will come
naturally over time, so it is worth reminding yourself every so often that
parenthood is not a race. As for the rest of the clichés, you're certain to hear
from others that babies grow big before you know it and how they're only
young once. Instead of elaborating, we thought we'd lighten things up a bit by
leaving you with a few thoughts that occurred to us while we were writing this
book—all of which relate to a concept that has become even more apparent
to us over the many years since we first wrote it: becoming a parent is really
quite a lot like writing a book on parenting.

- It seems as if everyone's doing it.
- It's a guaranteed adventure.
- If you're lucky, you fall right into your new role, but for most of us, this
  transition takes a good bit of time, effort, and patience.
- It has a way of taking over your life, but you find that you wouldn't want
  parenthood to be any other way.
- It serves as a reminder that almost everything is easier said than done.
- You are bound to run into obstacles along the way. You will be the excep-
  tion to the rule if you don't have days when you doubt yourself.
- Having faith and sticking with it pays off in the end.
- People are going to judge you. Regardless of what they think, if you do your
  best and remain committed to learning new things along the way, you'll
  always have something to be proud of.

- Striving for perfection is great, but expecting to achieve it is a setup for failure.
- Ultimately, it's always going to be a work in progress.
- And finally…

This end is only the beginning!

• • • • • •

index

• • • • • •

377

growth spurts and, 65
later feedings in, 62
leftovers from, 63
method for, 61
schedules and routines in, 64–67
sterilizing supplies for, 63–64
weighing in and, 62
Bottles. *See also* Formula feeding
angled, 58
BPA (bisphenol A)-free, 58
choosing, 57–58
disposable bags for, 58
heating of, 60–61
holding of, 61
size of, 57–58
slow flow, 58
sterilizing of, 63–64
Bouquets, dried, as birth keepsakes, 363–364
Boxes, play with, 196
Boys
circumcision of, 318
genitals in, 317–319
hydrocele in, 319
hypospadias in, 318
peeing during diaper changes, 144
penis care for, 317
undescended testicles in, 319
BPA (bisphenol A), 58
Brain, 179, 181–184
before birth, 182
hypothalamus of, 328
making connections in, 181–182
secret to smarter babies and, 182–183
"serve and return" interactions for, 183
Bras, nursing, 29–30
Breastfed babies
breathing room for, 16–17
first attempts at, 12–13
getting enough milk, 30–31
health of, 12
latching on, 17, 19
nipple confusion in, 36–37
poop in, 77–78
urine output by, 75
vitamin D for, 37
Breastfeeding, 3. *See also* Formula feeding
during air travel, 258
"breast is best" and, 5–7
caring for nipples and, 21–22

cost of, 4
cradle hold, 14
cramping with, 22–23
falling into bad habits with, 35
feeding intervals for, 32–33
football (or clutch) hold, 15
frequency of, 33
getting advice on, 9
getting started with, 9–12
on the go, 31–32
growing popularity of, 7
health insurance supports for, 39
in-hospital training in, xxix, 13, 18
legal rights regarding, 8
minimizing air swallowed during, 83–84
as natural act, 9
pain with, 19, 20
positioning for, 13–16
realistic expectations for, 5
settling into routine for, 31
side-by-side (or lying down) position for, 16
single- versus double-breasted approach to, 34–35
supplementing of, 37–38
support resources for, 10–11
"textbook" pattern in, xxii
waking babies at night for, 112–113
weighing babies in and, 33–34
Breast milk
benefits of, 6
coming in, 24, 26
hind milk, 34
letdown tingle with, 25
progressive production of mature, 25
pumping of, 38–39
storage of, 38–39
supply of, 23, 30–31
transitional, 17, 23, 24
Breasts
engorgement of, 26
leaky, 28–29
letdown tingle in, 25
mastitis in, 27
in newborns, 310
nursing bras for, 29–30
size of, 24
Breathing, 309
Brown Bear, Brown Bear, 197